Communications in Computer and Information Science 604

Commenced Publication in 2007
Founding and Former Series Editors:
Alfredo Cuzzocrea, Dominik Ślęzak, and Xiaokang Yang

More information about this series at http://www.springer.com/series/7899

Silvia Serino · Aleksandar Matic
Dimitris Giakoumis · Guillaume Lopez
Pietro Cipresso (Eds.)

Pervasive Computing Paradigms for Mental Health

5th International Conference, MindCare 2015
Milan, Italy, September 24–25, 2015
Revised Selected Papers

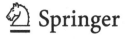 Springer

Editors
Silvia Serino
Istituto Auxologico Italiano
Milano
Italy

Guillaume Lopez
Aoyama Gakuin University
Tokyo
Japan

Aleksandar Matic
Telefonica I+D
Barcelona
Spain

Pietro Cipresso
Istituto Auxologico Italiano
Milano
Italy

Dimitris Giakoumis
The Centre for Research and Technology
Thessalomiki/Thermi
Greece

ISSN 1865-0929   ISSN 1865-0937 (electronic)
Communications in Computer and Information Science
ISBN 978-3-319-32269-8   ISBN 978-3-319-32270-4 (eBook)
DOI 10.1007/978-3-319-32270-4

Library of Congress Control Number: 2016935205

Printed on acid-free paper

This Springer imprint is published by Springer Nature
The registered company is Springer International Publishing AG Switzerland

Preface

The 2015 International Symposium on Pervasive Computing Paradigms for Mental Health – MindCare was held at the Istituto Auxologico Italiano, in Milan, Italy, during September 24–25, 2015. The symposium focused on the use of technologies in favor of maintaining and improving mental well-being and it brought together the community of researchers and practitioners from technological, medical, and psychological disciplines.

In its five editions, MindCare has gathered scientists from more than 30 countries creating a strong community that shares a common passion for building new computing paradigms and for addressing the multitude of challenges in mental healthcare. MindCare 2015 in Milan covered a diverse set of topics in psychiatric and psychological domains while featuring a wide span of new technologies, from video and audio technologies to mobile and wearable computing. Two distinguished keynote speakers, namely, Prof. Rosalind Picard and Prof. Giuseppe Riva, discussed the multidisciplinary challenges and potentials of using technologies in monitoring and maintaining mental health.

February 2016

Silvia Serino
Aleksandar Matic
Dimitris Giakoumis
Guillaume Lopez
Pietro Cipresso

Organization

MindCare 2015 was organized by the EAI in cooperation with ICST.

Steering Committee

Steering Committee Chair

Imrich Chlamtac   CREATE-NET, Italy

Technological Perspectives Chair

Anind K. Dey   Carnegie Mellon University, USA

Psychological Perspectives Chair

Giuseppe Riva   Istituto Auxologico Italiano, Italy

Organizing Committee

General Chairs

Aleksandar Matic	Telefonica I+D, Spain
Pietro Cipresso	Istituto Auxologico Italiano, Italy
Guillaume Lopez	Aoyama Gakuin University, Japan

Local Chair

Silvia Serino   Istituto Auxologico Italiano, Italy

Program Chair

Dimitris Giakoumis   The Centre for Research and Technology, Greece

Publicity Chairs

Mirco Musolesi	University College London, UK
Monica Tentori	CICESE, Mexico

Local Publicity Chair

Daniela Villani   Catholic University of the Sacred Heart of Milan, Italy

Publication Chair

Charalampos Doukas   CREATE-NET, Italy

Technical Program Committee

Agustin Ruiz	FundacioACE, Barcelona, Spain
Akio Nozawa	Aoyama Gakuin University, Japan
Anouk Kaiser	Universiteit Utrecht, The Netherlands
Atsushi Kimura	Tokyo Denki University, Japan
Chrysa Lithari	CIMeC, Università degli Studi di Trento, Italy
Cristina Botella	Jaume I University, Spain
Dai Hasegawa	Aoyama Gakuin University, Japan
Daniel Mestre	Centre de Réalité Virtuelle de la Méditerranée, France
Diego Hidalgo	Hospital Clinic, Barcelona, Spain
Dimitrios Tzovaras	Centre for Research and Technology Hellas, Greece
Elisa Pedroli	Istituto Auxologico Italiano, Italy
Federica Pallavicini	Università degli Studi Milano Bicocca, Italy
Francesc Colom	Hospital Clinic, Barcelona, Spain
Hao Zhang	University of Tokyo, Japan
Jean Marcel Dos Reis Costa	Cornell University, USA
Jongwa Kim	University of Augsburg, Germany
José Gutiérrez-Maldonado	University of Barcelona, Spain
Konrad Rejdak	Medical University of Lublin, Poland
Konstantinos Votis	Centre for Research and Technology Hellas, Greece
Kostas Karpouzis	National Technical University of Athens, Greece
Lida Mademli	Aristotle University of Thessaloniki, Greece
Lucian Georghe	NISSAN Research Laboratory, Spain
Mar Rus-Calafell	King's College London, UK
Margherita Antona	Foundation for Research and Technology Hellas, Greece
Martin Pielot	Telefonica Research, Spain
Mirco Musolesi	University of Birmingham, UK
Naoya Isoyama	Kobe University, Japan
Neal Lathia	University of Cambridge, UK
Nikolaos Laskaris	Aristotle University of Thessaloniki, Greece
Pedro Gamito	Universidade Lusófona de Humanidades e Tecnologias, Portugal
Rosa María Baños	University of Valencia, Spain
Sofia Segkouli	Centre for Research and Technology Hellas, Greece
Stefano Triberti	Università Cattolica del Sacro Cuore, Italy
Stelios Zygouris	Aristotle University of Thessaloniki, Greece
Willem-Paul Brinkman	Delft University of Technology, USA
Yasuhiro Kawahara	Open University of Japan, Japan
Yumi Kameyama	The University of Tokyo, Japan

Contents

Stay Positive and Well

Help Me If You Can: Tech-Interventions for Mental Health

All That Stress

Helping Women with Breast Cancer to Cope with Hair Loss: An e-SIT Protocol

Daniela Villani[1]([✉]), Chiara Cognetta[2], Davide Toniolo[2],
and Giuseppe Riva[1,3]

[1] Department of Psychology, Catholic University of Sacred Heart, Milan, Italy
{daniela.villani,giuseppe.riva}@unicatt.it
[2] Department of Medical Oncology,
"G. Salvini" Rho General Hospital, Milan, Italy
cognettachiara@gmail.com,
dtoniolo@aogarbagnate.lombardia.it
[3] Applied Technology for Neuro-Psychology Lab,
Istituto Auxologico Italiano, Milan, Italy

Abstract. The emerging convergence of technology and health care is offering new methods and tools to help people cope with stressful upcoming events. To address the distress of chemotherapy and of alopecia in particular, and to facilitate anticipatory coping, we developed a two weeks e-health protocol based on Meichenbaum's SIT intervention for helping women undergoing chemotherapy to cope with impeding hair loss. The paper aims to present the e-SIT protocol as a promising approach to facilitate coping and adjustment in breast cancer patients.

Keywords: e-health · SIT · Breast cancer · Hair loss · Coping · Well-being

1 Introduction

Chemotherapy treatment for breast cancer patients can have a profound impact on appearance, and is often experienced as distressing. Actually, hair loss is, for many patients, an unavoidable aspect of their chemotherapy treatment. According to a recent review [1], firstly, chemotherapy-induced hair loss is considered to be the most important side effect of chemotherapy. It is frequently ranked among the first three for breast cancer patients [2, 3], together with nausea and fatigue [4, 5]. Secondly, it is described by breast cancer women as causing distress and as being traumatizing [6–10] and may even be considered emblematic of the treatment and of cancer itself [7, 9, 11]. Thirdly, there might be an impact on body image [12] and self-esteem although not all studies reported this association. Indeed, while it is difficult to tease out whether differences in body image, self-esteem, or self-concept result from alopecia specifically, or more general adjustment to a cancer diagnosis and chemotherapy treatment, it is commonly recognized that many women experience a range of distressing side effects from chemotherapy treatment, including alopecia, which has a significant impact on their psychosocial well-being.

Some studies suggest that side effects are not experienced as distressing as patients can anticipate them [13–15]. However, up to now just a few studies have been focused

© Springer International Publishing Switzerland 2016
S. Serino et al. (Eds.): MindCare 2015, CCIS 604, pp. 3–12, 2016.
DOI: 10.1007/978-3-319-32270-4_1

on the anticipation and preparation for an altered appearance [13]. Thus, the process of preparing patients for hair loss is a significant challenge for healthcare professionals. This preparation could be seen as a form of anticipatory coping - coping which involves the preparation for managing the stressful consequences of an upcoming event, which is likely or certain to occur [16]. Anticipatory coping could involve some activities like resource accumulation (information etc.), initial appraisal (assessment of the impact of the event), initial coping efforts (activities to prevent or minimize the event) and elicitation and use of feedback.

This type of coping might be effectively integrated within interventions aimed to help people to manage stressful or difficult events related to illness, such as hair loss due to chemotherapy. Frith and colleagues [13] demonstrated that the active management in coping with impeding hair loss allows women to gain control over their situation. Control and management of negative emotions represent central concepts in psychological theories of well-being, adjustment and coping [17].

Stress inoculation training - SIT - [18, 19] represents a validated short, semistructured, and active approach to help people coping with difficult and specific situations. SIT is a type of training conceived to prepare individuals for stressful events by helping them in diminishing the potential for a negative cognitive, psychological, and behavioral reaction. SIT is based on the premise that to effectively manage stress, it is crucial to change the way people see the events and how to use their own coping skills. Thus, it is generally implemented through gradual and repeated exposure to the elements previously identified as stressors. The clinical rationale behind this approach is to "inoculate" the stressor in person's experience, in combination with the acquisition of effective coping skills, so that people could be prepared when they will encounter similar situations in daily life.

In fact, people experience stress when perception of their own skills does not balance the perception of difficulty of the environmental requirements. According to Cohen and colleagues [20], psychological stress occurs when people perceive that potential situational threats exceed their adaptive capacity.

SIT has been already validated in clinical contexts, to help patients in facing particularly strenuous conditions [21]. It has also been applied to cancer patients and post-treatment observations indicated that the stress inoculation techniques were beneficial in altering anxiety-related behaviors [22].

The general objectives of SIT are threefold and are related to the three phases of the protocol:

(1) SIT aims to change the maladaptive stress response of the individual, thanks to the acquisition of knowledge and the understanding of stress process. Thus, the first phase, named conceptualization, aims at making individual aware of the transactional nature of psychological stress [23] by giving general information about the main stress' effects and symptoms that could appear in specific stressful situations.

(2) SIT aims to develop an activity of self-regulation. Thus, the second phase, named skill acquisition and rehearsal, aims at teaching individual to manage emotions and maladaptive behaviors as well as learn new active coping skills. In accordance with Murphy [24], the combination of different strategies may yield better stress management than single-strategy programs. Specifically, relaxation practices [25] and breathing techniques, and mindfulness meditation programs [26] can be easily integrated in this phase.

(3) SIT aims to explore and modify dysfunctional cognitive appraisal related to stressful events. Thus, the last phase, named application and follow-through, aims at increasing self-efficacy [27] by helping individual to use the acquired coping skills in real contexts. The acquisition of specific skills of stress management during the mediated experience can promote the sense of personal self-efficacy and prepare people to cope with real stressful situations. According to Bandura's [28] theory, once established, self-efficacy tends to generalize to other situations. Indeed, once acquired, these competencies assigned to internal factors become a means to the management of stressful situations and they can be transferred and applied to other contexts.

2 Integrating Technologies in Psychological Interventions to Cope with Chemotherapy

The emerging convergence of technology and health care is offering new methods and tools to help people cope with stressful upcoming events. According to Botella and colleagues [29] computer assisted therapy [30] and Web 2.0 [31] have demonstrated their potentiality in supporting psychological interventions. More, as claimed by the Positive Technology approach, advanced technology offers several affordances for improving the quality of our personal experience to promote well-being [32]. Thus, the main objectives and the three stages of SIT have been recently implemented in cyber-interventions based on SIT methodology (cyber-SIT), which utilize advanced technologies to create simulations to teach individual how effectively cope with psychological stress [33].

Specifically, the use of advanced technology may efficiently support all the three phases of SIT. As far as the conceptualization phase, the multimedia presentations where information is enriched and distributed through images, animations, sound, voice, and written text can enhance the understanding of the transactional nature of stress, and its main causes and effects [34]. With respect to the skill acquisition and rehearsal phase, advanced technologies could guarantee participants meaningful experience in interactive environments and can help individuals in acquiring effective coping skills. Relaxation practices and meditation programs could be effectively integrated in mediated experiences characterized by natural and restorative settings where participants can do specific exercises [33, 35]. Finally, as far as the application and follow-through phase, digital environments can be used for patients' exposure to stressful stimuli with often equal therapeutic benefits to in vivo exposure [36] and/or superior to other methods such as guided imagery [37].

According to the results of a recent systematic review [38], cyber-SIT appears to be a promising clinical approach, and there are interesting researches that effectively combined traditional SIT clinical protocol within advanced technologies. Villani and colleagues tested the effectiveness of a cyber-SIT delivered through mobile phones by comparing it with a control group (neutral video through mobile phones) in a sample of oncology nurses [39]. Results showed psychological improvement of the experimental group in terms of anxiety state, anxiety trait reduction, and coping skills acquisition.

Computer-based approaches and imagery interventions, as well as patient education, have been found to be effective for a number of conditions suggesting the potential benefits of similar applications for alopecia [40–42]. Recently, the process of preparing patients for hair loss has been supported through a computerized hair imaging software which allowed women to see themselves with a new hairstyle/ without hair prior to change has been tested [43]. Based on concepts related to guided imagery and anticipatory grief, this intervention aimed to aid women in coping with anticipated treatment-related alopecia and promote self-acceptance. The HAAIR (Help with Adjustment to Alopecia by Image Recovery) system was assessed as a useful educational resource creating a realistic experience of hair loss and confrontation with baldness.

Integrating technologies in psychological interventions focusing both on the physical side effects and on the emotional and psychological aspects related to chemotherapy could represent a promising approach to facilitate coping and adjustment in breast cancer patients.

3 The e-SIT Protocol

In an effort to address the distress of chemotherapy and of alopecia in particular, and to facilitate anticipatory coping, we developed e-health protocol based on Meichenbaum's SIT intervention [19] for helping women undergoing chemotherapy to cope with impeding hair loss.

The e-SIT protocol last two weeks and details are presented in Table 1.

Table 1. e-SIT protocol: phases, objectives and proposed experiences

SIT phase	Objective	Proposed experience
Conceptualization phase (session 1)	The aim of this phase is to increase knowledge about the upcoming situation and its psychological impact.	At this stage breast cancer women are invited by the psychologist to reflect on the nature of the psychological stress due to disease and upcoming treatment in order to achieve a greater consciousness about its main components. Furthermore, in this session patients experience a live-video simulation of a chemotherapy session that they will receive within a few weeks. Patients are encouraged to pay attention to perceived threats, concerns and provocations as problems-to-be-solved and to identify which aspects of the situations and of their reactions are potentially changeable.

(Continued)

Table 1. (*Continued*)

SIT phase	Objective	Proposed experience
Skills acquisition and rehearsal phase (sessions 1–7)	The aim of this phase is to provide the opportunity to learn psychophysical coping strategies.	At this stage women start the online experience. The multimedia experience includes seven 25 min sessions to see once a day. Each session includes two parts. In the first one, patients can watch live-video interviews with women who have gone through breast cancer experience, with particular attention to their expectations and emotions, to chemotherapy side effects and to strategies to cope with changes. Specifically, interviews are focused on these areas: **Expectations:** the video investigates women' expectations and knowledge before starting chemotherapy; **Emotions:** the video explores women' emotional experiences related to disease and how women have managed them; **Chemotherapy side effects:** the video investigates the side effects women have to deal with after treatment; **Hair-loss:** the video explores the meaning of hair loss and related changes in the appearance perception; **Change:** the video explores the impact of illness and therapies on several aspects of women' life (physical, psychological, social, and working); **Activity:** the video focuses on the potential activities that women can do during the treatment; **Suggestions:** the video aims to offer a new perspective, highlighting that some women

(*Continued*)

Table 1. (*Continued*)

SIT phase	Objective	Proposed experience
		recognize also positive aspects related to disease experience. In the second part, a relaxation and meditation experience is proposed. Specifically, a natural relaxing video is integrated with narrative audio. Exercises are based on muscle progressive relaxation (focusing on legs, arms, abdome, shoulders, face, front, etc.) [25] and breathing. More, the narrative includes Mindfulness inspired strategies [26], such as thought contemplation and detached mindfulness, useful to be aware of one's thoughts and emotions associated with them, and to look at the problem from a different perspective.
Application and follow - through phase (sessions 8–10)	The aim of this phase is to expose women to the effects of the imminent chemotherapy and to verify their acquisition of coping skills to effectively manage the stressful upcoming event.	Women continue the online experience. Also in this case, each session includes two parts. First, video-live of breast cancer patients' interviews currently undergoing chemoterapic treatments - both with and without wigs - are presented. In this way women directly deal with changes due to illness, chemotherapy and related side effects. In addition, suggestions proposed by other patients offer the chance of anticipate possible solutions to problems they will have to cope with. Second, supported by a natural relaxing video integrated with narrative audio, women are encouraged to apply relaxation and meditation strategies acquired in the previous phase sessions.

The e-SIT protocol will be delivered by using a website (www.conilsenodipoi.it). Participants will be given access to the intervention for a period of 14 days. Upon log-in, a welcome page will appeared, providing information on what to expect within the online intervention. The psychologist researchers' personal contact will be provided for coping both with technical and psychological difficulties. Thanks to Internet, women can follow the intervention in their own comfortable, familiar surroundings [44].

Figure 1 shows the protocol flow.

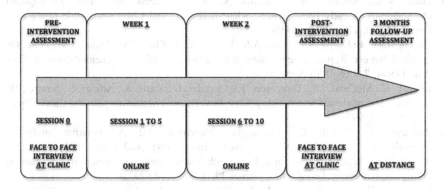

Fig. 1. E-SIT Protocol flow

Oncologists will propose the research to all breast cancer patients, which is offered chemotherapy, fulfilling the following inclusion criteria: diagnosis of breast cancer radically operated; negative staging for distant metastases; suitability for adjuvant chemotherapy with anthracyclines and taxanes. The trial will include fifty women with age between 30 and 70 years that will be randomized to two groups. The experimental group will follow the e-sit protocol as an adjunct to treatment as usual for two weeks. The control group will receive the usual care for two weeks.

The assessment will be realized in two moments. Before and after each online session, the emotional state of patients will be evaluated online through a Visual Analogue Scale (VAS). At the begin and at the end of the protocol the pre-intervention and post-intervention assessment will be performed. The psychologist will meet patients and will propose them several questionnaires aiming to assess their psychological well-being, adjustment to disease, emotion regulation skills and satisfaction about their body.

To conclude, the e-SIT protocol represents a promising approach to help women to cope with the stressful experience of chemotherapy and specifically with hair loss.

Nevertheless, controlled studies should test the effectiveness of the approach and compare it with treatment as usual.

Acknowledgments. This study has been supported by Catholic University of Sacred Heart of Milan (D3.2 Tecnologia Positiva e Healthy Aging - Positive Technology and Healthy Aging, 2014).

References

1. Lemieux, J., Maunsell, E., Provencher, L.: Chemotherapy-induced alopecia and effects on quality of life among women with breast cancer: a literature review. Psycho-Oncol. **17**(4), 317–328 (2008)
2. Carelle, N., Piotto, E., Bellanger, A., Germanaud, J., Thuillier, A., Khayat, D.: Changing patient perceptions of the side effects of cancer chemotherapy. Cancer **95**(1), 155–163 (2002)
3. Duric, V.M., Stockler, M.R., Heritier, S., et al.: Patients' preferences for adjuvant chemotherapy in early breast cancer: what makes AC and CMF worthwhile now? Ann. Oncol. **16**(11), 1786–1794 (2005)
4. Griffin, A.M., Butow, P.N., Coates, A.S., Childs, A.M., Ellis, P.M., Dunn, S.M., et al.: On the receiving end V: patient perceptions of the side effects of cancer chemotherapy in 1993. Ann. Oncol. **7**, 189–195 (1996)
5. Lindley, C., McCune, J.S., Thomason, T.E., Lauder, D., Sauls, A., Adkins, S., Sawyer, W. T.: Perception of chemotherapy side effects: cancer versus noncancer patients. Cancer Pract. **7**(2), 59–65 (1999)
6. Williams, J., Wood, C., Cunningham-Warburton, P.: A narrative study of chemotherapy-induced alopecia. Oncol. Nurs. Forum **26**(9), 1463–1468 (1999)
7. Richer, M.C., Ezer, H.: Living in it, living with it, and moving on: dimensions of meaning during chemotherapy. Oncol. Nurs. Forum **29**(1), 113–119 (2002)
8. Luoma, M., Hakamies-Blomqvist, L.: The meaning of quality of life in patients being treated for advanced breast cancer: a qualitative study. Psycho-Oncol. **13**(10), 729–739 (2004)
9. Rosman, S.: Cancer and stigma: experience of patients with chemotherapy-induced alopecia. Patient Educ. Couns. **52**(3), 333–339 (2004)
10. Browall, M., Gaston-Johansson, F., Danielson, E.: Post- menopausal women with breast cancer: their experiences of the chemotherapy treatment period. Cancer Nurs. **29**(1), 34–42 (2006)
11. Harcourt, D., Frith, H., Fussell, A.: "Chemo sucks": anticipating the impact of an altered appearance during cancer treatment on self and others. In: Appearance Matters Conference, Bath, UK (2006)
12. Fobair, P., Stewart, S.L., Chang, S., D'Onofrio, C., Banks, P.J., Bloom, J.R.: Body image and sexual problems in young women with breast cancer. Psycho-Oncol. **15**(7), 579–594 (2006)
13. Frith, H., Harcourt, D., Fussell, A.: Anticipating an altered appearance: women undergoing chemotherapy treatment for breast cancer. Eur. J. Oncol. Nurs. **11**(5), 385–391 (2007)
14. Lindley, C., McCune, J.S., Thomason, T.E., Lauder, D., Sauls, A., Adkins, S., Sawyer, W.T.: Perception of chemotherapy side effects: cancer versus noncancer patients. Cancer Practice **7**(2), 59–65 (1999)
15. Tierney, A., Taylor, J., Closs, S.J.: Knowledge expectations and experiences of patients receiving chemotherapy for breast cancer. Scand. J. Caring Sci. **6**(2), 75–80 (1992)
16. Aspinwall, L.G., Taylor, S.E.: A stitch in time: self-regulation and proactive coping. Psychol. Bull. **121**(3), 417–436 (1997)
17. Walker, J.: Control and the Psychology of Health. Open University Press, Buckingham (2001)
18. Meichenbaum, D.: Cognitive-Behavioral Modification: An Integrative Approach. Plenum Press, New York (1977)
19. Meichenbaum, D.: Stress inoculation training. Pergamon Press, New York (1985)

20. Cohen, S., Janicki-Deverts, D., Miller, G.E.: Psychological stress and disease. J. Am. Med. Assoc. **298**(14), 1685–1687 (2007)
21. Foley, F.W., Bedell, J.R., Larocca, N.G., Scheinberg, L.C., Reznikoff, M.: Efficacy of stress-inoculation training in coping with multiple-sclerosis. J. Consult. Clin. Psychol. **55**(6), 919–922 (1987)
22. Moore, K., Altmaier, E.M.: Stress inoculation training with cancer patients. Cancer Nurs. **4**(5), 389–394 (1981)
23. Lazarus, R.S., Folkman, S.: Transactional theory and research on emotions and coping. Eur. J. Pers. **1**, 141–169 (1987)
24. Murphy, L.R.: Stress management in work settings: a critical review of the health effects. Am. J. Health Promot. **11**(2), 112–135 (1996)
25. Jacobson, E.: Progressive Relaxation. University of Chicago Press, Chicago (1938)
26. Kabat-Zinn, J.: Mindfulness-based interventions in context: past, present, and future. Clin. Psychol. Sci. Pract. **10**(2), 144–156 (2003)
27. Bandura, A.: Health promotion from the perspective of social cognitive theory. Psychol. Health. **13**(4), 623–649 (1998)
28. Bandura, A.: Health promotion by social cognitive means. Health Educ. Behav. **31**(2), 143–164 (2004)
29. Botella, C., Riva, G., Gaggioli, A., Wiederhold, B.K., Alcaniz, M., Banos, R.M.: The present and future of positive technologies. Cyberpsychol. Behav. Soc. Netw. **15**(2), 78–84 (2012)
30. Proudfoot, J., Ryden, C., Everitt, B., Shapiro, D.A., Goldberg, D., Mann, A., Gray, J.A.: Clinical efficacy of computerised cognitive–behavioural therapy for anxiety and depression in primary care: randomised controlled trial. Br. J. Psychiatry **185**(1), 46–54 (2004)
31. Andersson, G.: Using the Internet to provide cognitive behaviour therapy. Behav. Res. Ther. **47**(3), 175–180 (2009)
32. Riva, G., Banos, R.M., Botella, C., Wiederhold, B.K., Gaggioli, A.: Positive technology: using interactive technologies to promote positive functioning. Cyberpsychol. Behav. Soc. Netw. **15**(2), 69–77 (2012)
33. Villani, D., Riva, G.: Does interactive media enhance the management of stress? Suggestions from a controlled study. Cyberpsychol. Behav. Soc. Netw. **15**(1), 24–30 (2012)
34. Mayer, R.: Multimedia learning. Cambridge University Press, New York (2009)
35. Villani, D., Riva, F., Riva, G.: New technologies for relaxation: the role of presence. Int. J. Stress Manage. **14**, 260–274 (2007)
36. Emmelkamp, P.M.G., Krijn, M., Hulsbosch, A.M., de Vries, S., Schuemie, M.J., van der Mast, C.A.P.G.: Virtual reality treatment versus exposure in vivo: a comparative evaluation in acrophobia. Behav. Res. Ther. **40**(5), 509–516 (2002)
37. Riva, G.: Virtual reality in psychotherapy: review. Cyberpsychol. Behav. **8**(3), 220–230 (2005)
38. Serino, S., Triberti, S., Villani, D., Cipresso, P., Gaggioli, A., Riva, G.: Toward a validation of cyber-interventions for stress disorders based on stress inoculation training: a systematic review. Virtual Reality **18**(1), 73–87 (2014)
39. Villani, D., Grassi, A., Cognetta, C., Toniolo, D., Cipresso, P., Riva, G.: Self-help stress management training through mobile phones: an experience with oncology nurses. Psychol. Serv. **10**(3), 315 (2013)
40. Freeman, L., Cohen, L., Stewart, M., et al.: Imagery intervention for recovering breast cancer patients: Clinical trial of safety and efficacy. J. Soc. Integr. Oncol. Spring. **6**(2), 67–75 (2008)
41. Lewis, D.: Computer-based approaches to patient education: A review of the literature. J. Am. Med. Inform. Assoc. **6**(4), 82–272 (1999)

42. Wofford, J.L., Smith, E.D., Miller, D.P.: The multimedia computer for office-based patient education: a systematic review. Patient Educ. Couns. **59**(2), 57–148 (2005)
43. McGarvey, E.L., Leon-Verdin, M., Baum, L.D., Bloomfield, K., Brenin, D.R., Koopman, C., Parker, B.E.: An evaluation of a computer-imaging program to prepare women for chemotherapy-related alopecia. Psycho-Oncol. **19**(7), 756–766 (2010)
44. Powell, J., Hamborg, T., Stallard, N., Burls, A., McSorley, J., Bennett, K., Christensen, H.: Effectiveness of a web-based cognitive-behavioral tool to improve mental well-being in the general population: randomized controlled trial. J. Med. Internet Res. **15**(1), e2 (2013)

Comparison of Machine Learning Techniques
for Psychophysiological Stress Detection

Elena Smets[1,2(✉)], Pierluigi Casale[3], Ulf Großekathöfer[3], Bishal Lamichhane[3],
Walter De Raedt[1], Katleen Bogaerts[4], Ilse Van Diest[4], and Chris Van Hoof[1,2,3]

[1] Imec, Kapeldreef 75, Heverlee, Belgium
Elena.Smets@imec.be
[2] Electrical Engineering-ESAT, KU Leuven, Kasteelpark Arenberg 10, Heverlee, Belgium
[3] Holst Centre/Imec, High Tech Campus 31, Eindhoven, The Netherlands
[4] Faculty of Psychology and Educational Sciences, KU Leuven, Dekenstraat 2, Leuven, Belgium

Abstract. Previous research has indicated that physiological signals can be used
to detect mental stress. There is however no consensus on the optimal algorithm
for this detection. The aim of this study is to compare different machine learning
techniques for the measurement of stress based on physiological responses in a
controlled environment. Electrocardiogram (ECG), galvanic skin response
(GSR), temperature and respiration were measured during a laboratory stress test.
Six machine learning techniques were investigated using a general and personal
approach. The results show that personalized dynamic Bayesian networks and
generalized support vector machines render the best average classification results
with 84.6 % and 82.7 % respectively.

Keywords: Stress monitoring · Physiology · Machine learning

1 Introduction

There is growing world-wide awareness of the problems caused by long-term stress,
such as depression, burn-out and cardiovascular disorders [1, 2]. To tackle these problems there is an urgent need for an objective, continuous and personalized stress measurement technique.

Currently, mainly questionnaires are used to measure stress in real-life and outside a
laboratory context. However, this technique does not allow for continuous monitoring and
often suffers from biases such as demand effects, response and memory biases. Therefore
the focus has shifted towards measuring bodily responses as indicators of stress. These
include biochemical responses such as cortisol and epinephrine, and physiological
responses such as galvanic skin response (GSR), heart rate variability (HRV), skin temperature, respiration and muscle tone. Although biochemical indicators have shown to correlate with stress [3], these are not ideal since the measurement techniques are intrusive and
can therefore not be done in a continuous manner. The physiological signals however can
be measured continuously and have gained great attention from the research community.
Karthikeyan et al. [4] classified stressful and not stressful events based on HRV features
achieving a classification accuracy of 79.2 %. Others apply a combination of different

© Springer International Publishing Switzerland 2016
S. Serino et al. (Eds.): MindCare 2015, CCIS 604, pp. 13–22, 2016.
DOI: 10.1007/978-3-319-32270-4_2

sensing modalities. Wijsman et al. [5] use a combination of HRV, respiration, GSR and muscle tone of the upper trapezius muscle to discriminate between states of stress and rest in working environments. Analysis using generalized estimating equations yielded a classification accuracy of 74.5 %. Healey and Picard [6] differentiate three levels of stress with an accuracy of over 97 % using a combination of HRV, GSR, respiration and electromyogram features extracted from the raw signals using a Fisher linear classifier.

Large differences exist among classification accuracies from different studies. This is mainly due to three aspects of the studies being the experimental design, the sensor quality and the analysis methods. The focus of the current study is on the latter aspect. In many research linear discriminants, generalized estimation equations or support vector machines have been used to classify rest and stress states [5–8]. Other, more recent, research has focused on probabilistic machine learning techniques such as Bayesian networks [9, 10]. Sharma and Gedeon [11] report an overview of different computational techniques for stress classification based on results from different studies conducted under different experimental designs, sensors and physiological parameters. Although this comparison can provide significant insight in which are good modeling techniques, up to our knowledge there is no direct comparison of modeling techniques that result in the optimal algorithm to employ for stress detection. Furthermore in most research one general model is developed for all subjects. Literature and experts however agree that physiological responses to a stressor differ among subjects, e.g., the difference according to gender [12].

This study sought to compare several computational techniques for classifying stress based on physiological parameters within the same study design. Additionally, both generic and personalized models will be compared.

The main contributions of this paper are

1. We set-up a representative experimental protocol with control for physiological responses due to speech
2. We evaluate and compare the results of different data analysis techniques for stress modeling in comparison to rest
3. We compare the results of generic and personalized models for stress detection.

2 Materials and Methods

A controlled experiment was conducted to investigate the effect of stress on physiological parameters. The Medical Ethical Committee of KU Leuven approved the protocol and analysis methods of the experiment. In this section, the protocol and the sensing modalities are described. Furthermore, the feature list used for detection is described.

2.1 Data Collection

Experimental Protocol – Twenty healthy participants, 10 males and 10 females volunteered to participate (mean age = 40 ± 10 years). Test subjects did not suffer from any psychological or physical disease. Experiments were conducted in a quiet room using a standard desktop computer.

Figure 1 presents the timeline of the experiment. During the preliminary phase the participant completed some general questionnaires and the sensors were attached. The test phase included three stress tasks of two minutes each. As a first task, a Stroop Color-Word test [13] was presented. Color words were written in an incongruously ink color, e.g., the word red was written in the color blue. Participants had to respond with the real ink color, e.g., blue in the previous example. A math test was performed as second task. In the third task, participants were instructed to tell about an emotional or stressful event in their life. To induce additional stress the experimenter could intervene by saying 'wrong' or 'faster' during the first two tasks. To control for the physiological response due to speaking, an additional counting task was included where the participant had to count out loud from zero to hundred. This task was performed twice: once before the Stroop test and once after the stress talk, separated by a two minutes rest phase. All parts during the test phase take two minutes, except for the counting blocks which are dependent of the participant's pace of counting and the first resting block which serves as a baseline and takes four minutes. During the finishing phase the participant completed a retrospective questionnaire where his/her stress levels during each task were rated on a five-point Likert scale.

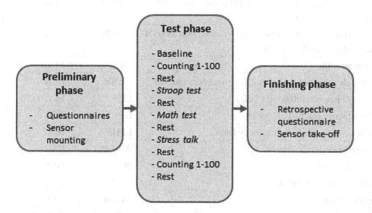

Fig. 1. Experimental protocol: three stress tasks and two counting tasks with a resting period between all tasks. Every task takes 2 min, except counting which is depending of the pace of counting and the first resting block which serves as a baseline.

Physiological Recordings – Two sensors were used. The first was the imec Necklace, a wireless electrocardiography (ECG) sensor for research use developed by imec [14]. With this sensor single-lead ECG in a lead-one configuration was recorded at a sampling frequency of 256 Hz. The second sensor was the NeXus 10 – MK II (Mind Media, Herten, The Netherlands). This sensor was used for the measurement of GSR and temperature at the fingertip and respiration using a chest belt. All NeXus signals were measured at a sampling frequency of 32 Hz.

2.2   Feature Computation

A comprehensive set of 22 features have been used, corresponding to features that have already been used in earlier publications on the expression of stress. For each sensing modality, features have been calculated on a sliding window of 30 s with 29 s overlap. ECG has been characterized with heart rate and heart rate variability, the latter considered in both time and frequency domain. GSR features are based on tonic and phasic responses. Temperature has been characterized using the mean value and standard deviation for each window, and the corresponding slope. Finally, respiration has been characterized as energy of several frequency bands. The complete list of features is reported in Table 1.

Table 1. List of features computed for each sensing modality

Nr.	Feature	Abbreviation	Extracted from	Ref.
1	The root of the mean of the sum of the squares of differences between normal to normal beat intervals	RMSSD	ECG	[4]
2	Proportion of the successive normal to normal beat intervals that differ more than 50 ms	pNN50	ECG	[4]
3	Proportion of the successive normal to normal beat intervals that differ more than 20 ms	pNN20	ECG	[4]
4	Mean heart rate	mHR	ECG	[5]
5	Standard deviation of the normal to normal beat intervals	SDNN	ECG	[5]
6	Low frequency band (0.04–0.15 Hz)	LF	ECG	[5]
7	High frequency band (0.15–0.4 Hz)	HF	ECG	[5]
8	Low frequency over high frequency band	LFHF	ECG	[5]
9	Absolute second difference	AbsDiff2	GSR	[5]
10	Skin conductance level	SCL	GSR	[5]
11	Ohmic perturbation duration	OPD	GSR	[5]
12	Number of peaks	Nrpeaks	GSR	[15]
13	Tonic component (0–0.16 Hz)	mTonic	GSR	[15]
14	Phasic component (0.16–2.1 Hz)	mPhasic	GSR	[15]
15	Mean temperature	mT	Temperature	[16]
16	Standard deviation of the temperature	stdT	Temperature	[16]
17	Slope of the temperature	slopeT	Temperature	[7]
18	Mean respiration frequency	meanRsp	Respiration	[5]
19	Energy band 0–0.1 Hz	EB1	Respiration	[6]
20	Energy band 0.1–0.2 Hz	EB2	Respiration	[6]
21	Energy band 0.2–0.3 Hz	EB3	Respiration	[6]
22	Energy band 0.3–0.4 Hz	EB4	Respiration	[6]

2.3   Analysis Methods

A binary classification problem was considered with classes corresponding to rest and stress periods. The reference stress profile contains stress during the three different stress tasks and rest in the remainder of the experiment, including the counting parts. A feature selection methodology based on correlation was used to eliminate features that are not useful but can negatively affect the classification performance. For every feature the correlation with the reference stress levels was calculated and all features with an absolute coefficient higher than 0.5 were retained. The feature selection procedure was performed only on the training set (see Sect. 2.4). Six machine learning algorithms were considered for evaluating the classification performance. The selection aims to cover a comprehensive set of algorithms with both conventional, linear techniques and more novel approaches. The algorithms are briefly described.

Logistic Regression (LR) – In LR the probability of the outcome of the stress vs rest classification is modeled as a function of the features weighed by coefficients [17]. To guarantee independent predictors, variables with an absolute correlation higher than 0.8 were eliminated.

Support Vector Machines (SVM) – SVM searches for an optimal hyperplane to separate the data between features of stress and rest [18]. SVM uses a geometrical transformation that projects the features into an infinite dimensional space where a linear separation is found.

Decision Trees (DT) – DT learn structures underlying the data using hierarchical partitioning [19]. Nodes of the tree represent splits, which test the value of an expression of the attributes. The final branches represent the outcomes of the test. Each leaf node has a class label associated with it.

Random Forests (RF) – RF is a combination of decision trees where each tree is built using a random selection of data and features [20]. To decide on the number of trees to be calculated the out-of-bag classification error is plotted in function of the number of trees. In our experiment, we set the number of trees to 20 for the RF model.

Bayesian Networks (BN) – BN are directed acyclic graphs, where each node represents a random variable, i.e., the features and stress levels, and edges represent direct correlations between the variables. Each node is characterized by a conditional probability distribution of the variable given its parents [21]. BN are static or dynamic. Dynamic BN are identical to the static BN, but additionally model the temporal relation of variables [10]. Therefore an additional edge is placed between the stress level at time $t - 1$ and time t. To learn the structure a greedy search algorithm was employed, the conditional distributions were calculated using maximum likelihood estimation. Junction three inference was used for classification of the test set.

2.4   Models Evaluation and Performance Measures

For every machine learning algorithm, two models were trained, one using data from all subjects, i.e., a *generalized* model, and one using only data of a specific subject, i.e., a *personalized* model.

For the generalized models, a leave-one-out validation procedure was used. The models were trained on the data of all, but one, participant and evaluated on the data of this participant. For the personalized models a different approach was used. Since stress accumulates over time and its physiological response does not return immediately to the original baseline [22], we have trained our models on the first two stress tests and evaluated their performance on the last stress test, including the stress talk. Using this validation approach instead of the usual cross-validation we have been able to take the time-dependent nature of stress into account and to provide more trustworthy performance indicators of the models.

Sensitivity (*Stress Detection Rate*) and specificity (*Rest Detection Rate*) were considered as performance measures. These two measures will give a good understanding of the classification performance in case of an unbalanced amount of rest and stress examples. As overall performance measure, the average of these two measures was taken instead of the usual classification accuracy. We define this measure as *Average Detection Rate* (ADR).

3   Experimental Results

First a correlation-based feature selection was performed. For generalized models, 4 features were selected, mHR from ECG and SCL, mTonic and mPhasic from GSR. For personalized models, the features selected varied according to person. On average 8 features were selected per person. The 5 features selected for the most participants are mHR and mPhasic (84 % of participants), SCL and mTonic (80 % of participants) and AbsDiff2 (74 % of participants). For no participant the following 5 features were selected: LF, LFHF, EB1, EB2 and EB4.

Figure 2 represents the GSR of one participant. The light grey bars indicate the counting periods, which have been included to control for the response due to speech, the dark grey bars indicate the stress tests. GSR reacts in both areas which underlines the importance of including a control for speech. The figure also highlights the time-dependent nature of stress as after each task the GSR does not return to baseline.

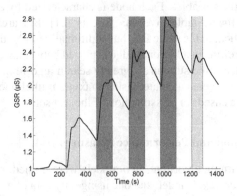

Fig. 2. GSR response of one participant. Light grey areas indicate a speech task, dark grey areas a stress task

The classification results obtained by generalized and personalized models are reported in Tables 2 and 3 respectively and graphically represented in Fig. 3. The average and standard deviation for rest detection rate (RDR), stress detection rate (SDR) and average detection rate (ADR) are presented. Most of the misclassifications for the rest condition are situated in the counting task, due to the physiological response to speech. Results indicate that overall the highest ADR is reached using personalized dBN (84.6 %) and generalized SVM (82.7 %). Besides for dBN the personal approach did not perform better than the general.

Table 2. Classification accuracy for generalized models (RDR = rest detection rate, SDR = stress detection rate, ADR = average detection rate).

	LR	SVM	DT	RF	sBN	dBN
RDR (%)	93.2 ± 2.8	93.4 ± 3.2	88.6 ± 4.4	90.7 ± 4.1	91.2 ± 3.6	58.3 ± 14.8
SDR (%)	68.2 ± 13.6	72.0 ± 10.4	65.4 ± 8.1	67.6 ± 8.4	70.5 ± 14.0	90.2 ± 14.1
ADR (%)	80.7 ± 7.3	82.7 ± 5.8	77.0 ± 4.9	79.2 ± 5.1	80.9 ± 7.8	74.3 ± 10.3

Table 3. Classification accuracy for personalized models (RDR = rest detection rate, SDR = stress detection rate, ADR = average detection rate).

	LR	SVM	DT	RF	sBN	dBN
RDR (%)	79.5 ± 20.4	77.5 ± 20.2	78.3 ± 18.7	79.1 ± 19.0	81.3 ± 21.2	87.7 ± 10.4
SDR (%)	72.5 ± 25.2	74.8 ± 25.8	69.2 ± 24.4	72.0 ± 25.4	77.0 ± 25.3	81.5 ± 21.9
ADR (%)	76.0 ± 10.7	76.1 ± 11.3	73.7 ± 12.6	75.6 ± 12.9	79.2 ± 13.7	84.6 ± 9.8

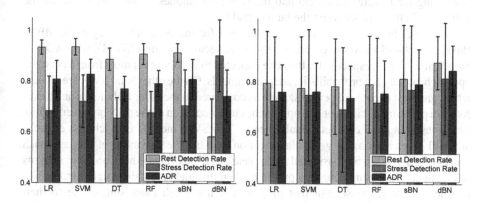

Fig. 3. Classification accuracy for generalized models (left) and personalized models (right)

4   Discussion

To correct for the inherent physiological response due to speech, a counting task was introduced before the first and after the last stress task. Experimental results show that most misclassifications for the rest condition were situated in this area. This emphasizes the importance of including regular speech in the experimental protocol. The feature selection procedure indicated that mainly GSR-based features together with the mHR are interesting with respect to the detection of stress in a controlled environment.

Comparison of the results in Tables 2 and 3 does not confirm the hypothesis that a personal approach renders higher average detection rates (ADR) than a general approach. This is only the case for dynamic Bayesian networks. However it can be observed that generalized models have relatively low stress detection rate, compared to rest detection rate. In most applications the main goal is to detect stress. Therefore models with higher stress detection rates should be preferred. Furthermore it can be observed that standard deviations for the personal approach are much higher than for the general approach. This means that for some participants a very high ADR could be reached, where for others the ADR was very low. Further analysis revealed that the datasets with high and low ADR are not the same for different modelling techniques. Future research should therefore investigate whether a further personalization in terms of machine learning algorithm selection could be beneficial. Another improvement could be made by merging the generalized approach with a subject-dependent feature calculation as suggested in [23]. Finally a personalized method is capable of giving more insight into the personal physiological stress response, e.g., the correlation-based feature selection can give an indication of the person's principal stress physiology. This can be interesting for targeted treatment and relaxation techniques in order to overcome the detrimental effects of stress on the human body.

The best classification results were obtained for the personalized dynamic (dBN) Bayesian networks and the generalized support vector machines (SVM), with ADR of 84.6 % and 82.7 % respectively. It can be expected that dBN profit most from a personal approach, as they are probabilistic, adapting models. On the other hand SVM are models which are most capable of generalization as compared to the other techniques and therefore can perform best in a general approach. The calculation of the dBN however is quite time consuming and computationally heavy. The SVM method is much less effortful and still gives reasonably good classification results. The downside of this approach however is that it can be considered a complete black-box. This is not a problem in terms of classification, but it becomes a problem when the goal is to gain insight in the physiological stress response. For that purpose BN are much more suited, due to their graphical character.

Therefore in the future a distinction should be made based on the purpose of the analysis. If the goal is to develop a fast algorithm for real-time stress detection, where only information about stress or no stress is required, the support vector machines technique should be considered the best choice. If the goal is to gain insight into a person's stress response a better option is to use dynamic Bayesian networks. Furthermore future research should investigate whether the conclusions drawn from this controlled study also hold for ambulatory studies.

5 Conclusion

The goal of the study was to identify the optimal computational methods for stress detection in a controlled environment. To this end an experiment was conducted in a laboratory environment where participants had to fulfill three different stress tests. To control for the physiological response to speech a counting task was introduced before the first and after the last stress task. Six machine learning techniques were investigated using a general and personal approach. It can be concluded that personalized dynamic Bayesian networks and generalized support vector machines render the best average classification results with 84.6 % and 82.7 % respectively. Based on characteristics inherent to the methods, it is suggested to use dynamic Bayesian networks when insight in the model is necessary and to use support vector machines when it is not.

Acknowledgements. Authors acknowledge the Institute for the Promotion of Innovation through Science and Technology in Flanders (IWT-Vlaanderen, Brussels, Belgium) for financial support.

References

1. Kawakami, N., Haratani, T.: Epidemiology of job stress and health in Japan: review of current evidence and future direction. Ind. Health **37**, 174–186 (1999)
2. Bakker, A., Demerouti, E.V.W.: Using the job demands-resources model to predict burnout and performance. Hum. Resour. Manag. **43**, 83–104 (2004)
3. Hoehn, T., Braune, S., Scheibe, G., Albus, M.: Physiological, biochemical and subjective parameters in anxiety patients with panic disorder during stress exposure as compared with healthy controls. Eur. Arch. Psychiatry Clin. Neurosci. **247**, 264–274 (1997)
4. Karthikeyan, P., Muragappan, M., Yaacob, S.: Analysis of Stroop Color-Word test-based human stress detection using electrocardiography and heart rate variability signals. Arab. J. Sci. Eng. **39**, 1835–1847 (2014)
5. Wijsman, J., Grundlehner, B., Hermens, H.: Wearable physiological sensors reflect mental stress state in office-like situations. In: Humaine Association Conference on Affective Computing and Intelligent Interaction (2013)
6. Healey, J., Picard, R.: Detecting stress during real-world driving tasks using physiological sensors. IEEE Trans. Intell. Transp. Sig. **6**, 156–166 (2005)
7. Zhai, J., Barreto, A.: Stress detection in computer users based on digital signal processing of noninvasive physiological variables. In: Proceedings of the 28th IEEE EMBS Annual International Conference, pp. 1355–1358 (2006)
8. Sano, A., Picard, R.: Stress recognition using wearable sensors and mobile phones. In: Humaine Association Conference on Affective Computing and Intelligent Interaction (2013)
9. Rigas, G., Goletsis, Y., Fotiadis, D.: Real-time driver's stress event detection. IEEE Trans. Intell. Transp. Syst. **13**(1), 221–234 (2012)
10. Liao, W., Zhang, W., Zhu, Z., Ji, Q.: A real-time human stress monitoring system using dynamic Bayesian networks. In: Computer Society Conference on Computer Vision and Pattern Recognition (2005)
11. Sharma, N., Gedeon, T.: Objective measures, sensors and computational techniques for stress recognition and classification: a survey. Comput. Methods Programs Biomed. **108**, 1287–1301 (2012)

12. Stoney, C., Davis, M., Matthews, K.: Sex differences in physiological responses to stress and in coronary heart disease: a causal link? Psychophysiology **24**(2), 127–131 (1987)
13. Van der Elst, W., Van Boxtel, P., Van Breukelen, J., Jolles, J.: The Stroop Color-Word test: influence of age, sex, and education; and normative data for a large sample across the adult age range. Assessment **13**, 62–79 (2006)
14. Brown, L., Grundlehner, B., van de Molengraft, J., Penders, J., Gyselinckx, B.: Body area network for monitoring autonomic nervous system responses. In: Pervasive Computing Technologies for Healthcare (2009)
15. Singh, R., Conjeti, S., Banerjee, R.: A comparative evaluation of neural network classifiers for stress level analysis of automotive drivers using physiological signals. Biomed. Sig. Process. Control **8**, 740–754 (2013)
16. Karthikeyan, P., Murugappan, M., Yaacob, S.: Multiple physiological signal-based human stress identification using non-linear classifiers. Elektronika ir elektrotechnika **19**(7), 80–85 (2013)
17. Hayes, A., Matthes, J.: Computational procedures for probing interactions in OLS and logistic regression: SPSS and SAS implementations. Behav. Res. Methods **41**(3), 924–936 (2009)
18. Burges, C.: A tutorial on support vector machines for pattern recognition. Data Min. Knowl. Disc. **2**(2), 121–167 (1998)
19. Murthy, S.: Automatic construction of decision trees from data: a multi-disciplinary survey. Data Min. Knowl. Disc. **2**(4), 345–389 (1998)
20. Breiman, L.: Random forests. Mach. Learn. **45**(1), 5–32 (2001)
21. Friedman, N., Geiger, D., Goldszmidt, M.: Bayesian network classifiers. Mach. Learn. **29**(2), 131–163 (1997)
22. Mezzacappa, E., Kelsey, R., Katkin, E., Sloan, R.: Vagal rebound and recovery from psychological stress. Psychosom. Med. **63**(4), 650–657 (2001)
23. Giakoumis, D., Tzovaras, D., Hassapis, G.: Subject-dependent biosignal features for increased accuracy in psychological stress detection. Int. J. Hum.-Comput. Stud. **71**, 425–439 (2013)

Stress Recognition in Daily Work

Yoshiki Nakashima[1]($\boxtimes$), Jonghwa Kim[2], Simon Flutura[2],
Andreas Seiderer[2], and Elisabeth André[2]

[1] Smart Energy Research Laboratories, NEC Corporation,
34 Miyukigaoka, Tsukuba, Ibaraki 305-8501, Japan
y-nakashima@bu.jp.nec.com
[2] Institute of Computer Science, University of Augsburg,
Universitätsstraße 6a, 86159 Augsburg, Germany

Abstract. Automatic detection of work-related stress has attracted an increasing amount of attention from researchers from various disciplines and industries. An experiment is discussed in this paper that was designed to evaluate the efficacy of multimodal sensor measures that have often been used but not yet been systematically tested and compared with each other in previous work, such as pressure distribution sensor, physiological sensors, and an eye tracker. We used the Stroop test and information pick up task as the stressors. In the subject independent case in particular, signals from the combined (chair and floor) pressure distribution sensors, which we consider the most feasible sensors in the office environment, resulted in higher recognition accuracy rates than the physiological or eye tracker signals for the two stressors.

Keywords: Stress · Activity recognition · Machine learning · Multi-modality

1 Introduction

Stress is the wear and tear that our minds and bodies experience as we attempt to cope with our continually changing environment. In particular, stress at work can be very expensive. It is identified as the second most frequently reported work-related health problem in the world and believed to be the cause of more than half of all lost working days.

The demands to office workers are sometimes too high and when they feel that they cannot handle all of the demands based on their capabilities, they become stressed [1]. However, if they have enough time to recover from their stressed state, they will less likely incur mental illness. So, it would be beneficial if the emotional states of office workers could constantly be monitored in order to detect their levels of stress, since this would make workers aware of their stress level and encourage them to have recovery time. Moreover, this would assist their employers in preventing them from demanding too much of them. For this purpose, the most important point is the feasibility of implementing a stress recognition system in the office environment.

Sometimes stress recognition means to differentiate between 'stressed' and 'relaxed' state, but office workers are normally concentrating on their work, and thus, are neither relaxed nor stressed. In other words, this is the state that people are in while

© Springer International Publishing Switzerland 2016
S. Serino et al. (Eds.): MindCare 2015, CCIS 604, pp. 23–33, 2016.
DOI: 10.1007/978-3-319-32270-4_3

doing a task without any stressors. So, we should add a new state, so-called 'concentrated' state, and be able to recognize between three states, which are 'relaxed', 'concentrated', and 'stressed'. If we are able to differentiate between these three states, we make an important step forward towards the automated recognition of stress states in daily work.

There have been various modalities that were proposed for stress recognition, including facial expression, speech expression (prosody), physiological signals, eye movements, and postures. Among them, using postures is significantly advantageous for long term daily use, especially in an office environment. First, they can be sensed non-intrusively [2] and unobtrusively, unlike physiological signals, which means the sensors themselves never make people stressed. Second, they can be sensed all the time while people are at work, unlike speech or eye movements. Most eye movement sensors can only detect eye gaze points which are inside the display. Third, postures can be analyzed at a relatively coarse level, in comparison to facial or speech expressions, which means they offer substantial benefits in terms of simplicity [2].

Pressure distribution sensor mats have garnered a lot of attention as sensor devices suitable for posture detection in office environments. They have also been tested as sensors for recognizing stress or emotions in publications [4, 7].

Stress and emotions are theoretically related to activities of the autonomic nervous system (ANS) [3]. ANS activities are largely involuntary and generally cannot be easily triggered by any conscious or intentional control. Therefore, physiological signals, which are the results of these ANS activities [3], are considered as reliable signals of stress and emotional activities. The same thing can also be said for some specific eye movements, such as fixation or saccades.

These three modalities are respectively interesting for long-term stress monitoring, in different reasons. These modalities have been used in previous work, but not yet been systematically tested and compared with each other. It is beneficial to know which modality or which combination of modalities is the best solution.

2   Related Work

In this chapter, we briefly review previous related work in terms of an argument about the stress states to be classified, stress stimuli, and the sensor modalities used for automatic detection.

Stress Stimuli. A Stroop test, especially a computer-based one, has been evaluated as an effective stressor in previous work on automatic stress recognition [5, 6]. There are two Stroop test versions, 'congruent' and 'incongruent'. In the congruent test, a screen containing a color name like "yellow" which is inked in the same color is shown to the participant. In the incongruent test, a color name is also shown to the participant, but in this case it is inked in a different color. For example the name of the color is "green" but it is inked "red". In both tests, the participant should answer with the name of the color the word is inked with. In the incongruent test, she/he should answer with a different word than she/he is looking at. This leads to stress resulting only out of the conflict between the recognition of the word and the color, and thus, does not depend on the participant's ability like it would be the case if calculations are used, so all participants should be stressed at a nearly equal level.

More natural-like tasks that mimic typical office work have been used as mental stressors. For example, text transcriptions, information pick up tasks, and expressive writings were designed as mental stressors in [8]. The office work stressors are more appropriately being evoked in these tasks. For these tasks, the stressors are also designed to be typical for office work, such as time pressure and interruptions (by phone calls or E-mails). These stressors force mental workloads on the participant. One research [9] classified the workload factors that are common in many kinds of work into [10] classes, and showed that the most important factor is time pressure. Relaxing videos are typically used for inducing a relaxed state [8].

Modalities. Several studies showed that pressure distribution sensors are an effective modality for recognizing stress by recognizing the participant's posture [4, 7]. Typically, the pressure distribution on a person's seat is sensed, and then the postures are recognized from the sensor data. Finally, the emotional and stress states can be determined using these recognized postures. Nevertheless, recent research has shown that the pressure distribution data itself can be used to recognize stress, without needing to first recognize the postures [4]. Furthermore, floor pressure distribution can be used for emotion recognition [10]. Peripheral physiological signals [11, 12] have been proven to be effective stress or emotion recognition modalities. Electro dermal activity (EDA) is one of the most effective signals from among the physiological signals used for stress or emotion recognition [12]. Blood volume pressure (BVP) and heart rate (HR) are also preferred as stress or emotion recognition features [13]. Involuntary eye movements, like saccades or fixations have also been investigated and shown to reflect the activities of the central nervous system, and are related to stress and emotions [14]. So, eye movement signals, which can be tracked by eye tracker sensors, can also be added as an effective modality for stress recognition.

3   Experimental Conditions

Stress Stimuli. We used the Stroop test and the information pick up task as the stress stimuli. For the Stroop test, a congruent test is used for the concentrated state and an incongruent one is used for the stressed state. The only difference between them is whether there is a mismatch between the color and the word. There are six colors to select. The time limit for an answer is three seconds and the whole duration of each test is three minutes (Fig. 1).

The participant reads an HTML page with around 900 words for the information pick up task. The participants are instructed to pick up 10 pieces of information from that page. There are two conditions. First is to induce a stressed state using a 3-min time limit as time pressure, emphasized by a timer shown on the display. The second task is for the concentrated state without stressors.

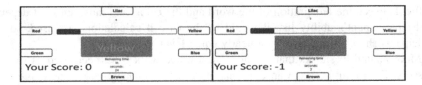

Fig. 1. Congruent (left) and incongruent (right) Stroop tests.

Sensors. Our setup includes three pressure distribution sensors (on the floor and on the seat and backrest of a chair), an eye tracker sensor, and a physiological sensor. We used SensingTex [15] sensors for the pressure distribution sensors. The seat and backrest chair sensors have a 4.5-cm resolution with 8×8 pressure detection cells, and the floor mat sensor is a 16×14 cells' sensor. The sampling rate for all of these SensingTex sensors was set to 20 Hz. With these three pressure sensors (chair seat, chair backrest and floor), we are able to monitor the whole body movement of a person in a sitting posture. Making these three sensors coalesce with other modalities is, at least in our knowledge, the first attempt. We selected the IOM [16] sensor for the physiological data. The sampling rate was 27 Hz. This sensor delivers BVP and EDA data. We can also obtain HR from the BVP signal by using signal processing. We used the Eye Tribe [17] as stationary eye tracker. Its sampling rate is 30 Hz. The setup of these sensors and photographs of the setup are shown in Fig. 2. The Social Signal Interpretation (SSI) framework was used for the synchronized recording of these multimodal sensor data [18].

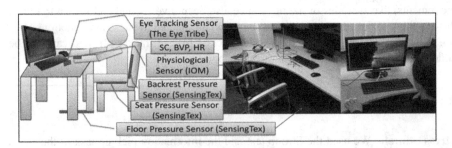

Fig. 2. Sensors used in our study (left), and photographs of set-up (center) and a participant doing task in set-up (right).

Participants. Ten healthy volunteers participated in our experiment. There were two women and eight men with an average age of 31 years. All of them were right handed and used the right hand to operate the computer mouse.

Experimental Procedure. We divided the participants into two groups, and set different schedules for each. Before the experiment, the participant was informed orally and through a document about the purpose of the experiment and the procedure that should be regarded. Then, each of them was connected to the physiological sensors. The eye tracker calibration also took place at this time. After that, each participant answered the first questionnaire. The questionnaire included the age, gender, dominant hand, and the hand she/he usually uses to operate a computer mouse. Afterwards, the participant shortly practices the congruent and incongruent Stroop tests to make sure they are understood correctly. Finally the experiment starts.

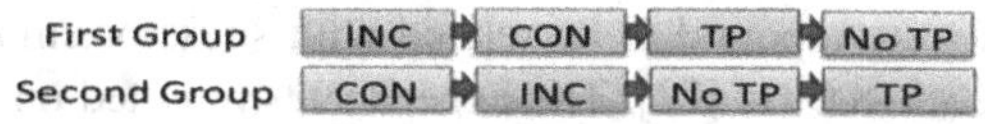

| First Group | INC → | CON → | TP → | No TP |
| Second Group | CON → | INC → | No TP → | TP |

Fig. 3. Time schedule for two groups. INC stands for the incongruent Stroop test, CON for the congruent Stroop test, TP for the information task with time pressure, and No TP for the information task without time pressure.

We begin with a 5 min relaxation session to relax the participant and to record the data of the relaxed state of the participant. During this session a video of landscapes accompanied with chill out music is shown. Then, a NASA TLX (Task Load Index) questionnaire [9] follows. The questionnaire consists out of six questions, asking their level of mental demand, physical demand, temporal demand, performance, effort, and frustration. We omitted asking the physical demand among these questions, because our purpose is to recognize the stress of office workers, who generally do not do physically demanding work.

The session with the Stroop tests begins after the questionnaire. For the first group, the incongruent test begins first, followed by the congruent test. For the second group the order is reversed, and then a 2 min relaxation video is shown followed by a NASA TLX questionnaire.

Then, the information tasks begin. A NASA TLX questionnaire follows each task. For the first group, the task with time pressure was done first. The second group starts with the task without time pressure. The 2 min relaxation video follows after the proceeding one. Ten pieces of information have to be gathered from around 900 words of text during the information pick up task. The text's context is related to fruit. The texts consisted out of adapted Wikipedia articles and were written in the mother tongue of the participants. The number of words was decided based on the known fact that the average reading speed is around 200 to 300 words per minute [19]. So 3 min is barely enough time for average readers.

4   Analysis

As we previously discussed, we used pressure distribution sensors, the eye tracker and physiological sensors. We calculated the features explained below within the time duration of 10 s, which we define as our event duration. Since we set the time duration of each stimulus (Stroop tests and information task) to 3 min or 180 s, we received 18 events for each stimulus.

Pressure Sensor. For the pressure distribution sensors, we focused on detecting the "Center of Pressure" or the weighted average point of distributed pressure loads for these sensors' two-dimensional coordinates. The two dimensions are AP (anterior-posterior) and LR (left-right). We used the euclidean distance (ED) to introduce a combined feature. Additionally we included the total intensity (TI) of each pressure distribution sensor mat. We calculated the statistical features and frequency features for these four values. The statistical features are the average, standard deviation, first and second difference, and the normalized first and second difference [20]. The frequency features are several body sway frequency bands that were reported to be related with stress or emotions: 0.1–0.7 Hz, 0.7–1.3 Hz [21], and 3.5–8.0 Hz [22]. The experiments reported on in these literatures were conducted with the participants standing, but these characteristic frequency bands depend on the time duration of the internal neural control system [21], so we also decided to use these frequency features. We also added the 1.3–3.5 Hz frequency band, which is in between the above bands, to see if there would be some relationship between the stress and this adjoining band.

Physiological Sensor. We calculated six statistical values (averages, standard deviations, first and second differences, and normalized first and second differences) [20] and the peak response time, peak amplitude, and energy [25] for EDA. We used the mean amplitude, skewness, and kurtosis [26] and the six statistical values of the signal for the blood volume pulse (BVP). Finally, we calculated the RMSSD [27], very low (0.05–0.15 Hz) and low (0.15–0.4 Hz) frequency bands and their ratio (low/very low), and the six statistical values for HR.

Eye Tracker Sensor. We calculated blinks, fixations, saccades, and scans [23, 24] from the eye tracker signals. We obtained the time duration, space distance (excluding blinks), and the number of occurrence of these four eye states, and calculated the maximum, mean, and summation values for these time durations and space distances as our features.

5 Classification

Feature Selection. We first try to select the features for each modality that we use, which are EDA, BVP, HR, floor, backrest, and the seat pressure distributions, and the eye tracker. We also set the physiological combined modality, which is the combination of EDA, BVP, HR, and the pressure distribution combined modality, which is the combination of the floor, backrest, and seat pressure distributions. We used sequential backward selection (SBS) as the method for the feature selections. The criterion for the SBS was pLDA.

Modality Level Classification. After selecting the features of each modality, we calculated the recognition accuracy rate of each modality for each state, using pLDA (pseudo LDA). We call the classification result of each modality for each state a 'decision'. Along with these modality decisions, we have also calculated the classification accuracy rate using all the modalities as a reference.

Decision Level Classification. The decision level classification [28] refers to the classification by combining the 'decisions' from multiple modalities. We used the recognition accuracy information for each state using the features of each modality first, and then, multiplied the accuracy rates as the weights of each decision for each modality. When the prediction accuracy for state j using the features extracted from modality i is defined as P_{ij}, and the 'decision' for state j using modality i is defined as X_{ij}, then the weight decision for state j can be expressed as X_j in Eq. (1).

$$X_j = \frac{\sum_i P_{ij} X_{ij}}{\sum_i P_{ij}}. \tag{1}$$

These weighted decisions for each state can be the features, and we made use of these 'decision level' features to train the classifiers. We used five classifiers in this 'decision level classification' phase, which are kNN (k = 1), pLDA, Linear SVM, RBF kernel SVM, and Fuzzy Logic.

6   Results

Modality Level Classification. We used pLDA to calculate the classification accuracy rates for each state. The results are listed in Table 2. Recall rates are shown in the table as accuracy rates. In the table, "Subject independent" means that we obtained training and test data set from different participants. "Subject dependent" means that we obtained the two kinds of data sets from the same participant. Leave one out cross validation method was used for calculating the recall rates.

Table 1. Classification accuracy rates for each state by each modality

| | Stroop Test | | | | | | | | Information Task | | | | | | | |
| | Subject independent | | | | Subject dependent | | | | Subject independent | | | | Subject dependent | | | |
Modality	Relax	Concen.	Stress	All	Relax	Concen.	Stress	All	Relax	Concen.	Stress	All	Relax	Concen.	Stress	All
EDA	76.7%	22.8%	28.9%	42.8%	100.0%	97.2%	95.6%	97.6%	64.4%	10.6%	47.8%	40.9%	100.0%	97.7%	100.0%	99.1%
BVP	42.2%	52.8%	36.7%	43.9%	77.2%	98.3%	62.8%	79.4%	47.8%	20.0%	49.4%	39.1%	90.3%	95.4%	94.0%	93.0%
HR	36.7%	26.7%	50.6%	38.0%	88.9%	83.9%	57.8%	76.9%	12.8%	38.3%	50.0%	33.7%	92.6%	63.9%	72.7%	75.7%
Floor	25.0%	35.6%	46.1%	35.6%	82.8%	74.4%	78.9%	78.7%	46.1%	52.8%	30.6%	43.1%	83.8%	84.7%	87.0%	84.1%
Backrest	62.8%	31.1%	29.4%	41.1%	100.0%	87.2%	82.2%	89.8%	62.8%	30.6%	31.1%	41.5%	94.4%	78.7%	73.6%	82.8%
Seat	38.9%	32.8%	53.9%	41.9%	100.0%	99.4%	93.9%	97.8%	42.2%	27.2%	52.8%	40.7%	96.8%	87.5%	91.2%	92.4%
Eye	66.1%	53.3%	21.1%	46.9%	95.0%	65.6%	63.9%	74.8%	46.1%	48.3%	40.6%	45.0%	87.0%	59.3%	61.6%	70.6%
Phys.	57.2%	40.0%	29.4%	42.2%	98.3%	98.9%	93.9%	96.9%	58.3%	32.8%	34.4%	41.9%	98.6%	95.8%	98.2%	97.0%
Pres.	45.6%	58.3%	46.1%	50.0%	99.4%	89.4%	85.6%	90.2%	73.9%	55.0%	49.4%	57.8%	86.6%	81.9%	81.5%	91.9%
All	70.0%	18.9%	60.6%	53.3%	100.0%	92.2%	93.9%	94.3%	80.6%	55.0%	32.2%	53.7%	96.3%	88.0%	87.5%	91.7%

Each column represents the two stressors, subject independent/dependent, and the three stress states. The *Relax, Concen.,* and *Stress* in the table represent the relaxed, concentrated, and stressed states, respectively, and *All* means all the states, which is the average of the three states. Each row represents the modality. *Floor, Backrest,* and *Seat* means the pressures distribution sensor signals from each place. *Eye* means the signals from the eye tracker sensor. *Phys.* means the combined physiological signals, and *Pres.*, the combined pressure distribution sensor signals. *All* means the signals from all the modality combined sensors.

The shadowed cells are for comparison between the combined pressure distribution signal, the combined physiological signal and eye movement signal. For the subject independent cases, the combined pressure sensor showed higher classification accuracy rates than the other two modalities, although this cannot be said for the subject dependent cases.

For further discussion, we also show the confusion matrix for *Eye*, *Phys.*, and *Pres.* The shadowed cells are for comparison. The precision rates show the same tendency: for the subject independent cases, the combined pressure sensor showed higher classification accuracy rates than the other two modalities.

Table 2. Confusion matrices for the three modalities

		Stroop Test								Information Task							
		Subject Independent				Subject Independent				Subject Independent				Subject Independent			
Eye		Predicted States Relax|Concen|Stress			Recall Rate	Predicted States Relax|Concen|Stress			Recall Rate	Predicted States Relax|Concen|Stress			Recall Rate	Predicted States Relax|Concen|Stress			Recall Rate
True States	Relax	119	39	22	66.1%	171	1	8	95.0%	83	52	45	46.1%	168	9	3	93.3%
	Concen.	45	96	39	53.3%|46.9%	4	118	58	65.6%|74.8%	37	87	56	48.3%|45.0%	14	94	72	52.2%|70.6%
	Stress	65	77	38	21.1%	7	58	115	63.9%	45	62	73	40.6%	5	56	119	66.1%
Precision Rate		52.0%	45.3%	38.4%	45.2%	94.0%	66.7%	63.5%	74.7%	50.3%	43.3%	42.0%	45.2%	89.8%	59.1%	61.3%	70.1%
Phys.		Predicted States Relax|Concen|Stress			Recall Rate	Predicted States Relax|Concen|Stress			Recall Rate	Predicted States Relax|Concen|Stress			Recall Rate	Predicted States Relax|Concen|Stress			Recall Rate
True States	Relax	103	42	35	57.2%	177	0	3	98.3%	105	42	33	58.3%	177	3	0	98.3%
	Concen.	67	72	41	40.0%|42.2%	1	178	1	98.9%|97.0%	76	59	45	32.8%|41.9%	3	171	6	95.0%|97.0%
	Stress	64	63	53	29.4%	3	8	169	93.9%	69	49	62	34.4%	0	4	176	97.8%
Precision Rate		44.0%	40.7%	41.1%	41.9%	97.8%	95.7%	97.7%	97.1%	42.0%	39.3%	44.3%	41.9%	98.3%	96.1%	96.7%	97.0%
Pres.		Predicted States Relax|Concen|Stress			Recall Rate	Predicted States Relax|Concen|Stress			Recall Rate	Predicted States Relax|Concen|Stress			Recall Rate	Predicted States Relax|Concen|Stress			Recall Rate
True States	Relax	82	43	55	45.6%	179	0	1	99.4%	133	38	9	73.9%	165	10	5	91.7%
	Concen.	21	105	54	58.3%|50.0%	2	161	17	89.4%|91.5%	43	99	38	55.0%|59.4%	6	145	29	80.6%|84.1%
	Stress	26	71	83	46.1%	6	20	154	85.6%	16	75	89	49.4%	2	34	144	80.0%
Precision Rate		63.6%	47.9%	43.2%	51.6%	95.7%	89.0%	89.5%	91.4%	69.3%	46.7%	65.4%	60.5%	95.4%	76.7%	80.9%	84.3%

Table 3. Classification accuracy rates for each state by each modality

Classifiers		Stroop		Inf. task	
		Subject independent	Subject dependent	Subject independent	Subject dependent
Decision level fusion	kNN	45.74 %	81.67 %	49.81 %	90.93 %
	pLDA	48.89 %	85.74 %	51.48 %	92.96 %
	Linear SVM	46.48 %	84.07 %	49.81 %	93.15 %
	RBF SVM	45.56 %	84.26 %	49.26 %	**93.52 %**
	Fuzzy Logic	45.93 %	80.00 %	**54.26 %**	87.59 %
Feature level fusion		**53.33 %**	**94.26 %**	53.70 %	91.67 %

Decision Level Classification. With the decision level fusion method using decision level features shown Eq. (1), we classified the three stress states using several classifiers for the four cases. The results are summarized in Table 3. Again, recall rates are shown in the table as accuracy rates. The feature level fusion results, using pLDA as the classifier, are also itemized in the table as reference.

For the information task states, our decision level fusion method worked well, showing higher rates than those of the feature level fusion. However, for the Stroop test states, our method could not obtain higher rates compared with the feature level fusion.

7 Discussions and Conclusion

Multi-modality is an effective method to recognize stress or emotion. In the state of the art of stress recognition, many modalities are used. However, the accuracy rates of each modality for each stress state have not yet been systematically tested and compared with each other, though this is important because it will provide the information for selecting and combining modalities to predict each state.

Therefore, the accuracy rates listed in Table 1, providing insights on the contribution of each single modality to stress state recognition, are important. Among them, one of the most remarkable results is that the pressure combined signal had higher prediction accuracy than the physiological combined signals or eye tracker signals in the subject independent case, for the two stressors (Stroop and Information Task) on average (*All* state). On the one hand, this is surprising because these two modalities (physiological signals and eye movement signals) are considered as involuntary modality and directly reflect neural activities which include emotion and stress. On the other hand, postures can be controlled voluntary. We will conduct further research to confirm the tendency shown in this research, and find the reason to underline the importance of using pressure distribution sensors. The confirmation of this result will make a new step towards the possibility of the usefulness of body placement for stress recognition in daily work, especially for unobtrusive, user independent systems.

The accuracy rates listed in Table 1 can be used not only for the selection or combination of modalities, but also for the fusion of the 'decision' of modalities to predict stress states. We demonstrated a decision level fusion; however, the result was not desirable. We will develop more advanced decision level fusion methods to take advantage of this information, especially for the subject independent case.

References

1. Demerouti, E., Bakker, A.B., Nachreiner, F., Schaufeli, W.B.: The job demands-resources model of burnout. J. Appl. Psychol. **86**(3), 499–512 (2001)
2. Grafsgaard, J.F., Boyer, K.E., Wiebe, E.N., Lester, J.C.: Analyzing posture and affect in task-oriented tutoring. In: 25th International Florida Artificial Intelligence Research Society Conference (2012)
3. Lang, P.J., Bradley, M.M., Cuthbert, B.N.: Emotion, motivation, and anxiety: brain mechanisms and psychophysiology. Biol. Psychiatry **44**(12), 1248–1263 (1998)

4. Arnrich, B., Setz, C., La Marca, R., Tröster, G., Ehlert, U.: What does your chair know about your stress level? IEEE Trans. Inf. Technol. Biomed. **14**(2), 207–214 (2009)
5. Frank, K., Robertson, P., Gross, M., Wiesner, K.: Sensor-based identification of human stress levels. In: International Conference on Pervasive Computing and Communications Workshops, pp. 127–132 (2013)
6. Calibo, T.K., Blanco, J.A., Firebaugh, S.L.: Cognitive stress recognition. In: Instrumentation and Measurement Technology Conference, pp. 1471–1474 (2013)
7. Meyer, J., Arnrich, B., Schumm, J., Tröster, G.: Design and modeling of a textile pressure sensor for sitting posture classification. IEEE Sens. J. **10**(8), 1391–1398 (2010)
8. Hernandez, J., Paredes, P., Roseway, A., Czerwinski, M.: Under pressure: sensing stress of computer users. In: SIGCHI Conference on Human Factors in Computing Systems, pp. 51–60 (2014)
9. Hart, S.G., Staveland, L.E.: Development of NASA-TLX (Task Load Index): results of empirical and theoretical research. Adv. Psychol. **52**, 139–183 (1998)
10. Giraud, T., Soury, M., Hua, J., Delaborde, A., Tahon, M., Antonio, D., Jauregui, G., Eyharabide, V., Filaire, E., Le Scanff, C., Devillers, L., Isableu B., Martin, J.C.: Multimodal expressions of stress during a public speaking task. In: 5th Biannual Conference of the Humaine-Association on Affective Computing and Intelligent Interaction, pp. 417–422 (2013)
11. Plarre, K., Raij, A., Hossain, S.M., Ahsan Ali, A., Nakajima, M., al'Absi, M., Ertin, E., Kamarck, T., Kumar, S., Scott, M., Siewiorek, D., Smailagic, A., Wittmers, L.E., Jr.: Continuous inference of psychological stress from sensory measurements collected in the natural environment. In: 10th International Conference of Information Processing in Sensor Networks, pp. 97–108 (2011)
12. Renaud, P., Blondin, J.P.: The stress of Stroop performance: physiological and emotional responses to color word interference, task pacing, and pacing speed. Int. J. Psychophysiol. **27**(2), 87–92 (1997)
13. Zhai, J., Barreto, A.: Stress detection in computer users based on digital signal processing of noninvasive physiological variables. In: 28th Annual Conference of IEEE Engineering in Medicine and Biology Society, vol. 1–15, pp. 1999–2002 (2006)
14. Di Stasi, L.L., Catenad, A., Cañasc, J.J., Macknike, S.L., Martinez-Condea, S.: Saccadic velocity as an arousal index in naturalistic tasks. Neurosci. Biobehav. Rev. **37**(5), 968–975 (2013)
15. SensingTex. http://sensingtex.com/
16. Wild Divine. http://www.wilddivine.com/
17. The EyeTribe. https://theeyetribe.com/
18. Wagner, J., Lingenfelser, F., André, E.: The social signal interpretation framework (SSI) for real time signal processing and recognition. In: 12th Annual Conference of the International Speech Communication Association, vol. 1–5, pp. 3252–3255 (2011)
19. Jackson, M.D., McClelland, J.L.: Sensory and cognitive determinants of reading speed. J. Verbal Learn. Verbal Behav. **14**(6), 565–574 (1975)
20. Picard, R.W., Vyzas, E., Healey, J.: Toward machine emotional intelligence: analysis of affective physiological state. IEEE Trans. Pattern Anal. Mach. Intell. **23**(10), 1175–1191 (2001)
21. Peterka, R.J., Loughlin, P.J.: Dynamic regulation of sensorimotor integration in human postural control. J. Neurophysiol. **91**(1), 410–423 (2004)
22. Krafczyk, S., Schlamp, V., Dieterich, M., Haberhauer, P., Brandt, T.: Increased body sway at 3.5–8 Hz in patients with phobic postural vertigo. Neurosci. Lett. **259**(3), 149–152 (1998)

23. Nodine, C.F., Kundel, H.L., Toto, L.C., Krupinski, E.A.: Recording and analyzing eye-position data using a microcomputer workstation. Behav. Res. Methods Instrum. Comput. **24**(3), 475–485 (1992)
24. Manor, B.R., Gordon, E.: Defining the temporal threshold for ocular fixation in free-viewing visuocognitive tasks. J. Neurosci. Methods **128**(1–2), 85–93 (2003)
25. Zhai, J., Barreto, A.B., Chin, C., Li, C.: Realization of stress detection using psychophysiological signals for improvement of human-computer interaction. In: Proceedings of IEEE SoutheastCon, pp. 415–420 (2005)
26. Mokhayeri, F., Akbarzadeh, M.R., Toosizadeh, T, S.: Mental stress detection using physiological signals based on soft computing techniques. In: 18th Iranian Conference of Biomedical Engineering (ICBME), pp. 232–237 (2011)
27. Koldijk, S., Sappelli, M., Verberne, S., Neerincx, M.A., Kraaij, W.: The SWELL knowledge work dataset for stress and user modeling research. In: 16th International Conference of Multimodal Interaction, pp. 291–298 (2014)
28. Kim, J.: Bimodal emotion recognition using speech and physiological changes. In: Grimm, M., Kroschel, K. (eds.) Robust Speech Recognition and Understanding, pp. 265–280. I-Tech Education and Publishing, Vienna (2007)

Hacking Alternatives in 21st Century: Designing a Bio-Responsive Virtual Environment for Stress Reduction

Mirjana Prpa(✉), Karen Cochrane, and Bernhard E. Riecke

School of Interactive Arts and Technology, Simon Fraser University, Surrey, Canada
{mprpa,kcochran,ber1}@sfu.ca

Abstract. In this paper we present the initial exploratory design of SOLAR, an immersive virtual environment (VE) that assists novice users to learn the stress reducing practice of mindfulness meditation. The VE is generated by the user's brain activity and respiratory rate. In addition, we provide an overview of previous work, outlining the elements we find effective and the gaps for each presented design. This is followed by a description of the design principles. Finally, we present the participatory design, design evaluation and iteration, followed by possible applications for the final design and future steps.

Keywords: Mindfulness practice · Virtual reality · Brain-computer interface (BCI) · Computer-supported mindfulness · Thought distancing

1 Introduction

It can be difficult to avoid the stresses of daily life. Meditation practice is known to reduce stress. Desbordes' research showed that practicing meditation can change the mental function even in non-meditative states [1]. Other studies have shown that meditation reduces stress levels and has a positive effect on stress-related disorders [2] such as anxiety and depression [3].

Mindfulness is a practice of meditation that is "a non-judgmental, non-conceptual, and accepting form of awareness of one's mental, emotional, and bodily sensory experience" [4]. The core practice focuses on breathing and letting go of strong thoughts of the past and future, especially those that trigger stress. The practice is about living in the present moment [4]. Recently, there is a trend in the mobile application market that offers a number of computer-supported mindfulness (CSM) [5] applications and devices that help support meditators in their practice. CSM is widely accepted in the research community and includes a range of different approaches to create mindfulness experiences. Examples include guided meditation videos posted on YouTube and Mindfulness-Based Stress Reduction (MBSR) therapy for war veterans implemented in Second Life [6]. However, it may be difficult to learn how to meditate independently without the guidance of a highly trained expert.

© Springer International Publishing Switzerland 2016
S. Serino et al. (Eds.): MindCare 2015, CCIS 604, pp. 34–39, 2016.
DOI: 10.1007/978-3-319-32270-4_4

In this paper, we present SOLAR, an immersive computer-supported virtual system for learning mindfulness meditation. We focus on investigating how we can design a support tool that will teach novice participants how to meditate. Presented virtual environment allows users to "stop, observe the thought, let the thought go and return to the practice" (SOLAR) [7]. The main part of the system is an audio-visual VE that reacts to the mediator's breathing and EEG data in real-time. SOLAR is an expansion of the Sonic Cradle [8] immersive audio environment, and as such it was built in Unity3D and Max6 while adding Emotiv EEG sensors to Thought Technology's ProComp2 and Respiratory Sensors. In SOLAR, the data is mapped to visual elements in VE and audio in Max6 in order to provide feedback to the user in real time. Though difficult, meditating with one's eyes open is the preferred practice. Therefore, our tool will assist novice mediators with keeping their eyes open while practicing meditation.

2   Design Principles

Our design objective for SOLAR was to accommodate the different needs of users, by following the design principles:

Thought Distancing. Thought distancing is one of the techniques widely used in mindfulness meditation to help practitioners experience negative thoughts as mental events rather than a self-critique or reflection of truth [9]. The goal is to reach a state of awareness in which internal mental events are not judged, analyzed or responded to [10]. When practitioners have a thought that is not related to the present moment, they are instructed to accept the thought and then let the thought go. However, many authors noted that for novice meditators thought distancing can be extremely difficult to achieve [11, 12] and may discourage further practice. As suggested by Chittaro and Vianello [5], a visual representation of thoughts incorporated into the system makes the thought distancing practice easier for novice practitioners. We believe that building a meditative environment with both visual and auditory feedback will support the practice of meditation for users with a range of needs.

Abstract Visual Elements. Chittaro and Vianello state that visual representations are recommended in meditation practice [5], however, definitive images may be distracting in certain situations. Abstract images and shapes are less distracting than concrete images (flowers, for instance) and will help participants relax [13]. The use of subtle visual elements as a reminder to focus on "positive coping strategies" is the preferred form of visible feedback [14]. In SOLAR we included a visual representation of one's breathing in the form of abstract elements such as particles, fog, and various lighting. The purpose was to create a pleasant visual feedback experience and to introduce an ambient quality to our computer-supported mindfulness system.

Rewarding System. Rewarding practice, we believe, can motivate users to meditate more often and for longer periods of time because of the enjoyment they feel. Some applications balance "reward" and "punishment" feedback by providing pleasant feedback when the meditation score is high, and unpleasant feedback when thoughts start wandering. Our design relies on pleasant sound and visuals only. We predict that the user's anticipation of an enjoyable soundscape that accompanies a proper meditation session will provide motivational feedback, signaling to the user that they are meditating properly, and will reinforce thought distancing techniques for longer periods of time.

Immersive and Attention Restorative Environments (ARE). Immersive environments can positively affect user's attention, which was explained by Kaplan [15] in his Attention Restoration Theory (ART) that focuses on the correlation between the type of stimuli and the restorative potential of different environments. The environments with stimuli that modestly capture attention are preferred (subtle nature sounds are preferred over traffic noise, for instance), and the design of our system relies on this principle.

3   Design Evolution

Designing a virtual environment for meditation came with many challenges. Our aim was to design an environment that will enhance the mediation experience. Following that rationale, we decided to keep a simple design and include elements that will directly provide feedback to its users. SOLAR was developed in phases. Following completion of the first prototype, we conducted a design activity to get feedback on the working elements. The feedback helped us reconsider some of the design decisions and redesign the model. In the following section, we explain the design decisions in more detail.

3.1   Exploratory Design of the Prototypes and Design Activity

Prototype One. For the first prototype, we did not use the EEG, respiration sensors, or the sounds from Sonic Cradle. We used the design activity to explore the idea of thought distancing. To implement thought distancing, we executed a simple visual element: a circle. We asked the user to push the "q" key when they were exhaling and press the "p" key when they were inhaling. When the user interacted with the keyboard, the circle expanded when the user inhaled and contracted when the user exhaled. SOLAR asked the user to focus their attention on the circle, and if any wandering thoughts occurred, we asked our participants to accept their thoughts then push their thoughts through the circle. For the audio we used Jon Kabat-Zinn's beginner meditation track.

Design Activity. We conducted the design activity with thirteen participants at Simon Fraser University's Surrey Campus open house. The participatory design activity was not an experiment and therefore did not include a control group. Instead, we used the activity to make changes to our prototype SOLAR. In the future, we plan to run a full experiment. Regardless, we did ask the participants to rate their calmness before and after the experience and to write down any comments they might have. The participants' answers were converted to a 0–100 score using linear transformation. The results showed that overall participants felt more relaxed after the session compared to before the session. We used a dependent t-test to analyze the relaxation means. The results showed that SOLAR had a statistically significant impact on the participants' reported relaxation levels. Relaxation before exposure to the meditation session (M = 53.23, SE = 7.105) improved substantially after experiencing the meditation session (M = 82.62, SE = 3.670), t(12) = 3.956, p = 0.002, r = 0.752). We felt that the thought distancing helped the participants feel more relaxed and we decided to keep the thought distancing design principle for the second prototype.

Comments from the participants were critical in the design of the second prototype. We will discuss these as we implement the design changes in the second version of SOLAR.

Prototype Two. The participants felt the instructional audio track through the whole meditative experience was distracting, therefore, we changed SOLAR to consist of two scenes. First, an introduction scene that included audio instructions on how the user's breathing and meditation score interacted with the visuals. In the second and main scene, the audio consisted of the Sonic Cradle soundscape and the visuals were mapped to breathing and EEG sensors. In addition, we added a burst of particles on the user's exhale.

Internal processes relevant to mindfulness meditation include a still posture, a focus on breathing and thought distancing. We aimed to create an embodied connectedness between the user and the user's virtual representation by positioning the user's silhouette in the center of the scene.

The participants in the activity felt it difficult to control their breathing with the keyboard. Therefore, the audio and visual elements of SOLAR were manipulated using two biofeedback input devices (Emotiv Epoc and Thought Technology's respiration sensors).

The participants felt that the animation of the circle was too simple and wanted more complex visuals. Therefore, we used the user's meditation scores during the session to provide a gentle feedback to the user when their mind started to wander. This meditation score was mapped to additional elements in our virtual environment: the "meditation" circle (positioned behind the silhouette) and the silhouette's opacity. If the user is focused and the meditation score is increasing, then the "meditation circle" appears blue and the silhouette becomes more transparent (Fig. 1 on the left). However, if the user loses focus and the meditation score decreases, then the colour of the circle will change to purple and the silhouette will become less transparent.

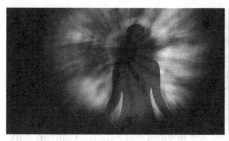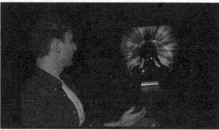

Fig. 1. Figure left: Silhouette's opacity decreased due to high meditation score. Figure right: The participant is meditating while using SOLAR.

The respiration sensors were placed on the user's thorax and diaphragm. The data received from the sensors was used for generating both audio and visual elements of SOLAR. In mindfulness meditation, it is suggested by the experts to practice deep diaphragm breathing [11]. In SOLAR, the user is rewarded with a complex soundscape when they are taking deep breaths from their diaphragm. If the user begins to breath from their chest (above their thorax) or starts taking shallow breaths, the soundscape becomes simplified. In the visuals, the respiration sensors are mapped to the "breathing circle" (in front of the silhouette). The breath circle becomes larger and smaller as the user inhales and exhales.

The participants commented that there should be soft lighting in the physical space and a comfortable chair. The room should be as dark as possible with no auditory or visual distractions so the user can fully focus on the screen (Fig. 1 on the right). Some of the participants did not feel comfortable with their eyes open. It was suggested that novice meditators meditate with their eyes open [11]. We realize that this aspect of SOLAR might not be appropriate for all participants.

4   Discussion and Conclusion

In this paper, we present the prototype SOLAR, an immersive virtual system created to serve as a training tool to teach mindfulness meditation. Our goal was to create a system with a unique design that will support novice meditators. The design of this system is grounded on four design principles (Thought Distancing, Abstract Visual Elements, Rewarding System, and Immersion and ARE) that emerged from current practices and experts' perspectives. The presented design is the result of a participatory design activity that we conducted with 13 participants.

Based on the feedback received from the participants, we iterated the prototype to address participant needs. In our iterations, we faced new challenges in the final design. We added an introduction scene that included audio instructions on how to use SOLAR, and in the main meditation scene we replaced the mindfulness meditation track with the Sonic Cradle soundscape. We focused on abstract visual elements, aiming to create a visually pleasing environment, and added complexity to user interactions. To address the issue of personal preference, we would like to add customizable visual and auditory elements in the next prototype.

In the future, we would like to consult with expert meditators and medical professionals working within the mental health and neurodevelopmental fields, and conduct user-centered design studies to create an effective system that would benefit their clients. After incorporating feedback from iterative user testing and refinement, we would like to conduct a more extensive usability study. More rigorous testing of the system's effectiveness is needed, specifically in supporting novices to learn mindfulness practice, testing for mental disorders (especially anxiety and depression), neurodevelopmental diseases (autism), and a comparison study between novices and experts. Concurrently with future studies, we will be working on system improvements to address recommendations and evaluate the effectiveness of visual elements. The design guidelines will continue to evolve.

Acknowledgements. We would like to thank all the participants, Amber Choo, Carman Neustaedter, Thecla Schiphorst, Marilyn Cochrane, and Moving Stories Project. This research was supported by the Social Sciences and Humanities Research Council of Canada.

References

1. Desbordes, G., Negi, L.T., Pace, T.W., Wallace, B.A., Raison, C.L., Schwartz, E.L.: Effects of mindful-attention and compassion meditation training on amygdala response to emotional stimuli in an ordinary, non-meditative state. Front. Hum. Neurosci. **6** (2012)
2. Barnes, V., Schneider, R., Alexander, C., Staggers, F.: Stress, stress reduction, and hypertension in African Americans: an updated review. J. Nat. Med. Assoc. **89**, 464 (1997)
3. Evans, S., Ferrando, S., Findler, M., Stowell, C., Smart, C., Haglin, D.: Mindfulness-based cognitive therapy for generalized anxiety disorder. J. Anxiety Disord. **22**, 716–721 (2008)
4. Frewen, P., Evans, E., Maraj, N., Dozois, D.A., Partridge, K.: Letting go: mindfulness and negative automatic thinking. Cogn. Ther. Res. **32**, 758–774 (2008)
5. Chittaro, L., Vianello, A.: Computer-supported mindfulness: evaluation of a mobile thought distancing application on naive meditators. Int. J. Hum.-Comput. Stud. **72**, 337–348 (2014)
6. Morie, J.F.: The healing potential of online virtual worlds. In: Brahnam, S., Jain, L.C. (eds.) Advanced Computational Intelligence Paradigms in Healthcare 6. SCI, vol. 337, pp. 149–166. Springer, Heidelberg (2011)
7. Burdick, D.E.: Mindfulness Skills Workbook for Clinicians and Clients: 111 Tools, Techniques, Activities & Worksheets. Pesi Publishing & Media, Eau Claire (2013)
8. Vidyarthi, J., Riecke, B.E., Gromala, D.: Sonic Cradle: designing for an immersive experience of meditation by connecting respiration to music. In: Proceedings of the Designing Interactive Systems Conference (2012)
9. Teasdale, J.D., Moore, R.G., Hayhurst, H., Pope, M., Williams, S., Segal, Z.V.: Metacognitive awareness and prevention of relapse in depression: empirical evidence. J. Consult. Clin. Psychol. **70**, 275 (2002)
10. Wells, A.: Detached mindfulness in cognitive therapy: a metacognitive analysis and ten techniques. J. Ration.-Emotive Cogn.-Behav. Ther. **23**, 337–355 (2005)
11. Kabat-Zinn, J.: Coming to Our Senses: Healing Ourselves and the World Through Mindfulness. Hachette, London (2005)
12. Segal, Z.V., Williams, J.M.G., Teasdale, J.D.: Mindfulness-Based Cognitive Therapy for Depression. Guilford Press, New York (2012)
13. Karamnezhad Salmani, M.: Virtual Reality and Health Informatics for Management of Chronic Pain (2014). http://summit.sfu.ca/item/14489
14. Cochrane, K., Schiphorst, T.: Developing design considerations for mobile and wearable technology: m-Health applications that can support recovery in mental health disorders. In: 9th International Conference on Pervasive Computing Technologies for Healthcare, 20 May 2015
15. Kaplan, S.: Meditation, restoration, and the management of mental fatigue. Environ. Behav. **33**, 480–506 (2001)

Listen and Watch: Audio and Voice Analysis in Mental Health

Validity of a Voice-Based Evaluation Method for Effectiveness of Behavioural Therapy

Shuji Shinohara[1(✉)], Shunji Mitsuyoshi[2], Mitsuteru Nakamura[2], Yasuhiro Omiya[1], Gentaro Tsumatori[3], and Shinichi Tokuno[2,3]

[1] PST Inc., Industry and Trade Center Building 905, 2 Yamashita-cho Naka-ku,
Yokohama, Kanagawa, Japan
{shinohara,omiya}@medical-pst.com
[2] Graduate School of Medicine, The University of Tokyo,
Industry and Trade Center Building 905, 2 Yamashita-cho Naka-ku, Yokohama, Kanagawa, Japan
{mitsuyoshi,tokuno}@m.u-tokyo.ac.jp,
NAKAMURAM-EME@h.u-tokyo.ac.jp
[3] National Defense Medical Collage, 3-2 Namiki, Tokorozawa, Saitama, Japan
{tsumagen,tokuno}@ndmc.ac.jp

Abstract. In this study, we used General Health Questionnaire 30 (GHQ30) and voice to evaluate the stress reduction effect of a stress resilience program, and examined the validity of stress evaluation by voice. We divided the subjects who participated in the program into two groups by the number of training sessions. The results showed a stress-reduction effect only in the group with more training sessions (more than 13 sessions) for both GHQ30 and voice-based indexes. Moreover, both indexes showed a highly negative correlation between the pre-training value and the difference between the post-training and pre-training values. This implies that the effect of the training is more evident for subjects with higher stress levels. The voice-based evaluation showed trends similar to those displayed by GHQ30.

Keywords: Stress check · Voice · Vitality · GHQ30 · Stress resilience program

1 Introduction

Mental health problems are serious issues in many developed countries [1], and economic costs such as medical expenses and poor performance at work are enormous [2]. Thus, there is a need for techniques that easily check depression state and stress, as well as ways to cure or reduce such conditions.

An example of screening methods for patients with mental health issues include self-administered psychological tests such as the General Health Questionnaire (GHQ) [3] and the Beck Depression Inventory (BDI) [4, 5]. Methods to check stress levels by using saliva and blood have also been proposed [6]. Self-administered psychological tests are effective for early detection and diagnostic aids but suffer from reporting bias issues. Additionally, stress-check methods using saliva and blood are not as simple due to issues related to test cost and burdens on the examinees.

© Springer International Publishing Switzerland 2016
S. Serino et al. (Eds.): MindCare 2015, CCIS 604, pp. 43–51, 2016.
DOI: 10.1007/978-3-319-32270-4_5

In contrast, analysis of patients' medical condition, stress and emotion using voice data has been attracting attention due to the widespread use of smartphones in recent years [7–9].

Voice-based evaluations with a smartphone are advantageous since they are non-invasive and can be conducted easily and remotely without any special equipment.

Studies on the relationship between mental disorders and voice characteristics include those which analysed depressed patients' speaking rates [10–12] and their switching pauses and percent pauses [12, 13]. Additionally, a study used chaos analysis to measure the Lyapunov exponents and Kolmogorov entropy in the voices of patients with depression [14]. Other research used frequency analysis to show that the shimmer and jitter values of vowel sounds made by patients with depression are higher than those of healthy individuals, while the first and second formant frequencies are lower for patients with depression [15]. A study proposed new features derived from Teager energy operator for stress classification [16]. Moreover, another report [17] proposed a method to measure mental health status based on the envelope information within pitch and voice waveforms.

While the above mentioned studies can be applicable for depression diagnosis and assessing stress levels, resilience programs that incorporate yoga and breathing techniques have been developed to reduce stress and depression, and have been implemented on a trial basis [18]. Additionally, a behavioural therapy called Smart, Positive, Active, Realistic, X-factor thoughts (SPARX), which utilises fantasy role-playing games, has also been developed and shown to be effective in treating younger-generation patients with depression [19, 20].

In this study, we used the GHQ30 and patients' voices before and after the stress resilience program to evaluate their stress levels, and examined the validity of the voice-based stress evaluation.

2   Materials and Methods

2.1   Samurai's Group and Individual Mental Training (S-Gim)

S-Gim is a stress resilience program developed by the Japan Self-Defence Forces [18]. S-Gim aims to acquire six skills, consisting of yoga stretches, breathing, imagery, viewpoint control, self-disclosure methods, and ways of supporting others to control stress. Yoga stretch and breathing can lead to control the mind by controlling the body. These give how to relax under the stress. Imagery is a method of controlling the image biased own. This is how to regain confidence. Viewpoint control fix a habit that is easy to catch negative. This is how to be taken to the positive things. Self-disclosure method is a training that represents the inside of your own mind. This is how to ask for help well. Way of supporting others is a technique to save the crisis of colleagues. This is how to control stress as a team.

The program entails 15 min a day, five times a week, for a total of 50 sessions, to become capable of demonstrating these skills easily.

2.2   Measuring Method for the Effectiveness of S-Gim

In this study, we measured the effect of S-Gim using the GHQ30 and a vitality score obtained from the voice-based analysis. GHQ30 is a self-administered psychological test with 30 questions, which provides scores for general disorder trends, physical conditions, sleep disorders, social activity disorders, anxiety and dysthymia, suicidal ideation, and depression [1].

A vitality score is one of the indices of mental health status that can be obtained by analysing patients' voices. The word "vitality" can have different definitions and implications. Here, it can be summarized as a measure that is low for patients with depression and strokes, and high for healthy individuals. The vitality score is calculated from the sound pressure level at the nadir of the amplitude envelope of the patient's voice between syllables, the change in the number of zero crossings in the waveform, and the pitch detection rate. Roughly speaking, clear, discernible, and fast voices usually correspond to higher vitality scores [17].

2.3   Acquisition of Voices

From 3rd October, 2012 to 18th February, 2013, S-Gim was carried out with approximately 100 members of the Japan Self-Defence Forces. We collected voice data and the self-administered GHQ30 psychological test data from the subjects before and after the program. Voices were recorded by an IC recorder ICR-PS502RM (Sanyo Electric, Osaka, Japan) placed about 15 cm from the subject's mouth. The recording format was as follows: linear PCM, a sampling frequency of 44.1 kHz, 16-bit quantization, low recording level, and ZOOM for directivity switching. Moreover, the microphone auto level control, low cut filter, recording peak limiter, VAS setting, and automatic soundless partitioning were turned off. The subjects were asked to read 11 types of passages.

There were 59 members from whom we were able to obtain both the voice and GHQ30 data before and after S-Gim. This paper targets these 59 members for the analysis.

3   Results

3.1   Evaluation of the Effect of S-Gim by GHQ30

The average GHQ30 score before S-Gim was 3.85 (SD = 5.57, n = 59). The average score after S-Gim was 2.85 (SD = 4.25). Additionally, there were 17 subjects whose score before S-Gim was zero. The purpose of this study is to measure the effect of S-Gim. The 17 subjects who scored zero before S-Gim were excluded from further analysis because no measurable decrease in their GHQ30 scores was possible. On the remaining 42 subjects, the average GHQ30 score before S-Gim was 5.40 (SD = 5.93, n = 42). The average score after S-Gim was 3.81 (SD = 4.66).

In order to examine the effect of S-Gim based on the number of sessions completed, we divided the 42 subjects into two groups: 22 subjects with fewer sessions completed (1–12 sessions), and 20 subjects more sessions completed (more than 13 sessions)[1]. The average number of sessions conducted for the two groups were 7.23 (SD = 3.80) and 31.50 (SD = 14.95), respectively.

Figure 1 shows the change in the GHQ30 scores for each group. The left group of bars shows the data for subjects who attended 1 to 12 sessions, while the right group of bars shows the data for subjects who participated in more than 13 sessions. The vertical axis shows the number of subjects who experienced each score change pattern (increased, unchanged, and decreased) before and after S-Gim. The proportions of subjects whose GHQ30 score decreased in each group were 50 % and 65 %, respectively. We performed a binomial test for the subjects whose scores increased and declined. The test results showed that there was no significant difference in the group that completed 1–12 sessions (p = 0.678)[2]. However, in the group that completed more than 13 sessions, there was a significant difference at the 5 % level (p = 0.0245).

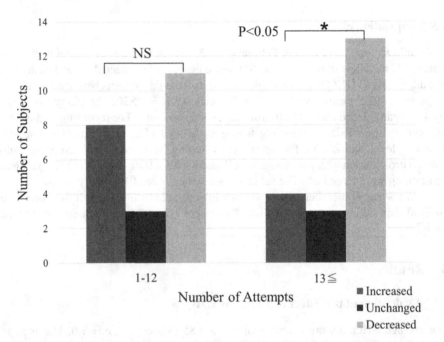

Fig. 1. Relationship between the number of S-Gim sessions attended and GHQ score change patterns. The bars on the left and the right represent the subjects who attended 1 to 12 sessions and more than 13 sessions, respectively. The vertical axis represents the number of subjects who experienced score change patterns (increased, unchanged, and decreased).

---

[1] We used 12 as cut-off criteria of two groups, because the value was the median of their training sessions.

[2] We assumed that increases and decreases in the score would occur with the same probability if the S-Gim were not performed.

Figure 2 shows the average GHQ30 scores for each group before and after conducting S-Gim. For the group that completed 1–12 sessions (n = 22), the average GHQ30 scores before and after S-Gim were 5.32 (SD = 7.17) and 4.00 (SD = 4.67), respectively. A paired t-test showed no significant difference between the scores before and after the training (t(21) = 0.904, p = 0.376). In the group of subjects who completed more than 13 sessions (n = 20), the average GHQ30 scores before and after S-Gim were 5.50 (SD = 4.15) and 3.60 (SD = 4.64). There was a significance difference at the 5 % level before and after the training (t(19) = 2.57, p = 0.018)[3]. Additionally, there was a highly negative correlation between the pre-S-Gim GHQ30 score and the difference between the scores before and after the training (n = 42, r = −0.662). That is, subjects with higher initial scores tended to show greater reductions in their scores.

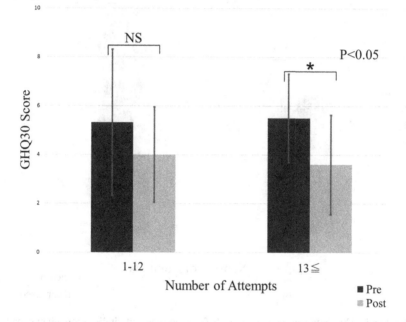

Fig. 2. Comparison between pre-and post-S-Gim GHQ30 average scores. The bars on the left and the right represent the subjects who attended 1 to 12 sessions, and more than 13 sessions, respectively. The vertical axis represents the GHQ30 score. The error bars represent the 95 % confidence intervals. For the group with more than 13 sessions, there was a significant difference at the 5 % level between the average scores before and after the training.

3.2 Evaluation of the Effect of S-Gim by Vitality Scores

The average vitality score before S-Gim was 7.15(SD = 1.66, n = 59). The average score after the training was 7.99 (SD = 1.38). The following comparison with the GHQ30

---

[3] We used the test function in Microsoft Excel 2010 for the tests.

results only targeted the 42 subjects whose GHQ30 scores were 1 or higher at the time of conducting the training.

Figure 3 shows the change in vitality scores in each group. The vertical axis represents the number of subjects who experienced each type of pattern (increased and decreased) of vitality score changes before and after S-Gim[4]. The proportions of subjects whose vitality score increased in each group were 45 % and 80 %, respectively. A binomial test comparing the subjects with increased vitality scores and those with decreased scores showed no significant difference for the group whose members completed 1–12 sessions (p = 0.832). In contrast, there was a significant difference at the 5 % level for the group whose members completed more than 13 sessions (p = 0.012).

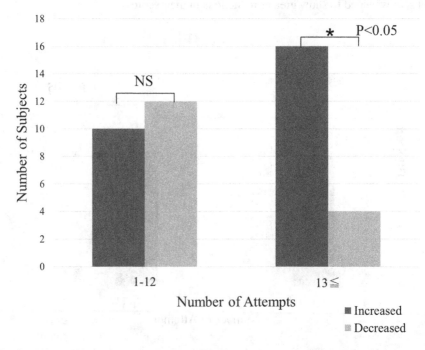

Fig. 3. Relationship between the number of S-Gim sessions and vitality score change patterns. The bars on the left and the right show the data for the subjects who attended 1 to 12 sessions and those who attended more than 13 sessions, respectively. The vertical axis represents the number of subjects who experienced each pattern of vitality score changes (increased and decreased).

Figure 4 shows a comparison of the average vitality scores before and after S-Gim. The bars on the left and the right show the subjects who attended 1 to 12 sessions, and those who attended more than 13 sessions, respectively. For those who attended 1–12 sessions (n = 22), the average vitality scores before and after S-Gim were 7.96 (SD = 1.83) and 7.99 (SD = 1.51), respectively. A paired t-test showed no significant

---

4 Since vitality scores are continuous values, there was no subjects whose vitality score did not change.

difference between the scores before and after the training (t(21) = −0.085, p = 0.933). For the subjects who completed more than 13 sessions (n = 20), the average vitality scores before and after S-Gim were 6.52 (SD = 1.22) and 7.59 (SD = 1.07), respectively. There was a significant difference at the 1 % level before and after the training (t(19) = −4.15, p = 0.00054). Moreover, there was a highly negative correlation between the pre-S-Gim vitality scores and the difference between the pre- and post-S-Gim scores (n = 42, r = −0.717). That is, subjects with lower vitality scores before training tended to increase their scores to a greater extent.

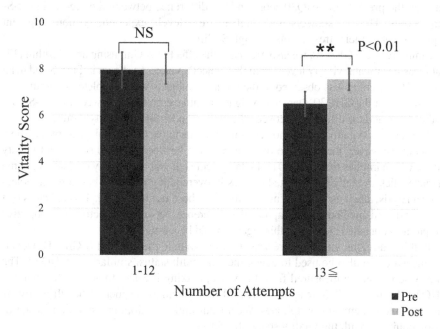

Fig. 4. Comparison of pre- and post-S-Gim vitality scores. The bars on the left and the right represent the subjects who attended 1 to 12 sessions, and those who attended more than 13 sessions, respectively. The vertical axis shows the vitality score. The error bars represent the 95 % confidence intervals. There was a significant difference at the 1 % level between pre- and post-S-Gim vitality scores for the subjects who attended more than 13 training sessions.

As these findings indicate, the subjects' vitality scores showed similar trends to the GHQ30 in terms of the effect of S-Gim. However, there was no direct correlation between GHQ30 scores and vitality scores (r = −0.022).

4   Discussion and Conclusion

In this study, we used a self-administered psychological test called the GHQ30, and vitality scores from a voice-based analysis, in order to evaluate S-Gim, a stress resilience program developed by the Japan Self-Defence Forces.

Figure 1 shows that there were more subjects whose GHQ30 scores decreased after S-Gim in the group whose members attended more than 13 sessions (average number of sessions attended = 31.50). Figure 2 also shows that the scores themselves declined after the training. That is, the effect of S-Gim was confirmed in terms of the number of subjects and the average score. However, there was no effect in the group of subjects whose members attended less than 12 sessions (average number of sessions attended = 7.23). This implies that a certain period of training is required to learn how to control stress through S-Gim. Additionally, there was a highly negative correlation between the pre-S-Gim GHQ30 score and the difference between the pre- and post-S-Gim scores. That is, subjects with higher stress levels experienced more apparent improvement in their stress levels through S-Gim.

Similarly to the GHQ30, we also evaluated the effect of S-Gim using an algorithm [17] that measures mental vitality levels from the subject's voice. As shown in Figs. 3 and 4, an effect of the training was observed in the group of subjects who completed more than 13 sessions. As for the GHQ30, there was a highly negative correlation between the pre-S-Gim vitality score and the difference between the pre- and post-S-Gim vitality scores.

The subjects' vitality scores showed similar trends to the GHQ30 in terms of the effect of S-Gim. However, there was no direct correlation between GHQ30 scores and vitality scores, which implies that GHQ30 and vitality scores do not necessarily evaluate the same characteristics. A study has reported success in overcoming reporting bias through voice-based analysis, albeit using different algorithms to those used here [21]. This indicates that the voice-based method might capture the difference between subjective and objective symptoms. A detailed analysis in this regard should be a future priority.

In this study, the vitality score was used to evaluate the effect of S-Gim. However, this measure can also be used to check mental health status, similarly to GHQ30. The vitality score can be measured from the voice, making it easier to administer than the GHQ30. Moreover, it is feasible to record daily changes in mental health easily by installing the system on smartphones. We are currently developing a smart phone application equipped with the vitality score algorithm.

Acknowledgements. We would like to express our sincere appreciation to Colonel Sota Shimozono of JGSDF Medical School and his staff members for their cooperation in sharing S-Gim and collecting data.

References

1. World Health Organization: The Global Burden of Disease: 2004 Update, pp. 46–49. WHO Press, Geneva, Switzerland (2004)
2. Kessler, R.C., Akiskal, H.S., Ames, M., Birnbaum, H., Greenberg, P., Hirschfeld, R.M.A., Jin, R., Merikangas, K.R., Simon, G.E., Wang, P.S.: Prevalence and effects of mood disorders on work performance in a nationally representative sample of U.S. workers. Am. J. Psychiatry **163**(9), 1561–1568 (2006)
3. Goldberg, D.P., Blackwell, B.: Psychiatric illness in general practice: a detailed study using a new method of case identification. BMJ **2**(5707), 439–443 (1970)
4. Beck, A.T.: A systematic investigation of depression. Compr. Psychiatry **2**(3), 163–170 (1961)

5. Beck, A.T., Ward, C.H., Mendelson, M., Mock, J., Erbaugh, J.: An inventory for measuring depression. Arch. Gen. Psychiatry **4**(6), 561–571 (1961)
6. Suzuki, G., Tokuno, S., Nibuya, M., Ishida, T., Yamamoto, T., Mukai, Y., Mitani, K., Tsumatori, G., Scott, D., Shimizu, K.: Decreased plasma brain-derived neurotrophic factor and vascular endothelial growth factor concentrations during military training. PLoS ONE **9**(2), e89455 (2014)
7. Arora, S., Venkataraman, V., Zhan, A., Donohue, S., Biglan, K.M., Dorsey, E.R., Little, M.A.: Detecting and monitoring the symptoms of Parkinson's disease using smartphones: a pilot study. Parkinsonism Relat. D. **21**(6), 650–653 (2015)
8. Rachuri, K. K., Musolesi, M., Mascolo, C., Rentfrow, P.J., Longworth, C., Aucinas. A.: EmotionSense: a mobile phones based adaptive platform for experimental social psychology research. In: Proceedings of the 12th ACM International Conference on Ubiquitous Computing, pp. 281–290 (2010)
9. Lu, H., Rabbi, M., Chittaranjan, G.T., Frauendorfer, D., Mast, M.S., Campbell, A.T., Gatica-Perez, D., Choudhury, T.: Stresssense: detecting stress in unconstrained acoustic environments using smartphones. In: Proceedings of the 2012 ACM Conference on Ubiquitous Computing, pp. 351–360 (2012)
10. Cannizzaro, M., Harel, B., Reilly, N., Chappell, P., Snyder, P.J.: Voice acoustical measurement of the severity of major depression. Brain Cogn. **56**, 30–35 (2004)
11. Moore, E., Clements, M., Peifert, J., Weisser, L.: Analysis of prosodic variation in speech for clinical depression. In: Proceedings of the 25th Annual International Conference of the IEEE EMBS, vol. 3, pp. 2925–2928. IEEE Press, New York (2003)
12. Mundt, J.C., Snyder, P.J., Cannizzaro, M.S., Chappie, K., Geralts, D.S.: Voice acoustic measures of depression severity and treatment response collected via interactive voice response (IVR) technology. J. Neurolinguist. **20**(1), 50–64 (2007)
13. Yang, Y., Fairbairn, C., Cohn, J.F.: Detecting depression severity from vocal prosody. IEEE Trans. Affect. Comput. **4**(2), 142–150 (2013)
14. Shimizu, T., Furuse, N., Yamazaki, T., Ueta, Y., Sato, T., Nagata, S.: Chaos of vowel /a/ in Japanese patients with depression: a preliminary study. J. Occup. Health. **47**(3), 267–269 (2005)
15. Vicsi, K., Sztaho, D.: Examination of the sensitivity of acoustic-phonetic parameters of speech to depression. In: IEEE 3rd International Conference on Cognitive Infocommunications, pp. 511–515. IEEE Press, New York (2012)
16. Zhou, G., Hansen, J.H.L., Kaiser, J.F.: Nonlinear feature based classification of speech under stress. IEEE Trans. Speech Audio Process. **9**(3), 201–216 (2001)
17. Shinohara, S., et al.: A mental health evaluation method using prosody information of voice. (in preparation)
18. Tokuno, S., et. al.: Usage of emotion recognition in stress resilience program. In: Proceedings of 40th ICMM World Congress on Military Medicine (2013)
19. Merry, S.N., Stasiak, K., Shepherd, M.: The effectiveness of SPARX, a computerised self help intervention for adolescents seeking help for depression: randomised controlled non-inferiority trial. BMJ **344**, 1–16 (2012)
20. Fleming, T., Dixson, R.: A pragmatic randomized controlled trial of computerized CBT (SPARX) for symptoms of depression among adolescents excluded from mainstream education. Behav. Cogn. Psychoth. **40**, 529–541 (2012)
21. Tokuno, S., Mitsuyoshi, S., Suzuki, G., Tsumatori, G.: Stress evaluation using voice emotion recognition technology: A novel stress evaluation technology for disaster responders. Proc. XVI World Congress of Psychiatry **2**, 301 (2014)

Prosodic Analysis of Speech and the Underlying Mental State

Roi Kliper[1], Shirley Portuguese[2], and Daphna Weinshall[1(✉)]

[1] School of Computer Science and Engineering, Hebrew University of Jerusalem,
91904 Jerusalem, Israel
kliper@cornell.edu, daphna@cs.huji.ac.il
[2] McLean Psychiatric Hospital, Boston 02478, USA
shirport@walla.com

Abstract. Speech is a measurable behavior that can be used as a bio-marker for various mental states including schizophrenia and depression. In this paper we show that simple temporal domain features, extracted from conversational speech, may highlight alterations in acoustic characteristics that are manifested in changes in speech prosody - these changes may, in turn, indicate an underlying mental condition. We have developed automatic computational tools for the monitoring of pathological mental states - including characterization, detection, and classification. We show that some features strongly correlate with perceptual diagnostic evaluation scales of both schizophrenia and depression, suggesting the contribution of such acoustic speech properties to the perception of an apparent mental condition. We further show that one can use these temporal domain features to correctly classify up to 87.5 % and up to 70 % of the speakers in a two-way and in a three-way classification tasks respectively.

Keywords: Schizophrenia · Machine learning · Mental health · Speech prosody · Jitter · Shimmer

1 Introduction

Psychiatry is a medical discipline in search of objective and clinically applicable assessment and monitoring tools. The acoustic characteristics of speech are a measurable behavior, hence can be used in the assessment and monitoring of disorders such as schizophrenia and depression. This observation has not gone unnoticed in the psychiatric community and previous attempts to quantify this acoustic effect in the psychiatric setting have been made. However, these attempts have been limited, in part by technical and technological limitations. Recent technological advancement has made the recording, storage and analysis of speech an available option for both researchers and practitioners.

The use of acoustic characteristics of speech in the description of pathological voice qualities has been studied in various contexts and with a variety of goals

© Springer International Publishing Switzerland 2016
S. Serino et al. (Eds.): MindCare 2015, CCIS 604, pp. 52–62, 2016.
DOI: 10.1007/978-3-319-32270-4_6

including mental health evaluation [1]. Studies have correlated acoustic features with perceptual qualities [2] and to a lesser extent with physiologic conditions at the glottis [3]. These studies looked at the use of syntactic structures, richness of vocabulary, time to respond and many other qualities.

Speech prosody is the component of speech that refers to the way words are spoken. It includes the rhythm, stress, and intonation of speech. Prosody may reflect various features of the speaker or the utterance: the emotional state of the speaker; the form of the utterance (statement, question, or command); the presence of irony or sarcasm; emphasis, contrast, and focus; or other elements of language that may not be encoded by grammar or choice of vocabulary. Changes in the acoustic characteristics of speech prosody in the course of mental disorders, notably depression and schizophrenia, are a well documented phenomenon [1,2, 4,5], and the evaluation of aspects of speech constitutes, today, a standard part of the mental status examination.

The acoustic changes in schizophrenia patients' speech are currently concep-tualized as a component of the negative symptoms [6]. The most accepted scale for negative symptoms is the Scale for the Assessment of Negative Symptoms (SANS) [7]. Negative symptoms are divided into five domains including blunted affect, alogia, asociality, anhedonia, and avolition [8], where speech acoustic changes are especially reflected in two different domains - blunted affect (dimin-ished expression of emotion) and alogia (poverty of speech).

Speech prosody is currently measured by subjective rating scales requiring highly trained staff. Several attempts at using speech cues for the automatic quantification of specific mental effects have been made in the past [2,4,9,10]. These attempts have made an effort to first correlate specific acoustic measures to their perceptual (clinical) counterparts, and second to quantify and asses different aspects of subjects' speech using different acoustic measures [5]. The advantage of automatic quantification of effects apparent in different mental states has been highlighted as early as 1938 [11] and is very well outlined in [12].

In [10] lexical analysis was proposed as a measure of mental deficits; but while some success has been shown, it has been claimed and shown that signifi-cant aspects of speech are missed when focusing on the lexical level [13]. In [4] several acoustic features were extracted from both structured speech and semi structured interview of depression subjects. A later study [5] showed high corre-lations between basic prosody measures (mainly inflection) and clinical ratings of negative symptoms of schizophrenia. In these and other studies results are highly task specific. Lastly, in [2] *Inflection* and *speech rate* were identified as discriminative features between schizophrenia patients and controls.

Our goal to develop automatic computational tools for the evaluation of mental state required two corresponding efforts. First, study the physical signal properties specific to schizophrenia and depression. We chose to focus on tem-poral domain features (see Sect. 3.1); these features, while not easy to extract or measure, provide a meaningful interpretation and may be referenced in the context of existing clinical evaluation scales.[1] Second, develop an automatic, real-time, reliable and objective assessment of the signal. We adopted a discriminative approach and trained a Support Vector Machine (SVM) classifier over the data (see Sect. 3.3).

2   Materials and Methods

Subjects. 62 subjects participated in the study, giving written consent approved by the McLean Hospital Institutional review board. The study subjects comprised of three groups, including schizophrenia patients (n = 22, 13 male, 9 female), patients with clinical depression (n = 20, 9 male, 11 female), and healthy participants (n = 20, 10 male, 10 female). The subjects were matched by age ($mean = 39.98, std = 11.37, p = 0.8489$), years of education ($mean = 14.8, std = 2.3, p = 0.063$), and gender ($\chi^2$ test of Independence, $q = 0.86$, $dof = 3, p = 0.65$).

Clinically Rated Symptom Measures. The subjects completed a clinical interview which included Semi structured Clinical Interview for DSM-IV (SCID IV) [14], Positive and negative Syndrome Scale for Schizophrenia (PANSS) [15], Scale for the Assessment of Negative Symptoms (SANS) [7], and the Montgomery and Absberg Depression Rating Scale (MADRS) [16] as well as the Hamilton Depression Scale (Ham-D) [17].

Acoustic Recordings. The recordings were made by a headset without sound isolation or calibration. To prepare the recordings for acoustic analysis, the audio tapes were digitized at a 44.1 kHz sampling rate. Acoustic analysis was conducted using MATLAB [18] (details are given in Sect. 2.1). Average length of a clinical interview was: schizophrenia - 57 m 13 s, depression - 30 m 31 s, healthy - 48 m 46 s. Silence was automatically removed at the beginning and end of each recording, while the remaining data was normalized to have 0 mean and variance 1, thus avoiding effects caused by the constellation of the headset. To enable efficient handling of the data each interview was divided into 2 min. segments, which were subsequently analyzed independently. All results from a single person's 2 min segments were later used together for classification.

---

[1] While it is possible to use existing automatic systems to produce a high dimensional non-specific description of the voice signal, we focus on a small set of meaningful features for two reasons: (i) These features appear to be ecologically relevant and correspond with psychiatrists' intuition about the characteristic features of the speech of Schizophrenia patients. (ii) Our application domain suffers from the problem of small sample, which necessitates the use of low dimensional representations to enable effective learning; this is accomplished by choosing a small set of relevant features. The alternative, which is to use a high dimensional representation followed by dimensionality reduction (like PCA), typically leads to the unfortunate outcome that the final result is hard to interpret in terms of the underlying features.

2.1 Speech Prosody and Feature Extraction

Two minutes segments of interview were used to measure nine diagnostic features. In this paper we focus on a very small and simple set of features extracted in the temporal domain. This choice was motivated by the fact that temporal domain features are, in general, easier to relate to perceptual properties of speech and thus provide better infrastructure for further use in the psychiatric community.

Alterations of the speech signal in abnormal conditions can occur at different time-scale levels, including the *macro-scale* level (above 1 s) which refers to variables such as speaking rate, the *meso-scale* (25 ms to 1 s), in which variables like pitch and its statistics are measured, and finally, the *micro-scale* (10 ms or less) level in which cycle to cycle measures are taken (this level appears to contribute to the naturalness of the speech sound). While *macro* and *meso* scales are influenced by voluntary aspects of speech, the *micro-scale* is involuntary in nature and, thus, can better serve as a reliable biomarker. All scales contribute to the prosodic structure of the speech signal, and thus using them as an ensemble may provide insight into the possible role of prosody in the characterization of pathological mental states. The focus on prosodic features follows reports showing the relevance of meso-scale and micro-scale levels to the tasks of mental evaluation and emotion detection [1–3].

Macro Scale Measures: Mean Utterance Duration, Mean Gap Duration, Mean Spoken Ratio. An utterance is any segment identified as speech that exceeds 0.5 s. A "gap" is any segment of recording with no subjects' speech. *Spoken ratio* is calculated as the ratio between the total volume of speech occupied by the speaker, that is the sum of the length of all utterances divided by the total conversation length.

Meso Scale Measures: Pitch Range, Pitch Standard Deviation, Power Standard Deviation. *Pitch range* was calculated as the difference between maximum estimated pitch and minimum estimated pitch normalized by the mean pitch over the entire 2 min segments. No significant between-group differences were observed for mean pitch, which was (Males: 112.3 Hz, 18.99 Hz; Females: 176.39 Hz, 18.53 Hz) ($F = 0.18, df = 2, 56, p = 0.83$) nor for interaction with gender ($F = 0.75, df = 2, 56, p = 0.47$). Between gender differences were strong as expected ($F = 182.9, df = 1, 56, p << 0.01$). Standard deviation (STD) of pitch was calculated for each utterance and was then averaged for each speaker. STD of pitch was again normalized by the mean pitch in each utterance. Mean active power and its variance were measured in decibels (dB) in reference to a calibration level and were 64 dB, with a standard deviation of 8.6 dB. Standard deviation of power within an utterance was measured, normalized by the mean power in the entire segment in order to avoid effects caused by noise in the location of the microphone.

Micro Scale Measures: Mean Waveform Correlation, Mean Jitter, Mean Shimmer. The mean of all correlation coefficients evaluated for every pair of consecutive periods was used as the acoustic measure termed *Mean Wave-form Correlation (MWC)*. It indicates the overall similarity between the cycles of the time signal. When applied to pitched segments it measures the level at which the speaker sustained its constant pitch.

Following [1] jitter and shimmer were calculated as the period perturbation quotient *PPQ* and the energy perturbation quotient *EPQ* respectively, where the locality parameter was chosen to be 5. Perturbation Quotient (PQ) measures the local deviation from stationarity of a given measure and is defined in (1). It measures the ratio of deviation of a given measure in a local neighborhood defined by the locality parameter K. Put in simple terms, the jitter measures the stability of the period in a 5-local cycles environment and the shimmer measures the stability of the energy in a given 5-local cycles environment.

$$PQ = \frac{100\%}{N-K} \sum_{v=\frac{K-1}{2}}^{N-\frac{K-1}{2}-1} \left| \frac{u(v) - \frac{1}{K}\sum_{k=-\frac{K-1}{2}}^{\frac{K-1}{2}} u(v+k)}{\frac{1}{K}\sum_{k=-\frac{K-1}{2}}^{\frac{K-1}{2}} u(v+k)} \right| \tag{1}$$

We chose to use the energy shimmer since it is expected to be considerably less susceptible to noise than the amplitude shimmer often used in acoustic analysis.

Discussion: We have previously observed that both macro-scale and meso-scale measures seem to incorporate a larger variability component due to the specific task: between task-variability S_b as compared to the within speaking-task variability (S_w). This task dependency is significantly reduced for micro-scale measures. This observation does not disqualify the larger scale measures from being useful in a classification task (as the task is known in advance); however, it highlights micro-scale features as candidates to be used by a robust general-purpose classifier.

2.2   Classification and Statistical Analysis

We used the extracted acoustic features and a basic linear classifier [19] to classify the different conditions: Healthy (HL), Schizophrenia (SZ) and Depression (DP) in a two-way classification task. For each classification scenario (e.g. HL vs. SZ), one subject was left out for testing and the rest were used to train a classifier. In a single classification setting all 2 min. segments of a given speaker were left out and later used for testing. The final decision was taken using a majority vote over all left out segments.

To check the statistical significance of the results over each of the individual features, we used 1-way ANOVA when the distribution was roughly normal, otherwise we used the nonparametric version of the 1-way ANOVA called the Kruskal-Wallis test. It is actually a more general test, in that it is comparing distributions rather than medians. Checking the statistical significance of the effects brings up the problem of multiplicity (multiple comparisons). We consider the problem of testing simultaneously 9 null hypotheses where within each 3 pair comparisons are nested. We therefore used a sequential Bonferroni type procedure, which is very conservative and assures the statistical soundness of the results. Specifically, the results were first tested for significance of main effect using a Bonferroni correction, and later multiple comparison was done using a second Bonferroni correction[2].

3   Results

In the following section we describe first an analysis of the individual features that were extracted as indicated above. We start by describing the distributions of the different features according to the different groups in Sect. 3.1. In Sect. 3.2 we describe the correlations between these features and standard clinical ratings, while in Sect. 3.3 we describe our efforts to train a an SVM classifier to predict the speaker's condition.

3.1   Isolated Features - Between Group Analysis

Figure 1 shows the mean and standard error of isolated features extracted from semi structured interview. Statistically significant deviations between any two groups are indicated with a horizontal bar. The analysis was performed while taking into consideration the issue of multiple comparisons as explained in Sect. 2.2, and is thus very conservative in nature.

Spoken Ratio. As seen in Fig. 1a, the ratio of spoken volume for healthy subjects (47.19 %,1.98 %) is larger than that of Schizophrenia subjects (37.16 %,2.4 %) and Depressed subjects (29.52 %, 2.4 %). The difference between the groups is indeed significant ($\chi^2 = 21.63; df = 2, 59; p < 0.001$) and possibly reflects the subject's initiative and willingness to engage in conversation.

Utterance Duration. Healthy subjects appear to speak in longer utterances ($\sim$1.35 s, 0.07 s) as compared to Schizophrenia subjects (1.26 s, 0.05 s) and depressed subjects (1.03 s, 0.05 s). Significant ($\chi^2 = 16.06; df = 2, 59; p < 0.001$) differences were observed between the depressed group and both the group of healthy subjects and schizophrenia subjects. Only a trend was observed between normal controls and schizophrenia subjects. In depressed recordings an average utterance length that exceeds 3 s (as averaged over a two minutes segment) never occurred, which is reflective of the reported difficulty of engaging in conversation. These results tend to agree with previous reports [20].

Gap Duration. Normal subjects tend to pause less and for less time (1.73 s, 0.1 s) as compared to schizophrenia subjects (2.44 s, 0.22 s) and depressed subjects (2.87 s, 0.29 s) ($\chi^2 = 14.63; df = 2, 59; p < 0.001$). Also, the pauses of healthy subjects are of more regular pattern as reflected by the small error bar.

---

[2] Note that with only three treatment groups, it's overly conservative to adjust the alpha levels with a Bonferroni method as with only 3 treatment groups, there is little risk in an increasing Type I error rate.

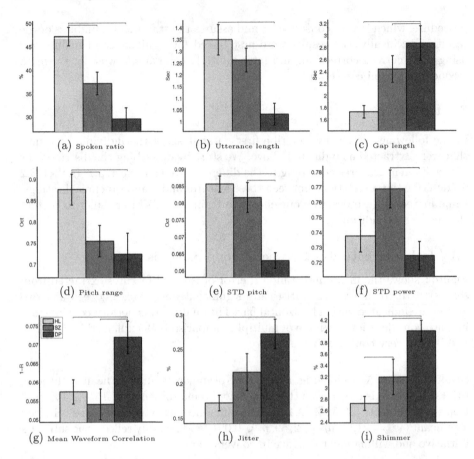

Fig. 1. Individual features: 9 features are analyzed showing mean and standard error (STE) bar for each feature in each group of patients. Significant differences are indicated with a horizontal bar. Significance was established using a Kruskal-Wallis procedure and a Bonferonni correction for multiple comparisons.

Pitch Range. Healthy subjects evidently displayed larger pitch range of ($\sim$0.88, $\sim$0.04) (mean, ste) of an octave, which is in agreement with reported literature [5,9,21]. Pitch range is significantly reduced for schizophrenia (0.75, $\sim$0.04) with an even lower pitch range of (0.67, $\sim$0.05) for depressed patients ($\chi^2 = 7.49$; $df = 2, 59$; $p < 0.05$).

Standard Deviation of Pitch. Our measure of standard deviation of pitch within an utterance represents a temporally local perception of inflection. healthy subjects display a wider dynamics of pitch (0.0992, 0.0024) within an utterance as compared to schizophrenia subjects (0.0924, 0.0044) and depressed subjects are significantly different (0.0629, 0.0023) ($\chi^2 = 21.28$; $df = 2, 59$; $p < 0.001$).

Power Standard Deviation. Differences in power standard deviation were evident between Schizophrenia subjects ($\sim$0.77, $\sim$0.01) and Healthy subjects (0.74, $\sim$0.01) on the one hand, and Depressed subjects (0.7244, 0.01) on the other hand ($\chi^2 = 6; df = 2, 59; p < 0.05$). Only differences between schizophrenia and depression remained significant after correction for multiple comparisons.

Mean Waveform Correlation. The results show a significant deviation of the depressed subjects ($\chi^2 = 10.42; df = 2, 59; p < 0.01$).

Mean Jitter. We see significant differences between healthy subjects (0.1722, $\sim$0.01) and both schizophrenia subjects ($\sim$0.22, 0.01) and depressed subjects ($\sim$0.27, 0.0212). The way jitter was calculated puts a focus on the physiological ability to maintain a constant period, and suggests a deficiency in this ability in both schizophrenia and depression subjects.

Mean Shimmer. Healthy subjects displayed the lowest shimmer (2.73 %, 0.12 %) whereas depressed subjects displayed an elevated shimmer (4 %, 0.18 %) with an intermediate level (3.22 %, 0.12 %) for schizophrenia subjects. Again these results may suggest some problem in spontaneous control of the glottal production mechanism. All post-hoc between-group comparisons were significant ($\chi^2 = 26.41; df = 2, 59; p << 0.01$).

3.2 Correlation

In order to compensate for excessive skew in the clinical measures we followed [2] and employed non-parametric statistics (Spearman's ρ correlation coefficient). Rank order correlations (Spearman) were computed between the acoustic and clinical based symptoms of the subjects (this data is omitted). More interestingly, we correlated the acoustic measures with the diagnostic rating as seen in Table 1. Here the correlation scores were only calculated within the relevant group, that is, Schizophrenia clinical ratings were correlated with acoustic measures of subjects diagnosed with schizophrenia, while depression clinical ratings were correlated with acoustic measures of depressed subjects only.

Some findings in Table 1 are worth special mention. Spoken ratio was defined to agree with the description of Alogia as a reduction in quantity of speech; we find it reassuring that it is highly correlated with the SANS-alogia clinical rating (0.64, $p << 0.01$). Contrary to reported results in [2], high correlations between STD of pitch and spoken ratio were observed.

3.3 Classification

The linear support vector machines (SVM) classifier [22] was employed to train discriminative models using the extracted measures. The task consists of either binary classification, where a model was trained to discriminate between two

Table 1. Acoustic features- psychiatric scales correlations.

	Schizophrenia scales				Depression scales	
	PANSS	SANS			MADRS	HAM-D
		(total)	(affect)	(alogia)		
1. Spoken ratio	−0.11	−0.5**	−0.58**	−0.64**	−0.11*	0.11
2. Utterance duration	−0.19	−0.44**	−0.55**	−0.49**	−0.27*	0.05
3. Gap duration	0.09	0.45**	0.45**	0.54**	−0.01*	−0.14
4. Pitch range	−0.16	0.04	0.13	0	−0.35*	−0.33*
5. STD pitch	0	−0.07	−0.17	−0.17	−0.18	−0.15
6. STD power	−0.14	−0.27	−0.39	−0.31*	−0.01	0.1
7. $1 - MWC$	0.03	0.24	0.4	0.32*	0.19	0.19
8. Jitter	0.34	0.38*	0.21	0.45*	−0.1	−0.3
9. Shimmer	0.41*	0.4*	0.18	0.31*	−0.01	0.2

* indicates $p < 0.05$,
** indicates $p \ll 0.01$.

distinct mental states, or multi-class classification, where a set of models was trained to identify the mental state of a specific speaker in a *1-vs.-all* approach. Our classifier obtained the following pair-wise classification success rates (chance at 50 %): control vs. Schizophrenia - 76.19 %, control vs. depression - 87.5 %, and Schizophrenia vs depression - 71.43 %. Multi-class classification success rate was at 69.77 (chance at 33.3 %).

4   Summary and Discussion

Speech acoustics is a measurable behavior that could be utilized as a biomarker in the clinical setting. The change in the acoustics of speech is not the only aspect of speech that changes in the course of various disorders [21], but these changes are a well documented phenomenon in both schizophrenia and depression. In both disorders speech acoustics often changes over time.

Our study was motivated by the desire to contribute to the search for a possible biomarker for schizophrenia and major depressive disorder. Clearly the development of reliable, objective, low-priced, and readily applicable assessment tools would enhance the accuracy of the clinical evaluation for diagnosis and monitoring. We focused on a relatively simple set of features extracted from the speech signal in the temporal domain. We divided the set of features into three groups of features, according to the time scale required for their extraction. We showed that while macro-scale features correlate with distinct components of the SANS rating scale, meso-scale features show poor correlations. Micro-scale features showed the highest promise as diagnostic measures both in terms of reliability and validity. Our findings that the acoustic features can separate schizophrenia from depression subjects, without reference to the content of the speech, provides converging evidence for the promise of this approach.

Acknowledgements. This work was supported in part by the Intel Collaborative Research Institute for Computational Intelligence (ICRI-CI), and the Gatsby Charitable Foundations.

References

1. Michaelis, D., Fröhlich, M., Strube, H.: Selection and combination of acoustic features for the description of pathologic voices. J. Acoust. Soc. Am. **103**, 1628–1639 (1998)
2. Cohen, A., Alpert, M., Nienow, T., Dinzeo, T., Docherty, N.: Computerized measurement of negative symptoms in schizophrenia. J. Psychiatr. Res. **42**, 827–836 (2008)
3. Moore, E., Clements, M., Peifer, J., Weisser, L.: Critical analysis of the impact of glottal features in the classification of clinical depression in speech. IEEE Trans. Biomed. Eng. **55**, 96–107 (2008)
4. Alpert, M., Pouget, E., Silva, R.: Reflections of depression in acoustic measures of the patient's speech. J. Affect. Disord. **66**, 59–69 (2001)
5. Alpert, M., Shaw, R., Pouget, E., Lim, K.: A comparison of clinical ratings with vocal acoustic measures of flat affect and alogia. J. Psychiatr. Res. **36**, 347–353 (2002)
6. American Psychiatric Association, American Psychiatric Association Task Force on DSM-IV: Diagnostic and Statistical Manual of Mental Disorders: DSM-IV-TR. American Psychiatric Publishing, Inc., Arlington (2000)
7. Andreasen, N.: Scale for the assessment of negative symptoms (sans). Br. J. Psychiatr. (1989)
8. Andreasen, N.: Negative symptoms in schizophrenia: definition and reliability. Arch. Gen. Psychiatr. **39**, 784–788 (1982)
9. Andreasen, N., Alpert, M., Martz, M.: Acoustic analysis: an objective measure of affective flattening. Arch. Gen. Psychiatr. **38**, 281–285 (1981)
10. Pennebaker, J., Mehl, M., Niederhoffer, K.: Psychological aspects of natural language use: our words, our selves. Ann. Rev. Psychol. **54**, 547–577 (2003)
11. Newman, S., Mather, V.: Analysis of spoken language of patients with affective disorders. Am. J. Psychiatr. **94**, 913–942 (1938)
12. Ishak, W.: Outcome measurement in psychiatry: a critical review. American Psychiatric Pub., Arlington (2002)
13. Kring, A., Bachorowski, J.: Emotions and psychopathology. Cogn. Emot. **13**, 575–599 (1999)
14. Dsm, I.: Diagnostic and Statistical Manual of Mental Disorders. American psychiatric association, Arlington (1994)
15. Kay, S., Flszbein, A., Opfer, L.: The positive and negative syndrome scale (panss) for schizophrenia. Schizophr. Bull. **13**, 261 (1987)
16. Montgomery, S., Asberg, M.: A new depression scale designed to be sensitive to change. Br. J. Psychiatr. **134**, 382–389 (1979)
17. Hamilton, M.: A rating scale for depression. J. Neurol. Neurosurg. Psychiatr. **23**, 56 (1960)
18. MATLAB: version 7.11.0 (R2010b). The MathWorks Inc., Natick, MA (2010)
19. Fan, R., Chang, K., Hsieh, C., Wang, X., Lin, C.: Liblinear: a library for large linear classification. J. Mach. Learn. Res. **9**, 1871–1874 (2008)
20. Alpert, M., Kotsaftis, A., Pouget, E.: Speech fluency and schizophrenic negative signs. Schizophr. Bull. **23**, 171–177 (1997)

21. Alpert, M., Rosenberg, S., Pouget, E., Shaw, R.: Prosody and lexical accuracy in flat affect schizophrenia. Psychiatr. Res. **97**, 107–118 (2000)
22. Fan, R., Chang, K., Hsieh, C., Wang, X., Lin, C.: LIBLINEAR: a library for large linear classification. J. Mach. Learn. Res. **9**, 1871–1874 (2008)

Quantifying Hypomimia in Parkinson Patients Using a Depth Camera

Nomi Vinokurov[1(✉)], David Arkadir[2], Eduard Linetsky[2], Hagai Bergman[2], and Daphna Weinshall[1]

[1] School of Computer Science and Engineering, Hebrew University,
91904 Jerusalem, Israel
Nomi.Vinokurov@mail.huji.ac.il
[2] Hadassah Medical School, Hebrew University, 91120 Jerusalem, Israel

Abstract. One of Parkinson's disease early symptoms is called hypomimia (masked facies), and timely detection of this symptom could potentially assist early diagnosis. In this study we developed methods to automatically detect and assess the severity of hypomimia, using machine learning tools and a 3D sensor that allows for fairly accurate facial movements tracking. To evaluate our prediction of hypomimia score for participants not included in the training set, we computed the score's correlation with hypomimia scores provided by 2 neurologists. The correlations in 4 conditions were $0.84, 0.69, 0.71, 0.70$. This should be compared with the correlation between the somewhat subjectives scores of the two neurologists, which is 0.78. When training classifiers to discriminate between people who suffer from hypomimia and people who do not, the area under the curve of the corresponding Receiver Operating Characteristic curves in the same 4 conditions is $0.90 - 0.99$. These encouraging results provide proof of concept that automatic evaluation of hypomimia can be sufficiently reliable to be useful for clinical early detection of Parkinson-related hypomimia.

Keywords: Parkinson's disease · Hypomimia · 3D camera · Facial expressions · Affect prediction

1 Introduction

Parkinson's Disease (PD) is the second most common neurodegenerative disorder with a prevalence rate exceeding $100/100,000$ among all American population and $1,588/100,000$ among population over the age of 65. This statistic might underestimate the problem because PD diagnosis is complicated. Since age is the single most important factor for PD and population is growing older, the prevalence rate could further increase in the not too distant future [1,2]. PD symptoms include tremor, rigidity and loss of muscle control in general, as well as cognitive impairment. The difficulty in reliable PD diagnosis has inspired researchers to develop decision support tools relying on algorithms aiming to differentiate healthy controls from people with PD [3,4].

© Springer International Publishing Switzerland 2016
S. Serino et al. (Eds.): MindCare 2015, CCIS 604, pp. 63–71, 2016.
DOI: 10.1007/978-3-319-32270-4_7

Hypomimia is a cardinal sign of the disease often presented in its early stages. The syndrome is characterized by a marked diminution of expressive gestures of the face, including brow movements that accompany speech and emotional facial expressions. Punctuation brow movements - very brief (~50 ms) contractions of the muscles of the upper face that occur during speech and appear to add semantic emphasis, are often absent. Additionally, hypomimia is commonly manifested in only one side of the face [5].

Research has shown that PD patients have lower expressivity ratings than the normal population while watching video clips, and that PD patients differ also in the frequency of smiles while watching a series of cartoons and in the degree of mouth opening while smiling [6,7]. In those studies ratings were performed with the assistance of human judges, while in our study we aim to measure these quantities automatically from video recordings, in order to compute an accurate prediction of hypomimia. Mergl et al. [8] investigated hypomimia in patients suffering from depression using ultrasonic markers placed on participants faces. New wearable technology could enable home monitoring of patients, but since the number of sensors that can be put on the patient's face is limited, the quality of assessing hypomimia severity is reduced.

The Unified Parkinson's Disease Rating Scale (UPDRS) is the most common scale used in clinical studies in order to follow the longitudinal course of PD. UPDRS defines hypomimia levels as follows:

0. Normal
1. Minimal hypomimia, could be called "poker face" (healthy subjects might get this score)
2. Slight but definitely abnormal diminution of facial expression
3. Moderate hypomimia; lips parted some of the time
4. Masked or fixed facies with severe or complete loss of facial expression; lips parted 1/4 inch or more

Quantitative assessment of hypomimia could assist early diagnosis of the disease, which could in the future (and with the development of new procedures) enable better treatment and slow down the progression of the disease. A home stationed application that enables quantitative assessment of hypomimia, with no need to meet the neurologist, would allow for better evaluation and monitoring of the treatment and could improve life quality of Parkinson's patients. Recent advances in computer vision allow for the reliable tracking of facial movements using simple devices that could be stationed in one's home. In this study we used a common depth camera - PrimeSense Carmine 1.09, which delivers depth video and audio information.

In the following we present an algorithm that utilizes depth sensor data to detect and scale hypomimia. In Sect. 2 we describe the data collection with some details of the recording procedure. In Sect. 3 we describe an algorithm that will assess hypomimia severity. In Sect. 4 we present the results, discussing the correlation between our algorithm's predictions and both neurologists scores, and presenting Receiver Operating Characteristic (ROC) curves for hypomimia detection.

2 Methods and Materials

Technology Overview. In recent years $3D$ sensors developed as part of the growth of the gaming market. Some of these sensors come with software support to track facial movements fairly reliably. In our study we chose to use the Carmine 1.09 camera developed by PrimeSense. The sensor depth acquisition is based on the "light coding" technology. The process codes the scene with near-IR light, light that returns distorted depending upon where things are. The solution then uses a standard off-the-shelf complementary metal-oxide-semiconductor image sensor to read the coded light back from the scene using various algorithms to triangulate and extract depth. The product analyzes scenery in 3 dimensions [9,10].

To generate features we used $Faceshift\copyright$, which is a commercial software that performs real time face tracking. The software gets as input data from the depth sensor with sampling rate of 19 Hz, and tracks points of interest on the participant's face. (see example in Fig. 1) After tracking it further analyzes facial movements and describes them as a mixture of basic expressions, as well as head orientation and gaze. Specifically, $Faceshift$ outputs the intensity level of 51 facial Action Units (fs-AU signals) over time, including eyes (blink, squint, up, down, in, out), brows (up, down), jaw (forward, left, right, open), mouth (left, right, frown, smile, dimple), lips (stretch, close, open, up, down, funnel, pucker), chin (raise), cheek (squint), sneer, and puff [11,12]. In the analysis below we use the fs-AU signal as raw data to generate features for our prediction algorithm.

Data Collection Protocol. The study was approved by the ethical committee of Hadassah Medical center. 14 Patients ages 58 to 84 with varying levels of hypomimia, and 15 Controls ages 48 to 84, were recruited at Hadassah Medical Center in Jerusalem. Each participant was given a short overview of the experiment, and then gave a written informed consent for study participation in accordance with the Helsinki Declaration. Each participant also indicated their consent for the whole procedure to be videotaped. The $3D$ camera was positioned 50 cm from the subject's face, 10 cm above eyes level.

First, the participant went through a short training stage (for the benefit of $Faceshift$) which included presenting different facial expressions to the camera. Afterwards each participant was recorded during 5 different sessions. The sessions were: Answering 5 interview questions, watching photographs as slide show, watching a funny short movie involving cats, watching a short movie involving humans, and staring at the camera for 60 s. The most discriminantive results were obtained when using the recordings of the $4th$ session (watching a short movie involving humans), and therefore only these results will be presented.

Two Movement Disorder specialists (denoted DA and ED) rated each participant for hypomimia using the recordings of the $1th$ session (an interview with 5 questions). DA scored participants with integer and half values in the range $[0, 4]$; he stated that as a matter of procedure he would round up the hypomimia score when his perception is that the hypomimia level is not an integer value. Neurologist ED scored all participants with only integer values in the range $[0, 4]$ as is the custom in such neurological evaluations.

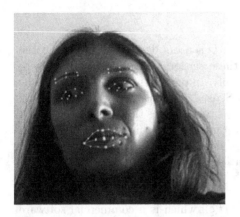

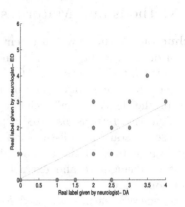

Fig. 1. Example of points tracking by *Faceshift©*

Fig. 2. Correlation of labels given by two neurologists, denoted DA and ED.

Data Representation. The *fs-AU* signal was used to generate the following representation for each recording, whose components included: (i) 4 moments of each *fs-AU* (mean, variance, skew and kurtosis). (ii) 4 moments of bilateral *fs-AU* differences (left vs. right side of the face). These comparisons were employed since hypomimia is also characterized by asymmetrical facial expressions [5]. (iii) Correlations between every pair of *fs-AU* signals (50*51/2). (iv) Quantization of the *fs-AU* signal to 4 discrete values, which were chosen using k-means for each *fs-AU* signal. Using this discretization, we could compute for each *fs-AU* signal the number of changes (a transition from one discrete value to another discrete value) and the number of fast changes (a change of 2 discrete values or more).

Methodology. To learn a predictor, the data was divided into train and test sets using the Leave One Out (LOO) procedure, where the data of each left out participant was kept for testing, while the data of all other participants was used to train the linear regressor. This was repeated for each participant. Given labeled data by two different neurologists, for each learning session we trained two predictors, one for each neurologist. We then tested the predictor on the test data from both movement Disorder specialists, giving us 4 different results (see below in Sect. 4). For lack of objective hypomimia score, by defition our gold standard is the Pearson Correlation Coefficient (PCC) between the subjective scores of the two expert neurologists when based on the same recordings as our algorithm, which is 0.78 (see Fig. 2).

3   Predicting Hypomimia Level

We shall now describe the procedure to obtain a prediction for hypomimia from each recording, using the data representation described above.

Learning Method: Supervised Learning Using Linear Regression. Linear regression is typically used to model the relationship between a scalar dependent variable Y and one or more explanatory variables X. Since our challenge is to predict an ordinal value in the range $[0, 4]$, we used linear regression slightly modified to construct such a predictor.

We start by noting that the data representation described in Sect. 2 lies in high dimension, while the size of our training data is rather small. Therefore training always started with greedy feature selection as described next. Subsequently we modeled the relationship between the selected features and the given labels in each training set. Finally, this model was used to predict a continuous hypomimia score for the left out recording of the test participant.

Note that this procedure outputs a continuous number, while the variable we aim to predict is integer following the UPDRS guidelines. Thus in the final step of the procedure, the output of the predictor is rounded to integer or half integer values. When the prediction value is lower than 0 or higher than 4, it is truncated to 0 or 4 respectively.

Feature Selection. The first step of the learning procedure reduced the dimensionality of the signal using forward greedy feature selection coupled with least squares regression [13]. The greedy selection procedure works as follow: in iteration i, the feature that mostly reduces the residual sum of squares (RSS) between the algorithm prediction and real labels is chosen, and improvement from the last iteration ($\Delta RSS = RSS_i - RSS_{i-1}$) is calculated. Features are added until the improvement is no longer statistically significant (under the null assumption that ΔRSS has a chi-square distribution with one degree of freedom).

When learning a predictor based on neurologist DA who typically used higher scores, we used all recordings in the train set with hypomimia score of 0 and all recordings with hypomimia score > 2, and ran forward greedy features selection using linear regression as the matched predictor. Similalry, when learning a predictor based on neurologist ED who used somewhat lower subjective scores, we used all recordings in the train set with hypomimia score of 0 and all recordings with hypomimia score ≥ 2.

Anecdotally, the Features that were selected by the greedy procedure using the data of each neurologist separately gave different results. When learning from DA, the features most often selected included the correlation between brows up movement and lower chin raise, the correlation between left side mouth smile and forward jaw movement, and the correlation between left side lips stretch and left side cheek squints (see Fig. 3a). When learning from ED, the features most often selected included the correlation between brows up movement and lower chin raise as above, the correlation between right eye squints and right side mouth press, and the mean value of the left side mouth press. In both cases, between 2 and 3 features were selected at each iteration of the algorithm (see Fig. 3b).

3.1 Learning Algorithm

We use the following notations: Let n denote the number of participants (in our case 29), $\mathcal{K}$ denote the set of participants whose scores were used to train

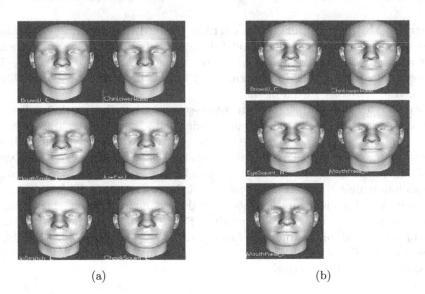

(a)   (b)

Fig. 3. Most frequently selected features: (a) when learning from DA, and (b) when learning from ED.

the greedy feature selection method, and $|\mathcal{K}| = m$. Let s_i denote subject i, y_i denote the label given by the neurologist to participant i, $\hat{y}_i$ the prediction of hypomimia score generated by our algorithm, and r_i the quantized hypomimia integer score generated by our algorithm. Let F_i denote the set of features that were selected using $\mathcal{K} \backslash s_i$ as the train set. Let V_{ji} denote the features vector of subject j according to the features in set F_i.

Algorithm 1. Predict Hypomimia Severity

1: **for** $i = 1..n$ **do**
2:     F_i = forward greedy features selection using $\mathcal{K} \backslash s_i$
3:     Generate V_{ji} for $j = 1 \ldots n$
4:     W_i = Linear regression(V_{ji}, y_j for $j \in \mathcal{K} \backslash s_i$)
5:     $\hat{y}_i = W_i^T * V_{ii}$
6:     $\hat{r}_i = \text{round}(\hat{y}_i)$
7: **end for**

---

4   Results

Predicting the Severity of Hypomimia. Using the algorithm described above, we predict a hypomimia score for each participant. We then test these predictions by correlating them with model scores. Specifically, recall that for each recording we have 2 predictions, based on two separate predictors trained for each neurologist. These 2 predictions are correlated with the scores of both neurologists (the one whose scores were used for training, and the other one), giving us 4 prediction graphs (see Fig. 4) and 4 correlation scores (see Table 1).

Binary Detection of Hypomimia. The predictors can be used to discriminate between healthy individuals (score ≤ 1) and people who suffer from hypomimia (score > 1). This is a binary classification task. We plot Receiver Operator Characteristic (ROC) curves to evaluate our algorithm in this discimination task, see Fig. 5. The area under the curve (AUC) is used to measure success, see Table 2.

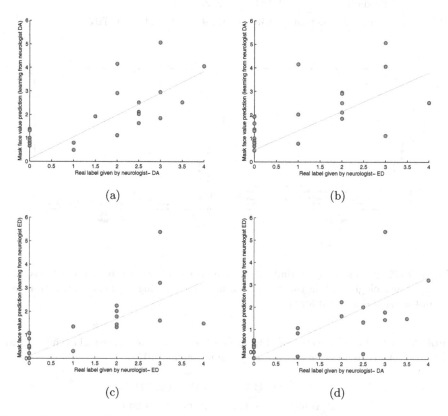

Fig. 4. Correlations between the scores given by each of 2 neurologists and our algorithm predictions in 4 conditions: (a) Scores of neurologist DA in the train data used for training, scores of neurologist DA in the test data used for testing. (b) Scores of neurologist DA in the train data used for training, scores of neurologist ED in the test data used for testing. (c) Same as (a), training with ED and testing with ED. (d) Same as (b), training with ED and testing with DA.

Table 1. Pearson Correlation Coefficient of our method's predictions with neurologists' scores in 4 conditions, each marked by a pair of initials. The first set of initial denotes the neurologist whose scores in the train data were used for training, while the second set of initials denotes the neurologist whose scores in the test data were used for correlation. In either case, correlation was computed with predicted values for unseen data from the test set. All correlation values are very significant $p < 3 * 10^{-4}$; The first row shows correlations based on the raw predictor values, while the second row shows correlations based on the integer predictor values. Since ED scored hypomimia with whole integer values, only the integer prediction values are shown when training on ED scores.

	DA - DA	DA - ED	ED - DA	ED - ED
Prediction	0.784	0.623		
Integer Prediction	0.836	0.686	0.711	0.707

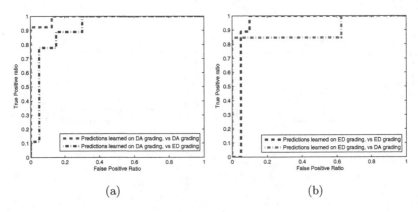

(a)   (b)

Fig. 5. ROC curves of hypomimia detection using our algorithm's predictions. (a) Scores of neurologist DA in the train data used for training.(b) Scores of neurologist ED in the train data used for training.

Table 2. AUC of ROC curves from Fig. 5. The 4 conditions are described in the caption of Table 1. All correlation values are very significant $p < 10^{-4}$.

	DA - DA	DA - ED	ED - DA	ED - ED
AUC	0.990	0.917	0.904	0.944

5 Discussion

We described a learning algorithm that detects and scores hypomimia with relatively high accuracy, when trained on other subjects. This kind of work may contribute to the goal of early detection of Parkinson, by providing an automatic tool which can be combined with other such tools to produce automatic scores correlated with symptoms of Parkinson. One attractive feature of the approach is its potential to provide a home-stationed diagnostic aid not requiring a trip to the neurologist's clinic. One drawback of our method is its reliance on the availability of a depth camera, which is less readily available to most people, and the use of the *Faceshift©* software which requires pre-training by all participants, a step which is not always straightforward for Parkinson patients.

Acknowledgements. This work was supported in part by the Intel Collaborative Research Institute for Computational Intelligence (ICRI-CI), and the Gatsby Charitable Foundations.

References

1. Willis, W.A., Evanoff, B.A., Lian, M., Criswell, S.R., Racette, B.A.: Geographic and ethnic variation in parkinson disease: a population-based study of us medicare beneficiaries. Neuroepidemiology **34**, 143–151 (2010)
2. von Campenhausen, S., Bornschein, B., Wick, R., Bötzel, K., Sampaio, C., Poewe, W., Oertel, W., Siebert, U., Berger, K., Dodel, R.: Prevalence and incidence of parkinson's disease in europe. Eu. Neuropsychopharmacol. **15**, 473–490 (2005)
3. Tsanas, A., Little, M.A., McSharry, P.E., Spielman, J., Ramig, L.O.: Novel speech signal processing algorithms for high-accuracy classification of parkinson's disease. IEEE Trans. Biomed. Eng. **59**, 1264–1271 (2012)
4. Guo, P.-F., Bhattacharya, P., Kharma, N.: Advances in detecting parkinson's disease. In: Zhang, D. (ed.) ICMB 2010. LNCS, vol. 6165, pp. 306–314. Springer, Heidelberg (2010)
5. Rinn, W.E.: The neuropsychology of facial expression: a review of the neurological and psychological mechanisms for producing facial expressions. Psychol. Bull. **95**, 52 (1984)
6. Simons, G., Pasqualini, M.C.S., Reddy, V., Wood, J.: Emotional and nonemotional facial expressions in people with parkinson's disease. J. Int. Neuropsychol. Soc. **10**, 521–535 (2004)
7. Katsikitis, M., Pilowsky, I.: A study of facial expression in parkinson's disease using a novel microcomputer-based method. J. Neurol. Neurosurg. Psychiatr. **51**, 362–366 (1988)
8. Mergl, R., Mavrogiorgou, P., Hegerl, U., Juckel, G.: Kinematical analysis of emotionally induced facial expressions: a novel tool to investigate hypomimia in patients suffering from depression. J. Neurol. Neurosurg. Psychiatr. **76**, 138–140 (2005)
9. He, G.F., Kang, S.K., Song, W.C., Jung, S.T.: Real-time gesture recognition using 3d depth camera. In: 2011 IEEE 2nd International Conference on Software Engineering and Service Science (ICSESS), pp. 187–190. IEEE (2011)
10. Zhang, Z.: Microsoft kinect sensor and its effect. IEEE MultiMedia **19**, 4–10 (2012)
11. Ltkebohle, I.: BWorld Robot Control Software (2015) (online). http://www.faceshift.com. Accessed 11 June 2015
12. Bouaziz, S., Wang, Y., Pauly, M.: Online modeling for realtime facial animation. ACM Trans. Graph. (TOG) **32**, 40 (2013)
13. Shalev-Shwartz, S., Ben-David, S.: Understanding Machine Learning: From Theory to Algorithms. Cambridge University Press, New York (2014)

Automated Facial Expressions Analysis in Schizophrenia: A Continuous Dynamic Approach

Talia Tron[1,4]([✉]), Abraham Peled[2,3], Alexander Grinsphoon[2,3], and Daphna Weinshall[4]

[1] ELSC Center for Brain Science, Hebrew University, Jerusalem 91904, Israel
Talia.Tron@mail.huji.ac.il
[2] Sha'ar Menashe Mental Health Center, Sha'ar Menashe 38706, Israel
[3] Rappaport Faculty of Medicine, Technion Institute of Technology, Haifa 3200003, Israel
[4] School of Computer Science and Engineering, Hebrew University, Jerusalem 91904, Israel

Abstract. Facial expressions play a major role in psychiatric diagnosis, monitoring and treatment adjustment. We recorded 34 schizophrenia patients and matched controls during a clinical interview, and extracted the activity level of 23 facial Action Units (AUs), using 3D structured light cameras and dedicated software. By defining dynamic and intensity AUs activation characteristic features, we found evidence for blunted affect and reduced positive emotional expressions in patients. Further, we designed learning algorithms which achieved up to 85 % correct schizophrenia classification rate, and significant correlation with negative symptoms severity. Our results emphasize the clinical importance of facial dynamics, and illustrate the possible advantages of employing affective computing tools in clinical settings.

Keywords: Schizophrenia · Machine learning · Mental health · Facial expressions · 3D cameras · FACS

1 Introduction

Both clinical observations and computational studies suggest that facial activity plays a major role in signaling people's emotional and mental state [8,13,14]. Accordingly, several mental disorders are manifested by reduced or altered facial activity, and facial observations are an integral part of psychiatric diagnosis. To date, there are no objective, quantitative methods to measure these alterations, and no clear relation between them and the underlying brain disturbances. This causes multiple interpretations of phenomenology and results in low reliability and validity of psychiatric diagnosis [2].

Schizophrenia is one of the most severe mental disorders, with lifetime prevalence of about 1 % worldwide. The disorder is characterized by negative symptoms, which involve the loss of functions and abilities (e.g. blunted affect), and by

© Springer International Publishing Switzerland 2016
S. Serino et al. (Eds.): MindCare 2015, CCIS 604, pp. 72–81, 2016.
DOI: 10.1007/978-3-319-32270-4_8

positive symptoms, which are pathological functions not present in healthy individuals (e.g. hallucinations). Studies have found that patients with schizophrenia demonstrate less positive emotions than controls [10], and lower congruity of emotional response [1]. Furthermore, there has been evidence for reduced upper facial activity [3] and reduced overall facial expressivity [5,7,12]. Nonetheless, these studies use a limited set of facial activity characteristic features, not necessarily ecologically relevant, and ignore information regarding facial dynamics and variability. An extensive use of computational methods together with clinical intuition is needed in order to obtain a more comprehensive description of patients behavior.

Our study combines descriptive methods with data-driven analysis. We use machine learning tools and cutting edge technology, in order to study a wide range of facial activity characteristic features, the relation between them, and the way they are manifested in clinical setting.

2   Materials and Methods

2.1   Study Design

Participants. The study was done in collaboration with Sha'ar Menashe mental health center. Participants were 34 patients and 33 control subjects. All patients were diagnosed as suffering from schizophrenia according to DSM-5, and the course of illness in these patients varied from 1.5 years up to 37 years, with mean of 16.9 years. All patients but one were under stable drug treatment (mood stabilizer, antidepressant, antipsychotic and/or sedatives). Informed consent was obtained from all individual participants included in the study.

Psychiatric Evaluation. Participants were evaluated by a trained psychiatrist using the *Positive and Negative Symptoms Scale* (PANSS), a 30 item scale especially designed to asses the severity of both negative and positive symptoms in schizophrenia [9]. The majority of patients suffered from post-psychotic residual negative signs (Type II) schizophrenia, namely, they showed severe negative symptoms (higher than 5 in the PANSS scale), while severe positive and general symptoms were rather rare (less than 10 % of patients). 16 of the symptoms did not vary enough for statistical analysis and learning; therefore, the analysis focused on the remaining symptoms: 3 positive symptoms (Delusions, Conceptual disorganization and Grandiosity), 2 general symptoms (Motor retardation and Poor attention) and 7 negative symptoms (Blunted affect, Emotional withdrawal, Poor rapport, Passive/apathetic social withdrawal, Difficulty in abstract thinking, Lack of spontaneity and flow of conversation and Stereotyped thinking). To test for diagnosis consistency, the PANSS evaluation was repeated independently by a second trained psychiatrist who watched the interview videos. Inter-rater reliability was calculated separately for each PANSS symptom using Pearson correlation test.

Experimental Paradigm. All subjects were individually recorded using a 3D structured light camera (carmine 1.09), during a 15 min long interview conducted by a trained psychiatrist. The interview was constructed out of one general question ('Tell me about yourself'), and three emotionally evocative questions regarding subject's current mood and recent emotional events. The camera was placed on the table between subject and interviewer, in a way that did not interfere with eye contact and none of the subjects reported discomfort from being recorded. All procedures performed in the study were in accordance with the ethical standards of the institutional research committee and with the 1964 Helsinki declaration and its later amendments or comparable ethical standards.

2.2 Facial Activity Features

The Facial Action Coding System (FACS). Scores the activity of 46 individual facial muscles called Action Units (AUs) based on their intensity level and temporal segments [4]. Scoring is traditionally done manually, one frame at a time, by certified FACS coders, and automated FACS coding poses a major challenge in the field of affective computing. The advantage of the coding system is that it does not interpret the emotional value of specific features, and allows for a continuous and dynamic facial activity analysis.

Facial Activity Extraction. For AUs activity extraction we used the *Faceshift©* commercial software which provides real time 3D face and head tracking, and which is typically used for animating avatars in film and game industry (www.faceshift.com). The software automatically analyzes data from 3D cameras based on structured light technology. These cameras capture facial surface data, which is less sensitive to head pose and to lightning conditions than 2D data, and yields a better recognition rate of AUs [11]. *Faceshift* outputs the intensity level over time for 48 AUs. The output was manually evaluated for tracking sensitivity and noise level. Subsequently, 23 *Faceshift* Action Units (AUs) were selected for further analysis and learning, including Brows-up (center, left and right), Mouth-side (left or right), Jaw-open, Lips-up, Lips-Funnel, Eye-In-Right (looking left), Chin-raise, Sneer and both sides (left and right) of Blink, Smile, Frown, Dimple, Lips-Stretch, and Chick-squint (see Fig. 1).

Characteristic Features Computation. In order to obtain a detailed characterization of facial behavior, which captures both the dynamics and intensity of the activity in a clinically relevant manner, we calculated 5 characteristic features separately for each AU. First, the raw *Faceshift* signal was quantized using k-means (k=4) clustering. Then a transition matrix was generated, measuring the number of transitions between quantization levels. 5 facial activity characteristic features were then computed:

1. *Activation Ratio* - Fraction of segment during which the AU was activated
2. *Activation Level* - Mean intensity of AU activation

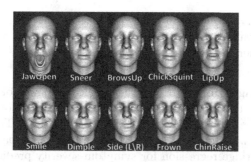

Fig. 1. Illustration of *Faceshift* facial Action Units (AUs) used for learning.

3. *Activation Length* - Number of frames that the AU activation lasted
4. *Change Ratio* - Fraction of the period of AU activation when there was a change in activity level
5. *Fast Change Ratio* - Fraction of fast changes (>1) in activation level

Activation Level and *Change Ratio* were calculated using frames with non-zero activity only, so that they will not overlap with the *Activation Ratio*. For *Fast Change Ratio*, we normalized the number of fast changes frames by the total number of frames with activity change.

3   Analysis and Learning

The first part of our analysis was descriptive, and was aimed to obtain detailed characterization of facial activity in patients in comparison with controls. In the second part, we applied machine learning tools to generate predictions. We tested whether facial features have predictive power for patients vs. control classification, and for evaluating symptoms severity. To exclude possible confounds such as gender, education level, age and religion, we performed one-way ANOVA; a variable that was found to be different between groups, was further investigated for its effect on facial activity within groups.

Descriptive Data Analysis. In the descriptive part of the analysis, we explored how the facial activity is altered in different parts of the face, paying special attention to smiles. This was done using two tail student's t-tests on the *Activity Level* of each AU separately. For smiles, we further analyzed the difference in all characteristic features, using separate t-test for each feature type. The AU activity was given an emotional interpretation (e.g. high smile level indicates positive emotion), based on the *Emotional Facial Action Coding System* (EMFACS) developed by Paul Ekman, which systematically categorizes combination of AUs to specific emotional categories [6].

To study the way blunted affect is manifested in patients, we performed a regularized ridge regression between symptom severity and all features over all AUs.

Feature selection (n = 10) was done using f-regression, based on d' scores. Regression results were evaluated by *Pearson's R*, and the output regression weights were used for further feature type analysis.

Machine Learning Tools. To test the predictive power of our features we trained a learner on train data and evaluated its performance on one test patient at a time, following the Leave-One-Out (LOO) procedure. The basic learning algorithm we used was Support Vector Machine (SVM) for patients vs. control classification, and ridge regression for symptom severity prediction. Before the regression, principle component analysis (PCA) was performed on train data separately for each feature type, resulting in a mixture of AUs. Feature selection was performed based on train data using f-regression (for SVM), or by selecting the highest PCA components (for regression).

To increase learning robustness, we employed a two step prediction algorithm, where each stage is learned separately from train data (see Fig. 2). Interview data of each individual subject was divided into 30 seconds long segments, and 5 representative features were computed separately for each segment ($F1$). In step 1, a learner was trained on the segments of all train subjects, giving as output the first model weights ($W1$) and a prediction for each segment. In step 2, prediction mean and standard deviation over all segments were calculated for each subject ($F2$), and a second learner was trained to predict a participant's label from these moments ($W2$).

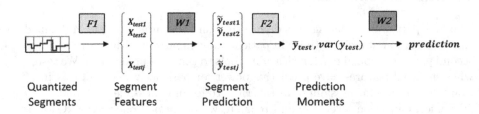

Fig. 2. Illustration of the 2-step algorithm.

Performance evaluation was done between-subjects, namely, all segments of one subjects were left out for testing the algorithm. The SVM classifier was evaluated by the area under the Receiver Operator Curve (AUC), a combined measure for the learner's sensitivity (true positive rate) and specificity (true negative rate) with 1 signaling perfect separation and 0.5 signaling chance. Regression results were evaluated by *Pearson's R* between the psychiatrist score and the algorithm prediction, separately for each PANSS symptom.

4   Results

4.1   Inter-rater Reliability

All negative symptoms scores were at high agreement between raters (with an average of $R = 0.850$, $p << 0.01$), and so was 3 positive symptoms ($R = 0.630$, $p = 0.021$ for Delusions, $R = 0.880$, $p << 0.01$ for Conceptual disorganization) and one general symptoms ($R = 0.671$, $p << 0.01$ for Motor Retardation). Poor Attention and Grandiosity were not significantly correlated between raters.

4.2   Facial Activity, Descriptive Analysis

Facial Parts Analysis. We found a significant difference in the *Activation Level* of 16 out of 23 *Facefhit*-AUs (see Fig. 3). Specifically, patients demonstrated lower level of activity in Smile, Dimple, Lip-stretch and Lip-up ($p << 0.01$), AUs which are typically in correspondence with positive emotional state. Frowns, Brows-Up and Chin-raise, on the other hand, were at much higher level in patients than in controls, which may indicate the presence of negative valance emotions (sadness, surprise and fear). Although those facial expressions were more intense, they changed more slowly, with reduced *Change Ratio* ($p = 0.004$ for Chin-raise) and *Fast Change Ratio* ($p << 0.01$ for both Chin-raise and Frowns). Blink *Activation Level* was reduced in patients, which in the *Faceshift* framework could mean that they closed their eyes less than controls. Sneer *Activation Level* was also significantly reduced. The level of Cheek-Squint activation was surprisingly enhanced in patients.

Smiles Analysis. A closer look at smile activation (Fig. 4) reveals that in comparison with controls, smile *Activation Level* was reduced, while *Activation Length* and *Fast Change Ratio* were significantly enhanced in patients. These results suggest that in clinical settings, patients may not necessarily smile less, but rather their smiles are at lower intensity, longer, and with faster onset and offset (aka frozen or fake smiles).

Blunted Affect. Regression results (Fig. 5) suggest a significant correlation between AUs activation features and psychiatric evaluation of blunted affect severity ($R_{Pearson} = 0.686$, $p << 0.01$). Based on the regression weights, the two most discriminative AU features were *Activation Level* and *Activation Ratio*, which were in negative correlation with symptom's score. *Change Ratio* and *Fast Change Ratio* were also given negative weights, while *Activation Length* seemed to be positively correlated with the severity of the symptom. These Results are consistent with clinical observations.

Possible Confounds. One-way ANOVA on patients and controls data revealed significant difference between groups for gender ($F = 16.77$, $p << 0.01$) and education level ($F = 6.42$, $p = 0.014$). Neither of these variables was found to

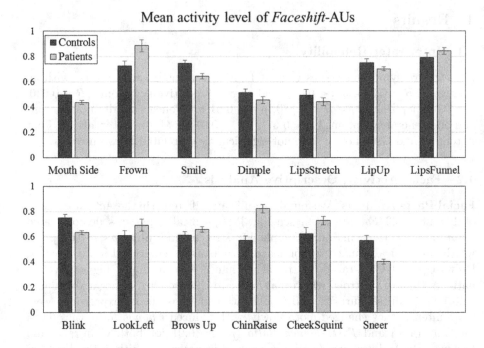

Fig. 3. Mean *Activation level* of facial Action Units in patients and controls. Only significantly different results are presented ($p < 0.05$ in student's t-test).

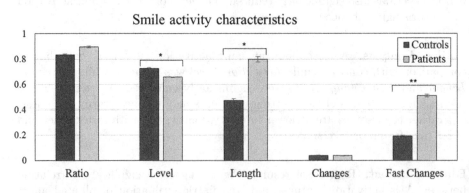

Fig. 4. Smile activation characteristic features for patients and controls.

have a significant effect on facial activation characteristic within each group. The possible effect of neuroleptic drugs on observed facial activity could not be excluded, since all of our patients were under drug treatment, and additional control is needed.

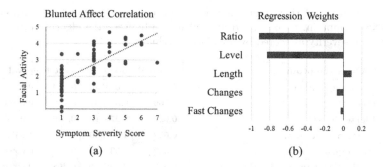

Fig. 5. (a) Regression between blunted affect severity and facial activity features. (b) Weights given to each feature by the regression model.

4.3 Facial Expression Predictive Power

Patients vs. Controls Classification. We employed the 2-step learning algorithm one feature type at a time, and using all features together. Each of the feature types was distinctive on its own on test data with AUC significantly better than chance (Fig. 6). *Activation Length* gave out the best classification results $(AUC = 0.887)$, followed by *Fast change ratio* $(AUC = 0.815)$ and *Fast change ratio* $(AUC = 0.814)$. This indicates the importance of looking at the duration and dynamic of facial activity, rather than general intensity measures. The predictive power of using all features together was slightly lower $(AUC = 0.799)$, most likely as a result of small sample and subsequent over-fitting.

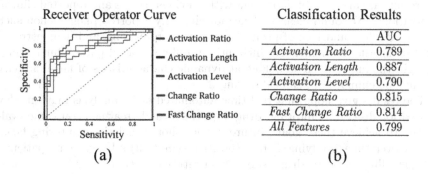

Fig. 6. a) ROC curves of each feature type for patients vs. control classification. (b) Classification results summarized as Area Under the ROC Curve (AUC).

PANSS Severity Regression. For all negative symptoms, the prediction of the algorithm was significantly correlated with the score given by the psychiatrist $(R > 0.3, p \leqslant 0.01)$. No such significance was found for any of the positive symptoms, which can be explained by the small variability of positive symptoms scores in our data. We got an unexpected result for general symptoms, with

Table 1. Summary of ridge regression results on train and test data, separately for each PANSS symptom. *Pearson's* R was calculated between the algorithm prediction and symptom severity as scored by a trained psychiatrist.

Code	PANSS symptom	Train R	p-val	Test R	p-val
G11	Motor retardation	0.463	1.023E-03	0.154	0.213
G7	Poor attention	0.566	9.35E-07	0.292	0.0166
N1	Blunted affect	0.686	8.27E-10	0.530	4.042E-06
N2	Emotional withdrawal	0.652	4.52E-09	0.510	1.045E-05
N3	Poor rapport	0.550	2.53E-06	0.315	0.00949
N4	Passive/apatheticsocial withdrawal	0.548	2.89E-06	0.368	0.00216
N5	Difficulty in abstract thinking	0.585	3.83E-07	0.369	0.00211
N6	Lack of spontaneity and conversation flow	0.555	1.58E-06	0.301	0.0133
N7	Stereotyped thinking	0.539	3.86E-06	0.369	0.00211
P1	Delusions	0.344	0.005	0.017	0.891
P2	Conceptual disorganization	0.332	0.007	0.065	0.600
P5	Hallucinations	0.306	0.013	0.055	0.660

significant correlation only for Poor attention ($R = 0.292$, $p < 0.05$), which outperform the inter-rater correlation for this symptom. Train and test results are summarized in Table 1.

5   Discussion

Our results are in excellent agreement with previous studies and reported clinical observations. We found clear evidence for clinically reported phenomenon such as blunted affect and lack of positive emotional expressions, and demonstrated how the disorder is manifested differently in different facial parts. Our findings highlight the importance of looking at dynamic characteristics of facial activity and may be employed in clinical settings.

The results give hope that real time automated facial analysis may one day be used for disease monitoring, drug adjustment and treatment outcome evaluation. To achieve these goals, future studies should include monitoring facial activity over time, studying Type-I (positive symptom) schizophrenia patients, and controlling subjects' drug usage. Other future directions include broadening facial activity research to other disorders such as depression and autism, and investigating the relation to neural mechanisms and cognitive performance.

Acknowledgements. This work was supported in part by the Intel Collaborative Research Institute for Computational Intelligence (ICRI-CI), and the Gatsby Charitable Foundations.

References

1. Bersani, G., Polli, E., Valeriani, G.: Facial expression in patients with bipolar disorder and schizophrenia in response to emotional stimuli: a partially shared cognitive and social deficit of the two. Neuropsychiatric Dis. Treat. **9**, 1137–1144 (2013)
2. Cohn, J.F., Kruez, T.S., Matthews, I., Yang, Y., Nguyen, M.H., Padilla, M.T., Zhou, F., De la Torre, F.: Detecting depression from facial actions and vocal prosody. In: 2009 3rd International Conference on Affective Computing and Intelligent Interaction and Workshops, pp. 1–7. September 2009
3. Ekman, P., Friesen, W.V.: The repertoire of nonverbal behavior: categories, origins, usage, and coding. In: Nonverbal Communication, Interaction, and Gesture, pp. 57–106 (1981)
4. Ekman, P., Rosenberg, E.L.: What The Face Reveals: Basic and Applied Studies of Spontaneous Expression Using the Facial Action Coding System (FACS). Oxford University Press, New York (1997)
5. Falkenberg, I., Bartels, M., Wild, B.: Keep smiling!. Eur. Arch. Psychiatry Clin. Neurosci. **258**(4), 245–253 (2008)
6. Friesen, W.V., Ekman, P.: Emfacs-7: emotional facial action coding system. University of California at San Francisco, 2: 36 (1983) (Unpublished manuscript)
7. Gaebel, W., Wölwer, W.: Facial expressivity in the course of schizophrenia and depression. Eur. Arch. Psychiatry Clin. Neurosci. **254**(5), 335–342 (2004)
8. Gunes, H., Pantic, M.: Automatic, dimensional and continuous emotion recognition. Int. J. Synth. Emotions **1**(1), 68–99 (2010)
9. Kay, S.R., Flszbein, A., Opfer, L.A.: The positive and negative syndrome scale (panss) for schizophrenia. Schizophr. Bull. **13**(2), 261–276 (1987)
10. Lotzin, A., Haack-Dees, B., Resch, F., Romer, G., Ramsauer, B.: Facial emotional expression in schizophrenia adolescents during verbal interaction with a parent. Eur. Arch. Psychiatry Clin. Neurosci. **263**(6), 529–536 (2013)
11. Sandbach, G., Zafeiriou, S., Pantic, M., Yin, L.: Static and dynamic 3D facial expression recognition: a comprehensive survey. Image Vis. Comput. **30**(10), 683–697 (2012)
12. Simons, G., Ellgring, J.H., Beck-Dossler, K., Gaebel, W., Wölwer, W.: Facial expression in male and female schizophrenia patients. Eur. Arch. Psychiatry Clin. Neurosci. **260**(3), 267–276 (2010)
13. Trémeau, F., Malaspina, D., Duval, F., Corrêa, H., Hager-Budny, M., Coin-Bariou, L., Macher, J.-P., Gorman, J.M.: Facial expressiveness in patients with schizophrenia compared to depressed patients and nonpatient comparison subjects. Am. J. Psychiatry **162**(1), 92–101 (2005)
14. Valstar, M., Schuller, B., Smith, K., Eyben, F.: AVEC - the continuous audio/visual emotion and depression recognition challenge (2013). cs.nott.ac.uk

When Reality Bites Try Virtual Reality: Virtual Reality for Mental Health

Home-Based Virtual Reality Exposure Therapy with Virtual Health Agent Support

Dwi Hartanto[1(✉)], Willem-Paul Brinkman[1], Isabel L. Kampmann[2],
Nexhmedin Morina[2], Paul G.M. Emmelkamp[3,5], and Mark A. Neerincx[1,4]

[1] Delft University of Technology, Delft, The Netherlands
{d.hartanto,w.p.brinkman,m.a.neerincx}@tudelft.nl
[2] University of Amsterdam, Amsterdam, The Netherlands
{i.l.kampmann,n.morina}@uva.nl
[3] King Abdulaziz University, Jeddah, Saudi Arabia
p.m.g.emmelkamp@uva.nl
[4] TNO Human Factors, Soesterberg, The Netherlands
[5] Netherlands Institute for Advanced Study, Wassenaar, The Netherlands

Abstract. To increase the accessibility and efficiency of virtual reality exposure
therapy (VRET) this paper proposes a system for home-based use where patients
with social phobia are supported by a virtual health agent. We present an overview
of our system design, and discuss key techniques such as (1) dialogue techniques
to create automated free speech dialogue between virtual characters and patients
in virtual reality worlds; (2) a multi-modal automatic anxiety feedback-loop
mechanism to control patients' anxiety level; and (3) motivational techniques
applied by a virtual health agent. The system was evaluated in a pilot study where
five patients with social phobia utilized our home-based VRET system. The
results showed that the system was able to evoke the required anxiety in patients
and that over time self-reported anxiety and heart rate gradually decreased as
expected in exposure therapy.

Keywords: Virtual reality therapy · Virtual coach · Virtual health agent ·
Behaviour change support system · Social anxiety disorder · Self-therapy

1 Introduction

Social phobia is one of the most often occurring mental disorders, with reports that estimate
this to affect around 13.3 % of the US population [1] during their lifetime. Patients with
social phobia fear social situations in which they may be scrutinized by others [2], for
example when having a conversation with someone, being observed, meeting someone new,
or giving a presentation. Exposing patients in virtual reality to these social situations has
been suggested [3] as a treatment for this disorder. As for other anxiety disorders, the development of virtual reality exposure therapy (VRET) systems mainly focuses on systems that
can be used in a health clinic where a therapist directly controls the system when the patient
is exposed [4]. However, with an ever-increasing demand for more efficiency and accessibility, it is desirable to be able to offer this treatment at the patient's home. We therefore

© Springer International Publishing Switzerland 2016
S. Serino et al. (Eds.): MindCare 2015, CCIS 604, pp. 85–98, 2016.
DOI: 10.1007/978-3-319-32270-4_9

propose a home-based VRET system where social phobia patients are also supported by a virtual health agent. In the design of this system three specific challenges were addressed that are discussed in this paper. First, how to create a long conversation with a virtual character to let patients experience the required social anxiety? Second, how do you automatically control the patient's anxiety throughout a conversation with virtual characters? Third, how could a virtual health agent motivate a patient to continue with the therapy? We also present the results of a pilot study in which individuals with social phobia utilized our home-based VRET system.

2   Related Work

Providing treatment for social phobia over the Internet is possible. For example, in a randomized controlled trial, Gallego et al. [5] found a significant improvement in patients receiving a remotely delivered treatment using non-interactive exposure video over the internet. The patients' fear of public speaking, work impairment, and avoidance behavior decreased. Instead of using video exposure, others [6] have suggested a system that allowed the therapist to control VRET from a remote location over the internet. Still, this set up required the therapist to be actively involved.

At least part of the exposure does not require the presence of a therapist. In cognitive-behavioral therapy (CBT), homework exposure exercises have been employed as an integral component in the treatment for several anxiety disorders such as obsessive-compulsive disorder, post-traumatic stress disorder and social phobia [7]. Even though effective for some intervention [8], lack of an active involvement of the therapist during treatment has been associated with reduced therapeutic efficacy, such as in relation to depression [9]. In self-therapy settings, patients usually rely on persuasive power of the homework-exercise itself. Whereas when therapists are involved, patients are often also influenced by the therapeutic alliance, even with virtual exposure therapy [10]. This brings forward the questions whether such an effect could also brought about with a virtual health agent?

The presence of a virtual health agent can have a positive effect on treatment outcome [11]. These agents often aim to guide individuals through a specific task thereby stimulating positive behaviour, increasing motivation and adherence [11, 12]. Typically, the health agent applies persuasive techniques to change people's attitude and behaviors [13].

3   System Design

The entire concept of the home-based VRET system was review in a series of discussions with eight clinical psychologists. Based on their input, a number of scenarios were written and again reviewed by eight clinical psychologists, leading eventually to an implemented system called the Memphis system [14]. The system consists of three main entities: (1) the virtual health agent, (2) the virtual reality system and (3) the therapist application.

3.1   The Virtual Health Agent

The main objective of the virtual health agents (Fig. 1) was to guide the patient through the various steps of the therapy and motivate them to continue with the therapy. Guiding the patients through the therapy involved explaining patients how to assemble the system so it could be used. Patients received a set of video's and instructions manuals on how to connect the various hardware elements such as: head mounted display (HMD), head tracker, heart rate device, internet dongle, security dongle, and microphone. Once the Memphis system was started, the virtual health agent helped the patient to calibrate and test the system, for example, training the speech recognizer, calibrating the anxiety measurement, testing sound and internet connection, wearing the heart rate device and finally setting up the HMD and the head position tracker.

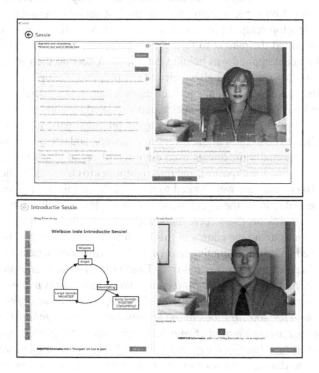

Fig. 1. The female virtual health agent guiding patient to set the therapy goals (top), and the male virtual health agent providing interactive psycho-education (bottom)

Besides guiding patients through the technical aspect of the system, the virtual agent also introduced the patients to the therapy itself. The first motivational strategy the agent applied was to help patients to formulate an achievable treatment goal. After explaining the purpose of setting goals and also giving some example, the agent asked patients to enter their goal. Interpreting this textual formulated goal and providing feedback by the agent was regarded as no achievable. Instead the agent used the strategy of empowering the patients to do this themselves. In other words, after entering the goal, the agent gave patients criteria to evaluate their own goal, for example, achievable, concrete, but also not too easy. Again, it provided this with some examples. Afterwards patients were asked again to reflect on their goal. This procedure was repeated when helping patients to formulate specific sub goals. This information together with information the agent asked about anxiety for specific social situations, and avoidance behaviors were automatically sent through a server to the therapist, who could use the information to create the anxiety hierarchy for social situations and a treatment plan. The second motivation strategy the agent applied was psycho-education. The agents explained what social anxiety disorder is, and the mechanisms underlying it. The agents also explained the therapy and what patients could expect. Besides this general information, the agent also explained in each session all the steps, e.g. filling out questionnaires, conducting virtual reality exposures, and reflecting on the outcome and progress. In the last session, the agents also helped the patients to develop relapse prevention strategies in a similar manner as the agent initially had supported the patient to formulate a treatment goal. The third motivation strategy that the agent applied was helping patients to reflect on their reactions during the virtual reality exposures, and also their overall progress during the treatment. For this the agent used an expert system approach using a therapeutic social anxiety knowledge base. The knowledge base was written and validated by clinical therapists. After patients were exposed in a virtual world, the agent provided patients with an interpretation of the collected heart rate data, self-reported anxiety, and stress level manipulation in virtual world. Internally the agents used eight templates to characterize the data of anxiety progress during the exposure, and three templates to characterize the stress level manipulation. Interpretations were linked to the 24 cells of this a 8×3 matrix. When formulating the reflections, the agent started with explaining what information was shown by the graphics on the screen. This was followed by the data interpretation, possible speculations about the causes of this result and elements of psycho-education. The agent finished with an encouraging remark aiming to improve patient's self-efficacy. The following is an example translated from Dutch of what the agent said: *"After the exercise in the virtual world we can now look together at the results that were collected. At the screen you can see several graphs....The last graph shows how difficult the system has tried to make it for you...if I look at the graphs, there are two things I notice. First, your anxiety level, the combination of your heart rate and self-reported anxiety, started relative high but reduced during the exercise. Secondly, the number of social challenges remained constant during the entire exercise. This exercise nicely demonstrates that after a while your anxiety naturally deceased. This is exactly what we try to achieve with this exercise. Very good! Nice result!"* To avoid repetition of agent reflection over time, each cell include several alternative formulations of what the agent could say.

The last motivation strategy the agent applied was to provide patients with a reflection of their overall treatment progress. For this, the agent looked at the overall anxiety level of the last three sessions and the sessions before this. As with the reflection after the exercises in the virtual world, the agent used a number of templates to characterize the recorded anxiety level across the sessions. Important was also that given the number of exercises scheduled and completed, the agent could recommend patients to contact the therapist if the therapy does not seem to work. Again, an example of a reflection that the agent could offer: *"Let's look at a number of things. First, if I look at the list with exercises, I can see that you have already completed 10 exercises, you are working currently on a new exercise, and that eight other exercises have been planned for you. This is very good! Secondly, if I look at the averages of the self-reported anxiety scores for the last 3 sessions I see scores that are relatively low. In the sessions before that, the anxiety scores were relative low. ...Because you have finished more that 60 % of the anxiety hierarchy, is might be a good idea to discuss this with your therapist. It is important to find exercises that evoke anxiety. Also, it is important that you do not use anxiety avoidance strategies during the exercise..."*.

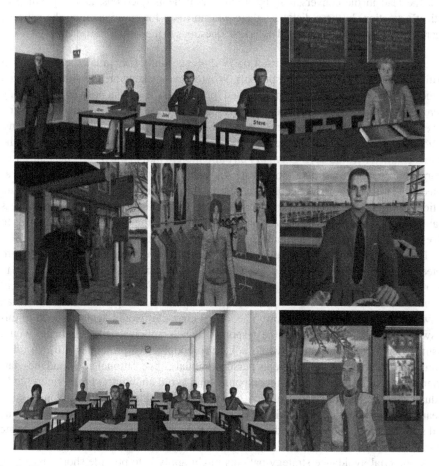

Fig. 2. Examples of seven virtual scenarios supported by the Memphis system (left to right). Top: Participating in an English class, having appointment in a restaurant, middle: being ask to participate in a survey, buying t-shirt in a shop, meeting a blind date in a restaurant, and bottom: having presentation in a class, meeting a stranger in a bus stop

3.2   The Virtual Reality System

Virtual Social Scenario. The Memphis system provided 19 different virtual reality social scenarios, such as meeting a blind date in a restaurant, a job interview, visiting a doctor, talking to a stranger at a bus station, buying a t-shirt, and meeting a stranger at a party (Fig. 2). All social scenarios were selected and developed to elicit social anxiety. They are also often used and suggested for exposure exercise in real life [15].

Dialogue Techniques. A key component of the system was to expose patients to free natural dialogues. As this was a home-based system, a dialogue should unfold without the need for direct human control, which is often not the case in current systems. Our system therefore employed key word recognition and speech detection technology. Each dialogue lasted around 18 min. To avoid an ever-broadening dialogue, the virtual characters always took the lead in the conversation, by asking the patients questions, and responding to patient's reaction. In these dialogues there was no room for questions from the patients. Therefore, patients were instructed not to ask questions to the virtual characters.

On average, each dialogue consisted of 78 dialogue units (i.e. [avatar's question] → [patient's answer] → [avatar's response]). Where obvious keywords could be expected in the patient's answer, the system searched for them in the patient answers. When they were detected, the virtual character gave a response directly related to patients' answers, for example: [foreigner character] *"when traveling with a train, how do I know I have to get out of the train?"* If answer of patients included the word "announcement", the virtual character would say: *"Ok than I pay attention to that in the train"*. In some cases characters' response was not appropriate, for example, when the wrong keyword was detected. This was however considered acceptable, as the objective was to exposure patients to social situations that would evoke anxiety, and not to expose them to flawless dialogues. By using keyword detection at some places in the dialogue, the hope was to give patients the illusion that character reacted intelligently towards their answers.

The majority of the virtual characters' responses however were not based on keyword detection. Instead, the characters provided responses that patients might think related to their answer, but were in fact independent of their answer. For example, [shop assistance] *"Can you also specify to me the price range that you're aiming for?"* After which an answer of the patient would follow. The virtual character would again respond to this answer *"Well, that's fine"*. For the responses it was anticipated that patients would assume that virtual characters would adhere to cooperative principles [16]. In other words, virtual characters and patients pursued mutual conversational goals and the character would try to provide relevant responses and avoid ambiguity. Furthermore, individuals often heavily rely on the process of interfering. In other words, they would assign meaning to the response of the virtual characters in light of the context of the dialogue and social setting. Table 1 provides a list of specific strategies that were used to create character responses.

A potential avoidance strategy patients might apply is to provide short answers to avoid exposure. To address this behavior the system monitored the length of patients' answers. Hence, when a patient gave a short answer, the virtual character engaged the patients into a dialogue that encouraged the patient to provide longer answer, for

Table 1. List of dialogue techniques employed in the Memphis VR dialogue system

Dialogue techniques	Example
Create topic blocks in the story line to avoid repetition in questioning. Blocks start with a monolog where the avatar provides information about him or herself, followed by questions the topic	Block 1: [avatar talking about his family extensively] → [continue with questions about patient family] → Block 2: [avatar talking about his holiday last summer extensively] → [continue with questions about patient summer holiday] → etc.
Create generic avatar's respond that fit to any participant's answer	Avatar: "Hi, it seem that you're looking for someone, may I join you?" → Patient: [answer] → Avatar: "okay"
(Dis)agree on what the patient said	Avatar: "What do you think about the climate change now days?" → Patient: [answer] → Avatar: "Great! I agree with you in this case"
State an attitude or emotion towards the answer	Avatar: "I've been waiting for my food for 20 min now. The service is really slow here, what do you think?" → Patient: [answer] → Avatar: "Ah, I see. I am glad that you mention that!"
Reflect on your original question, e.g. it was not relevant	Avatar: "Do you have OHRA health insurance or do you have another private health insurance?" → Patient: [answer] → Avatar: "OK, I understand that, it does not matter anyway."
State an opinion	Avatar: "What do you think is the most interesting thing to see in the Netherland?" → Patient: [answer] → Avatar: "Yeah, I think visiting a traditional cheese factory, or clogs shop is a nice experiences."
State (mis)understanding of patient answer, and extend response with own information	Avatar: "What do you think about Amsterdam public transport right now?" → Patient: [answer] → Avatar: "Ok, I see your point. I also have pretty similar thoughts since I used it a lot the last couple of years."
State an opinion based on your beliefs, emotion or perceptions	Avatar: "What make you a good team leader?" → Patient: [answer] → Avatar: "Yeah, but honestly I feel that you're not ready yet to become a good team leader by judging your answer and your current experience"
Makes a statement that is always true in relation to the topic	Avatar: "Are you feeling under any pressure or stress lately?" → Patient: [answer] → Avatar: "Okay, please remember that too much stress can affects your health."

example, "*It is not quite clear to me. Can you explain further?*", "*What do you mean by that?*", "*I have plenty of time here, can you explain it to me a bit more?*", or "*Now you make me curious, tell me something more.*"

The Phobic Stressors. As a patient's anxiety response towards fear stimuli varies, the system deployed several phobic stressors in each virtual world. First, the dialogue units could either be positive or negative. Controlling the ratio of positive and negative dialogue units has been demonstrated as a key function to induce different level of anxiety [17]. A positive dialogue unit meant a dialogue that consisted of a friendly, affirmative or enthusiastic type of question and avatar response, such as "*I like to know your taste music, what kind of music do you like?*" and was followed by the avatar's response to the patient's answer "*Cool! Nice taste of music!*". On the other hand, the negative dialogue unit meant that the dialogue was formulated in an unfriendly, unenthusiastic and criticizing question and response, for example "*I don't think that you have a good taste of music, but in case I'm wrong, can you tell me what type of music you like?*" followed by the avatar's response "*Mmm... as I have expected, you know nothing about good music!*". A second type of phobic stressors was the avatar gestures, for example the gaze of the avatar. As mentioned in other studies [18], (intense) direct eye gaze can evoke anxiety. Therefore the virtual characters also have the capability to stare at patients, look away, or simulate turn taking gaze behavior in a conversation. Besides gaze behavior, body posture of an audience [19], e.g. an interested audience or an audience that is bored, were used in public speaking scenarios.

The Anxiety Feedback-Loop. The system regulates patients' anxiety level by monitoring their anxiety and in a real-time fashion adjusting phobic stressors in the virtual world to reach the desired anxiety level as set by the therapist prior to a session. To monitor anxiety level, the system used both self-reported anxiety and a physiological measurement in the form of an automatically collected Subjective Unit of Discomfort (SUD) scale using speech recognition technology [20], and heart rate (bpm unit) using Zephyr HxM heart rate monitoring device. Both measurements were collected every four minutes during the exposure. Furthermore, using an individualised linear regression function, these two different modality measures were internally, at run time, combined into a single anxiety measure on which the system acted. As patients vary on how their anxiety is expressed in the two anxiety measures, a calibration procedure was used in the first session of the therapy. Imaginary exposure was used to determine a patient anxiety response in a low anxiety and high anxiety situation. Using relaxing sounds clips, a patient was asked to relax for four minutes while SUD and hear rate data was collected. Next, the patient was asked to imagine giving a presentation and push him or herself to the highest, but still tolerable, level of anxiety using various sound clips of an audience (i.e. from a nice, quiet audience to a loudly boing audience). Again anxiety data was collected for again a period of four minutes.

The automatic feedback loop used the personalised anxiety measure to regulate the patient's anxiety level. Before a session, therapists set the patient's initial target range for the patient's anxiety by defining the lower and upper bounder. At the start of a virtual reality (VR) exposure, the system increased or decreased the patient's anxiety to a level within the target range. The system did this by gradually increasing or decreasing the number or the degree of the phobic stressors in the virtual world. Once the patient's anxiety was within the target range, phobic stressors remained constant, or were reduced if patient's anxiety exceeded the target range. This regulation mechanism allowed patients to experience that their anxiety would naturally decline over time, and ensured that patients would not experienced an undesirable high level of anxiety for a long time.

3.3 The Therapist Application

The therapist application was a standalone application used by the therapist to interact with their patients. Using this application, therapists were able to create a personalized treatment plan for a patient, monitor the patient's progress during the treatment by evaluating the questionnaires, SUD score and heart rate results (Fig. 3), exchange personal messages with the patient using integrated e-mail services, creating and adjusting the treatment schedule, write a patient log book and relapse prevention strategy, and find the Memphis helpdesk contact information in case there is a technical problem. Once a therapist registered a session schedule and a treatment plan in the system, patients could start their treatment at home using the Memphis system.

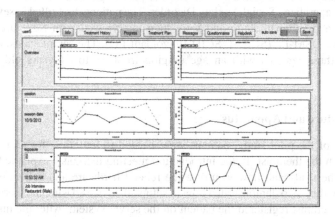

Fig. 3. Monitoring the patient's progress during the treatment by evaluating the SUD score and heart rate results in the therapist application

To support the interaction and communication between the therapist application and the virtual coach application, a secure and centralized database server was established. This database server records all occurring events during the treatment, for example: recording the psychological measurement data, store all questionnaires data, store therapist – patient messaging activities. To ensure security ISO standards on the medical informatics security, such as ISO27001, ISO9001, ISO14001, but also the national guideline (NEN7510) were consulted and work procedures were formulated. Also, prior to treatment both therapist and patients received personalized encryption and decryption keys, which they had to plug into their computer. All data stored on the server and data exchange between server and the therapist and patient application was encrypted using these keys.

4   Evaluation

System operation and testing the usability of the system was done with a group of 5 university students and staff (non-patients) and an experimenter acting as a therapist. This test was conducted on a single set of hardware (Dell Inspiron 7720 laptop running

Windows 7 64 bits). The tests revealed no serious operational or usability problems. The next step, therefore, was to examine the system in a small pilot study with actual patients, a first step towards larger scale clinical trial. The aim of the pilot study was to examine whether the system could evoke social anxiety and resulted over time in anxiety reduction when social phobic patients were exposed in virtual reality. The pilot study was approved by the ethics committee of the University of Amsterdam (Approval number: 2014-CP-3660).

4.1 Subjects

The pilot study was conducted with five social phobia patients who met DSM-IV [2] criteria for generalized Social Anxiety Disorder. The patients first filled in several questionnaires on psychopathology and were then interviewed with Structured Clinical Interview for DSM-IV (SCID-I, SCID-II/avoidant PD). The sample consisted of two males and three females with an age ranging from 38 to 64 years old ($M = 49$, $SD = 10.63$).

4.2 Procedure and Apparatus

At the start of the pilot study, patients were invited to the clinic for an introduction meeting with the therapist. In the introduction meeting therapists explained the background of the study and how to utilize the related hardware and software involved. Furthermore they also demonstrated how to setup all devices. Using the therapist application, the therapist registered the patient on the server system. After the introduction, patient received a suitcase with all equipment and a manual that they brought home. Each patient was scheduled to receive 10 treatment sessions. From the 10 sessions planned, 8 sessions (sessions 2 to 9) included exposure in the virtual reality, while session 1 served as an introduction session and session 10 as a relapse prevention session. At the start of each session, the therapist called the patient by phone. During the session the therapist would listen and advice the patient over the phone while the patient was using the system at home.

4.3 Measures

SUD scores and average heart rate were recorded every four minutes during VR exposure. The level of presence in the virtual reality during the first two treatment sessions was measured using Igroup Presence Questionnaire (IPQ) [21].

4.4 Results

Due to technical glitches that arose unexpectedly during treatment sessions, only one patient, who used the same hardware set that was used in the usability test, was able to complete all 10 sessions successfully. For the other four patients, who used another brand of laptop, it was decided to stop the trial and offer them face-to-face treatment.

This meant that for one patient data was collected from only the first six sessions, from two patients from only the first three sessions, and from one patient only the first two sessions.

The overall IPQ results were compared with online IPQ dataset[1] (downloaded on March 2nd, 2015) for stereo HMD visual stimuli. The overall IPQ rating ($N = 5, M = 60.4$, $SD = 4.51$) was significantly higher ($t(40) = -2.79, p = .008$) than the overall rating of the online IPQ dataset ($N = 37, M = 38.16, SD = 17.53$). The system therefore seems to have been successful in establishing significant levels of presence.

A total of 204 SUD scores were collected from the five patients. This data was analyzed with linear mixed-effect models (*lme*) in R taking the SUD scores as response variable and session number (2–9) and order number of the exposure exercise in a session (1–3) as factors nested within random effect variable participant. The objective of the analysis was not to generalize findings to a larger population, but instead to examine how SUD progressed for this sample, which for session 7 to 9 only included data from a single patient. The analysis showed that sessions ($\chi^2(1) = 24.2, p. < .001$) and exposure order number ($\chi^2(1) = 11.5, p. = .007$) had a significant effect on the SUD scores. No interaction effect between these two factors was found ($\chi^2(1) = 2.9, p. = .087$). As Fig. 4 shows, patients self-reported anxiety level decreased over the 22 (8 session × 3 exercises – 2 as first and last session only included 2 exercises) exposures exercises.

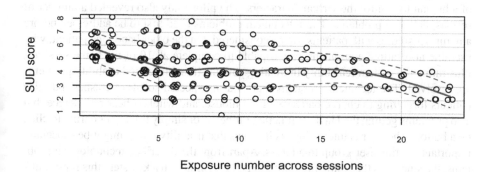

Fig. 4. Self-report anxiety across the treatment sessions including .25 and .75 quantiles spread.

Similar models were fitted on heart rate data ($n = 204$). Both session ($\chi^2(1) = 37.0$, $p. < .001$) and exposure order number ($\chi^2(1) = 71.5, p. < .001$) had significant effect on the heart rate data. Again no significant ($\chi^2(1) = 0.3, p. = .62$) two-way interaction was found. As Fig. 5 shows also heart rate decreased over 22 exposure exercises.

---

[1] Data available at http://www.igroup.org/pq/ipq/data.php.

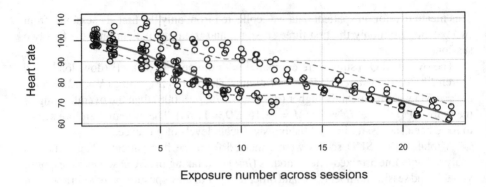

Fig. 5. Heart rate across the treatment sessions including .25 and .75 quantiles spread.

5 Discussion

The pilot study findings show that for this sample (1) the system could evoke anxiety and (2) over time the expected habituation sets in as anxiety levels dropped. Furthermore, the patients reported to have experienced a substantial level of presence, which is encouraging given that the 18 min dialogues were fully automated without intervention of a human to control the virtual characters. The pilot study also revealed a number of serious technical problems. These technical problems need first to be addressed before any further studies with patients can be considered. On the other hand, one patient, who used the non-failing equipment, was capable to complete all 10 of the home sessions, illustrating the system feasibility in treating patients if technical and usability problems are resolved. The technical problems included unexpected software crashes, but also patients forgetting to charge batteries of the mouse, and wireless hear rate device, but also problems getting the HMD to function properly, or simply finding or daring to click on a button. The later is interesting, as it shows that usability issues might be especially important for this user group to address. Apart from the described technological problems, the study has the following limitations. First, although a key step, this represent a pilot study with only a small sample and without a control condition to compare the findings with. Second, because of the technical glitch, patients did not do the exercise completely on their own. Often the therapist also had to provide technical support on the phone. Third, because of ethics considerations it was necessary at this stage to have a therapist listening in over the phone while patients conducted their exercises at home. Besides the insights the pilot study offered into the feasibility of home-based VRET, the scientific contribution of the work presented in this paper lies in the techniques proposed to address three key challenges, namely, (1) techniques a virtual health agent could apply to motivate a patient, (2) dialogue techniques to create 18 min long conversation with virtual characters, and (3) an automatic feedback loop to control the anxiety of a phobic patient. These contributions are not limited to the psychotherapy domain, but might also be beneficial for application domains that require a level of controlled stress in the form of conversation such as serious gaming or as part of stress test, for example Trier Social Stress Test.

Acknowledgments. This research is supported by the Netherlands Organization for Scientific Research (NWO), grant number 655.010.207. The funders had no role in study design, data collection and analysis, decision to publish, or preparation of the manuscript.

References

1. Kessler, R.C., McGonagle, K.A., Zhao, S., Nelson, C.B., Hughes, M., Eshleman, S., Wittchen, H.-U., Kendler, K.S.: Lifetime and 12-month prevalence of DSM-III-R psychiatric-disorders in the United States - results from the national-comorbidity-survey. Arch. Gen. Psychiatry **51**(1), 8–19 (1994)
2. American Psychiatric Association. Diagnostic and Statistical Manual of Mental Disorders, 4th edn., Text Revision, Washington (2000)
3. Anderson, P.L., Price, M., Edwards, S.M., Obasaju, M.A., Schmertz, S.K., Zimand, E., et al.: Virtual reality exposure therapy for social anxiety disorder: a randomized controlled trial. J. Consult. Clin. Psychol. **81**(5), 751 (2013). doi:10.1037/a0033559
4. Meyerbroker, K., Emmelkamp, P.M.G.: Virtual reality exposure therapy in anxiety disorders: a systematic review of process-and-outcome studies. Depress. Anxiety **27**(10), 933–944 (2010)
5. Gallego, M., Emmelkamp, P.M.G., van der Kooij, M., Mees, H.: The effects of a Dutch version of an internet-based treatment program for fear of public speaking: a controlled study. Int. J. Clin. Health Psychol. **11**, 459–472 (2011)
6. Brinkman, W.P., Hartanto, D., Kang, N., de Vliegher, D., Kampmann, I.L., Morina, N., et al.: A virtual reality dialogue system for the treatment of social phobia. In: CHI 2012 on Human Factors in Computing Systems, pp. 1099–1102 (2012)
7. Emmelkamp, P.M.G.: Behavior therapy with adults. In: Lambert, M.J. (ed.) Bergin and Garfield's Handbook of Psychotherapy and Behavior Change, 6th edn. Wiley, New York (2013)
8. Craske, M.G., Barlow, D.H.: Mastery of your Anxiety and Worry: Client Workbook, 2nd edn. Oxford University Press Inc., New York (2006)
9. Haeffel, G.J.: When self-help is no help: traditional cognitive skills training does not prevent depressive symptoms in people who ruminate. Behav. Res. Ther. **48**(2010), 152–157 (2009)
10. Meyerbroker, K., Emmelkamp, P.M.G.: Therapeutic processes in virtual reality exposure therapy: the role of cognitions and the therapeutic alliance. CyberTherapy Rehabil. **1**, 247–257 (2008)
11. Henkemans, O.A.B., van der Boog, P.J.M., Lindenberg, J., van der Mast, C.A.P.G., Neerincx, M.A., Zwetsloot-Schonkc, B.J.H.M.: An online lifestyle diary with a persuasive computer assistant providing feedback on self-management. Technol. Health Care **17**, 253–267 (2009)
12. Andrade, A.S., McGruder, H.F., Wu, A.W., Celano, S.A., Skolasky, R.L.J., Selnes, O.A., et al.: A programmable prompting device improves adherence to highly active antiretroviral therapy in HIV-infected subjects with memory impairment. Clin. Infect. Dis. **41**(6), 875–882 (2005)
13. Fogg, B.J.: Persuasive Technology: Using Computers to Change What We Think and Do. Morgan Kaufmann Publishers, Amsterdam (2003)
14. Hartanto, D., Brinkman, W.-P., Kampmann, I.L., Morina, N., Emmelkamp, P.G.M., Neerincx, M.A.: Design and implementation of home-based virtual reality exposure therapy system with a virtual eCoach. In: Brinkman, W.-P., Broekens, J., Heylen, D. (eds.) IVA 2015. LNCS, vol. 9238, pp. 287–291. Springer, Heidelberg (2015)

15. Hofmann, S.G., Otto, M.W.: Cognitive Behavioral Therapy for Social Anxiety Disorder: Evidence-Based and Disorder Specific Treatment Techniques. Routledge, New York (2008)
16. Grice, H.P.: Logic and conversation. In: Studies in Syntax and Semantics III: Speech Acts, pp. 183–198. Academic Press, New York (1975)
17. Hartanto, D., Kampmann, I.L., Morina, N., Emmelkamp, P.M.G., Neerincx, M.A., Brinkman, W.-P.: Controlling social stress in virtual reality environments. PLoS ONE **9**(3), e92804 (2014). doi:10.1371/journal.pone.0092804
18. ter Heijden, N., Brinkman, W.-P.: Design and evaluation of a virtual reality exposure therapy system with automatic free speech interaction. J. CyberTherapy Rehabil. **4**(1), 44–55 (2011)
19. Kang, N., Brinkman, W.-P., Riemsdijk, B.M., Neerincx, M.A.: An expressive virtual audience with flexible behavioral styles. IEEE Trans. Affect. Comput. **4**(4), 326–340 (2013)
20. Hartanto, D., Kang, N., Brinkman, W.-P., Kampmann, I.L., Morina, N., Emmelkamp, P.M.G., et al.: Automatic mechanisms for measuring subjective unit of discomfort. Ann. Rev. Cybertherapy Telemedicine 192–197 (2012)
21. Schubert, T., Friedmann, F., Regenbrecht, H.: The experience of presence: factor analytic insights. Presence: Teleoperators Virtual Environ. **10**(3), 266–281 (2001)

Feeling Ghost Food as Real One: Psychometric Assessment of Presence Engagement Exposing to Food in Augmented Reality

Irene Alice Chicchi Giglioli[1(✉)], Alice Chirico[1], Pietro Cipresso[1], Silvia Serino[1], Elisa Pedroli[1], Federica Pallavicini[1], and Giuseppe Riva[1,2]

[1] Applied Technology for Neuro-Psychology Lab, IRCCS Istituto Auxologico Italiano, Milan, Italy
alice.chicchi@gmail.com
[2] Department of Psychology, Università Cattolica del Sacro Cuore, Milan, Italy
giuseppe.riva@unicatt.it

Abstract. In the last decade, the use of technology is considerably increased. A propriety that makes technologies effective tools is to elicit high levels of sense of presence similar to real one experience. Augmented Reality is a new paradigm involving virtual elements in the real world enriching reality with valuables information. This study investigated the flux of the sense of presence and the state anxiety to food stimuli exposure across reality, pictures, and Augmented Reality in twenty-two healthy subjects. The results showed that subjects were clearly able to distinguish the three types of domains, reporting high levels of presence engagement both in reality and Augmented Reality condition. Furthermore, all food stimuli were able to relax subjects, regardless the exposure condition.

In conclusion, our preliminary findings suggest initial evidences of the potential of AR in a variety of experimental and clinical settings, representing a new challenge for the assessment and treatment of psychological disorders.

Keywords: Augmented reality · Sense of presence · Presence engagement · Anxiety · Psychological disorders

1 Introduction

In the last decade, the use of technology for the assessment and treatment of psychological disorders is considerably increased [1–6]. With this regard, Virtual Reality (VR) emerged as an effective tool for the evaluation and treatment of psychological disorders. In details, several studies showed that VR is one of the most used and effective therapeutic tools in the field of anxiety treatment [2–5]. Several researches showed that exposure therapy through VR is effective for reducing and regulating negative affective symptoms, while exposure to emotional situations and prolonged trial result in the regular activation [7]. Therefore, repeated exposure to similar stimuli results in a decrease of psychophysiological activation, reducing the subjects' anxiety and stress.

© Springer International Publishing Switzerland 2016
S. Serino et al. (Eds.): MindCare 2015, CCIS 604, pp. 99–109, 2016.
DOI: 10.1007/978-3-319-32270-4_10

Furthermore, a property that makes VR an effective therapeutic tool is that it is able to elicit high levels of sense of presence. According to Riva [8] presence is the spontaneous (non mediated) awareness of fruitfully turning intentions into actions within an external world. Hence, a high sense of presence in a mediated experience provides a greater realistic perception of the experience and involvement assuring a similar experience to the real one. Indeed, Gorini et al. [9] compared virtual stimuli with the real ones and with pictures for exploring changes in psychophysiological reaction to food in a sample of eating disorder patients and healthy volunteers. The results showed that the virtual and reality foods elicited a similar significant degree of presence. To increase the sense of presence, another technology is proving its potential in the assessment and treatment psychological disorders: Augmented Reality (AR).

AR is a new paradigm involving virtual elements in the real world. The AR concept is that synthetic objects can be add to the real world in real time enriching reality with helpful and relevant information [10, 11]. AR user sees the real world, except that in this real world the virtual objects are placed or superimposed over it forming a part of what the user is seeing with the sensation that the virtual and real objects coexist in the same space without distinguishing the difference between real and virtual objects. In other words, AR allows to add-on "ghost" elements to reality that user can perceive as similar to the real one.

To date, AR systems have been developed for several applications, above all in the field of entertainment [12], maintenance [13], architecture [14], education [15, 16], medicine [17], and cognitive and motor rehabilitation [18–21]. Nevertheless, a very few applications of AR has been developed in the treatment of psychological disorders [22, 23]. In particular, the main AR applications for the psychological disorders' assessment and treatment included the phobia for small animals and acrophobia [24] and among these a few but remarkable studies assessed the degree of presence in an AR system for the treatment of psychological disorder [24–31].

Purposely, Botella et al. [24] and Juan et al. [26], for the first time, evaluated the sense of presence and reality judgment and anxiety experienced in an AR system in patients affected by cockroach and spider phobia. Data showed high level of presence and reality judgment and at the beginning of the exposure the virtual cockroaches were able to arouse anxiety that after one hour of exposure significantly reduced it.

In 2010, Bretón-Lopez et al. [25] assessed the ability of an AR system to rise anxiety and elicit sense of presence and reality judgment in six patients affected by cockroach phobia.

An another study of Juan and Joele [29], using an AR visible marker-based versus an AR invisible marker-based system for the treatment of small animals phobia, assessed the levels of sense of presence and anxiety in twenty-four non-phobic subjects. Data showed that the AR invisible marker-based elicited a higher sense of presence compared to the AR visible marker-based system.

Finally, other AR studies [27, 28, 30, 31], using similar anxiety and sense of presence measures, reported encouraging results in regards to the AR as a promising tool in the treatments of anxiety disorders.

Starting from these premises, and aiming to enlarge the AR applications to other psychological disorders, such as eating disorders, we developed an AR system in order to primarily investigate the fluctuation of the sense of presence across three conditions: (i) reality; (ii) pictures; (iii) AR. Our secondary aim was to explore changes in subject's state anxiety according to the type of medium used to display food stimuli.

2   Methods

2.1   Subjects

The experimental sample included 22 healthy subjects (14 females). The mean age was 42.55 (SD = 12.432), mean body mass index (BMI) was 21.431 (SD = 1.707) (See Table 1). Subjects were randomly recruited from through local advertisements among college students and workers. The inclusion criteria were: no Axis 1 disorders as defined in the Diagnostic and Statistical Manual of Mental Disorders, fourth edition (DSM-IV-TR) [32], age between 18 and 60 years, no history of neurological diseases, psychosis, no headache, or vestibular abnormalities, and no food allergies on intolerances. Moreover, in order to exclude the presence of any psychiatric diseases, such as eating disorders or anxiety disorders, we administered to subjects the Mini International Neuropsychiatric Interview Plus (MINI) [33].

Table 1. Age, weight, height and body mass index (BMI) averages of experimental group

Variable	N	Mean	SD
Age	22	42.55	12.432
Weigh	22	63.41	8.567
Height	22	1.7168	.081
BMI	22	21.432	1.707

Finally, subjects did not receive any compensation for their time and who gave their written informed consent to participate were included in the study.

2.2   Psychological Assessment

Subjects were administered the following questionnaires:

- **State-Trait Anxiety Inventory Form Y-1 (STAI-Y1)** [34]. The STAI-Y is a validated and largely used measure of state and trait anxiety. STAI-Y1 consists of twenty items self-report questionnaire based on a four-point Likert scale, which assesses trait anxiety levels.
- **ITC-Sense of Presence Inventory (ITC-SOPI)** [35]. The ITC-SOPI is a validated questionnaire focusing on users' experiences of virtual reality (and media, in general), which evaluates the degree to which the subject experienced the "sense of being in the virtual environment", how far the virtual environment was the dominant reality, and how far it is recalled as a "place". More specifically, forty-two items, divided in two parts, A (6 items) and B (36 items), composed the ITC-SOPI. Furthermore, the ITC-SOPI provides four subscales, which correspond to the sense of

physical space, engagement, ecological validity, and negative effects. A five-point Likert scale (1 = strongly disagree; 5 = strongly agree) was chosen as the response option for all items.

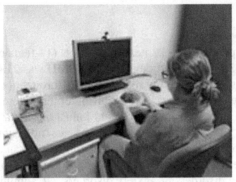

Real Food

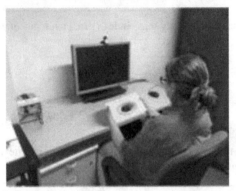

Picture Food

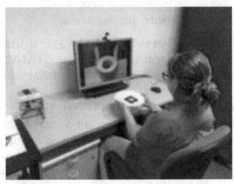

AR Food

Fig. 1. Experimental exposure conditions.

2.3 Food Stimuli

According the nutrition facts (such as total fat and saturated fat), we elected nine foods divided in three categories, as follows:

- Three high salty calorie foods – potato chips, crackers, and salami – with total fats amounting to >20 g/100 g and saturated fats equal to >6,25 g/100 g;
- Three high sweet calorie foods – chocolate, muffins, and cookies – with total fats amounting to >10 g/100 g and saturated fats equal to >5 g/100 g;
- Three low-calorie foods – pears, tomatoes, and carrots – with low total fats amounting to <4 g/100 g and saturated fats equal to <1.25 g/100 g.

The three categories food stimuli were presented to subjects in real, picture, and in AR (Fig. 1).

2.4 Experimental Procedure

All subjects were assigned to the following three exposure conditions:

1. **Real food stimuli:** the nine real foods were presented for 30 s each on a plate in front of the subject. Each stimulus presentation was interspersed with 30 s of pause. During the pause, the foods were hid with red plastics covers so that the subjects could not see them.
2. **Picture food stimuli:** The same nine foods presented in the real condition were presented in picture format. Subjects were asked to watch each food picture for 30 s, followed by 30 s of pause. Pictures were taken by the real food plates and, then, settled with Photoshop software in order to control the brightness and contrast. The picture's sizes were 180×260 mm and were printed, centered horizontally, on A4 paper (210×297 mm).
3. **Augmented Reality stimuli:** In the AR condition subjects were asked to hold a plate marker-based. A camera positioned on the pc display recognized the plate marker-based, projecting each food on the plate for 30 s. Subjects were able to move and turn the plate exploring and observing the foods. The AR setting included the following hardware units: (a) Microsoft's HD LifeCam camera, which offers true HD capture in 720p resolution, able to capture 30 frames per second (Microsoft, Redmond, WA, USA); (b) the marker to decode the AR stimulus; and (c) a portable computer (ACER ASPIRE with Intel® CoreTMi5, graphics processor Nvidia GeForce GT 540M and Bluetooth support).

The order of presentation of each experimental condition, as well as the order of appearance of each food within the different conditions, was counterbalanced for each subject. All subjects were tested at least 2 h after a meal in order to avoid effects related to excessive hunger or overeating. The experiment was composed of three sessions. First, subjects' level of anxiety was assessed using STAI-Y1 [34] questionnaire. Next, subjects were assigned to each of the above-mentioned condition (Real food stimuli; Picture food stimuli; and Augmented Reality stimuli). At the end of each condition, subjects' levels of sense of presence (ITC-SOPI) [35] and anxiety (STAI-Y1) [34] were assessed.

3   Results

This research aimed to investigate the differences (i) in the sense of presence and (ii) in anxiety, in function of the three experimental conditions (Real food stimuli vs. Picture food stimuli vs. Augmented Reality food stimuli).

Hence, Normality test (i.e. Kolmogorov-Smirnov) was carried out to determine if variables were normally distributed. Because this condition was not satisfied, a Wilcoxon test for each of the ITC-SOPI [35] and STAI-Y1 [34] subscales, and regarding each condition (Real food stimuli; Picture food stimuli; and AR food stimuli), was carried out.

Results showed that all food stimuli, regardless the type of medium used (i.e. reality, picture or augmented reality), were able to relax subjects (Baseline vs. Reality: $Z = -2,596$, $p = .009$; Baseline vs. Picture: $Z = -2,509$, $p = .012$; Baseline vs. Augmented Reality: $Z = -2,460$, $p = .014$) (Table 2).

Table 2. Descriptive statistics of STAI scores pre (baseline) and post (reality/picture/augmented reality) food exposure.

Subject	Baseline	Reality	Pictures	Augmented reality
1	33	33	29	34
2	33	28	27	30
3	24	21	23	26
4	24	20	20	20
5	39	32	22	20
6	27	20	20	20
7	32	20	20	20
8	50	41	47	46
9	31	30	31	31
10	40	37	33	32
11	44	48	51	45
12	33	31	28	28
13	21	20	20	20
14	20	20	20	20
15	38	33	34	32
16	20	20	20	20
17	24	22	22	22
18	22	20	22	20
19	30	30	20	20
20	25	31	33	33
21	25	21	21	29
22	31	32	29	27

On the other hand, it is possible to note significant differences regarding the sense of presence, among the three conditions.

In details, the sense of engagement perceived during picture condition was significantly different, compared to other two conditions (Reality vs. Pictures: $Z = -4,075$, $p < .001$; AR vs. Pictures: $Z = -3,880$, $p < .001$). Moreover, subjects experienced a similar level of engagement in the two conditions of reality and augmented reality (Reality: mean = 3.548; SD = .418; Augmented Reality = 3.478; SD = .688). Furthermore, ecological validity in the picture food stimuli condition was significantly higher than that perceived (i) in Real food stimuli condition ($Z = -4.116$, $p < .001$) and (ii) in Augmented reality food stimuli condition ($Z = 2.939$, $p = .003$). No significant difference was found regarding the other two dimensions of ITC-SOPI (i.e. sense of physical safe and negative effect) across the three conditions.

In other words, only food presented in AR condition was able to elicit levels of sense of engagement similar to reality. However subjects were able to clearly recognize that food stimuli displayed in pictures, and by mean of AR were artifacts.

4 Discussion

The aim of this preliminary research was to investigate the phenomenon of presence across three domains: (i) reality; (ii); pictures and (iii) augmented reality. In details, subjects were exposed to food stimuli, which were effectively present, showed in pictures or displayed by an augmented reality system. In addition, we also explored changes in subject's state anxiety according to the type of medium used to display food stimuli. In accordance with the first aim of this study, our data showed that AR food, compared with food presented in pictures, could elicit a sense of presence similar to reality. More interesting, the ITC-SOPI [35] scoring showed similar significant levels of sense of presence on the Engagement subscale both in AR food stimuli presentation and in reality. The sense of engagement in a media experience can be defined as the user's involvement and relevance in the content and the general pleasure of the experience [36–38]. Then, content, attention and involvement are three essential factors that impact on user's engagement evaluation of a media experience. Indeed, the engagement ITC-SOPI [35] subscale includes items relate to how appealing the user found the content and arousal and emotionality, determining the engagement measure both by the media content and the media form variables.

Furthermore, the data of the ITC-SOPI [35] scoring on the Ecological Validity subscale showed that all subjects were able to clearly distinguish the three types of domains.

Regarding our second aim, we found that all food stimuli were able to relax subjects, regardless the type of medium used. According to this result, food stimuli in healthy subjects seem to be able to produce positive psychological pattern for reducing anxiety. Indeed, there is growing evidence on the close interaction between anxiety and emotional eating in order to regulate emotions [39–41]. According to the emotional regulation strategy, the individuals' experiencing anxiety or other emotional states affects their eating behaviour for decreasing an unpleasant or lessening negative feelings

[42]. In general, food can provide some relief from negative emotion or mood states, producing reward, gratification and positive emotions [43, 44].

Despite the clearness of the present findings, this study presented some limitations. First, the small number of subjects makes us careful about the generalization of the results. A future randomized controlled study including a larger sample and a eating disorder patient's sample will address this issue. Second, presence is a subjective condition and the use of retrospective measures as the ITC-SOPI [35] to assess it could not be able to capture the occurrence of the phenomenon of presence in its totality. In order to address this issue, future researchers should focus also on physiological measures (such as the wearable physiological sensors), which can lead to a deeper comprehension of it.

5   Conclusion

In conclusion, this preliminary study showed that, even though subjects were able to clearly distinguish the three types of domains, they reported high levels of sense of presence engagement both in reality and in augmented reality condition, whereas food displayed in pictures elicited a lower sense of presence engagement. On the other hand, all food stimuli were able to relax subjects, regardless the type of medium used.

More generally, the present results provided initial evidences of the potential of AR in a variety of experimental and clinical settings, representing a new challenge for the assessment and treatment of psychological disorders. In particular, according to a therapeutic perspective the use of AR could simplify the arrangement of specific contexts to help patients to cope with their conditions in a very controlled stimulation.

Finally, if this paradigm would be associated to more traditional methods such as biofeedback [45, 46], we could expect a better management of anxiety both in lab environments and real life, helping patients to deal with critical situations.

Acknowledgements. The Authors wish to thanks the Company Regola S.r.l. of Torino – Italy, which programmed the software for augmented reality based on our specific requirements and ideas.

References

1. Côté, S., Bouchard, S.: Virtual reality exposure for phobias: a critical review. J. CyberTherapy Rehabil. **1**, 75–91 (2008)
2. Gorini, A., Riva, G.: The potential of virtual reality as anxiety management tool: a randomized controlled study in a sample of patients affected by generalized anxiety disorder. Trials **9**, 1745–6215 (2008)
3. Parsons, T.D., Rizzo, A.A.: Affective outcomes of virtual reality exposure therapy for anxiety and specific phobias: a meta analysis. J. Behav. Ther. Exp. Psychiatry **39**, 250–261 (2008)
4. Riva, G.: Virtual reality in eating disorders and obesity: state of the art and future directions. Cyberpsychology Behav. **8**, 351 (2005)
5. Riva, G., Bacchetta, M., Baruffi, M., Molinari, E.: Virtual reality-based multidimensional therapy for thetreatment of body image disturbancesin obesity: a controlled study. Cyberpsychology Behav. **4**, 511–526 (2001)

6. Rizzo, A., Buckwalter, J.C., Van der Zaag, C.: Virtual environment applications in clinical neuropsychology. In: Stanney, K.M. (ed.) The Handbook of Virtual Environments, pp. 1027–1064. Erlbaum Publishing, New York (2002)
7. Parsons, T.D., Rizzo, A.A.: Affective outcomes of virtual reality exposure therapy for anxiety and specific phobias: a meta-analysis. J. Behav. Ther. Exp. Psychiatry **39**, 250–261 (2008)
8. Riva, G., Waterworth, J.A., Waterworth, E.L., Mantovani, F.: From intention to action: the role of presence. New Ideas Psychol. **29**, 24–37 (2011)
9. Gorini, A., Griez, E., Petrova, A., Riva, G.: Assessment of the emotional responses produced by exposure to real food, virtual food and photographs of food in patients affected by eating disorders. Ann. Gen. Psychiatry **9**, 30 (2010)
10. Azuma, R., Baillot, Y., Behringer, R., Feiner, S., Julier, S., MacIntyre, B.: Recent advances in augmented reality. IEEE Comput. Graph **21**, 34–47 (2001)
11. Azuma, R.T.: A survey of augmented reality. Presence Teleoperators Virtual Environ. **6**, 355–385 (1997)
12. Özbek, C.S., Giesler, B., Dillmann, R.: Jedi training: playful evaluation of head-mounted augmented reality display systems. In: SPIE Conference Medical Imaging, San Diego, vol. 5291, pp. 454–463 (2004)
13. Schwald, B., Laval, B.: An augmented reality system for training and assistance to maintenance in the industrial context. In: Proceedings of the International Conference in Central Europe on Computer Graphics, Visualization and Computer Vision, pp. 425–432 (Year)
14. Grasset, R., Decoret, X., Gascuel, J.D.: Augmented reality collaborative environment: calibration and interactive science editing. In: VRIC, Virtual Reality International Conference, Laval Virtual 2001 (2001)
15. Arvanitis, T.N., Petrou, A., Knight, J.F., Savas, S., Sotiriou, S., Gargalakos, M., et al.: Human factors and qualities pedagogical evaluation of a mobile augmented reality system for science education used by learners with physical disabilities. Pers. Ubiquit. Comput. **11**, 1–8 (2009)
16. Kerawalla, L., Luckin, R., Seljeflot, S., Woolard, A.: "Making it real": exploring the potential of augmented reality for teaching primary school science. Virtual Reality **10**, 163–174 (2006)
17. De Buck, S., Maes, F., Ector, J., Bogaert, J., Dymarkowski, S., Heidbüchel, H., et al.: An augmented reality system for patient-specific guidance of cardiac catheter ablation procedures. IEEE Trans. Med. Imaging **24**, 1512–1524 (2005)
18. Assis, G.A., Corrêa, A.G., Martins, M.B., Pedrozo, W.G., Lopes, R.D.: An augmented reality system for upper-limb post-stroke motor rehabilitation: a feasibility study. Disabil. Rehabil. Assist. Technol. **4**, 1–8 (2014)
19. Chang, Y.J., Kang, Y.S., Huang, P.C.: An augmented reality (AR)-based vocational task prompting system for people with cognitive impairments. Res. Dev. Disabil. **34**, 3049–3056 (2013)
20. Hervás, R., Bravo, J., Fontecha, J.: An assistive navigation system based on augmented reality and context awareness for people with mild cognitive impairments. IEEE J. Biomed. Health Inform. **18**, 368–374 (2014)
21. Hondori, H.M., Khademi, M., Dodakian, L., Cramer, S.C., Lopes, C.V.: A spatial augmented reality rehab system for post-stroke hand rehabilitation. Stud. Health Technol. Inform. **184**, 279–285 (2013)
22. Baus, O., Bouchard, S.: Moving from virtual reality exposure-based therapy to augmented reality exposure-based therapy: a review. Front. Hum. Neurosci. **8**, 112 (2014)
23. Chicchi Giglioli, I.A., Pallavicini, F., Pedroli, E., Serino, S., Riva, G.: Augmented reality: a brand new challenge for the assessment and treatment of psychological disorders. Comput. Math. Methods Med. (in press)

24. Botella, C., Banos, R., Guerrero, B., Juan, M., Alcañiz, M.: Mixing realities?: an augmented reality system for the treatment of cockroach phobia. CyberPsychology Behav. **8**, 305–306 (2005)

25. Bretón-López, J., Quero, S., Botella, C., García-Palacios, A., Baños, R.M., Alcañiz, M.: An augmented reality system validation for the treatment of cockroach phobia. Cyberpsychol. Behav. Soc. Netw. **13**, 705–710 (2010)

26. Juan, M.C., Alcañiz, M., Botella, C.M., Baños, R.M., Guerrero, B.: Using augmented reality to treat phobias. IEEE Comput. Graph. Appl. **25**, 31–37 (2005)

27. Juan, M.C., Baños, R., Botella, C., Pérez, D., Alcañiz, M., Monserrat, C.: An augmented reality system for acrophobia. the sense of presence using immersive photography. Presence Teleoperators Virtual Environ. **15**, 393–402 (2006)

28. Juan, M.C., Calatrava, J.: An augmented reality system for the treatment of phobia to small animals viewed via an optical see-through HMD. Comparison with a similar system viewed via a video see-through. Int. J. Hum. Comput. Interact. **27**, 436–449 (2011)

29. Juan, M.C., Joele, D.: A comparative study of the sense of presence and anxiety in an invisible marker versus a marker augmented reality system for the treatment of phobia towards small animals. Int. J. Hum. Comput. Studi. **69**, 440–453 (2011)

30. Juan, M.C., Pérez, D.: Using augmented and virtual reality for the development of acrophobic scenarios. Comparison of the levels of presence and anxiety. Comput. Graph. **34**, 756–766 (2010)

31. Wrzesien, M., Alcañiz, M., Botella, C., Burkhardt, J.-M., Bretón-López, J., Ortega, M., et al.: The therapeutic lamp: treating small-animal phobias. IEEE Comput. Graph. Appl. **33**, 80–86 (2013)

32. American Psychiatric Association: Diagnostic and Statistical Manual of Mental Disorders, 4th edn., Text review, Washington, DC (2000)

33. Rossi, A., Alberio, R., Porta, A., Sandri, M., Tansella, M., Amaddeo, F.: The reliability of the MINI-international neuropsychiatric interview - Italian version. J. Clin. Psychopharmacol. **24**, 561–563 (2004)

34. Spielberger, C.D., Gorssuch, R.L., Lushene, P.R., Vagg, P.R., Jacobs, G.A.: Manual for the State-Trait Anxiety Inventory. Consulting Psychologists Press, Palo Alto (1983)

35. Lessiter, J., Freeman, J., Keogh, E., Davidoff, J.D.: A cross-media presence questionnaire: the ITC sense of presence inventory. Presence Teleoperators Virtual Environ. **10**, 282–297 (2001)

36. Barfield, W., Weghorst, S.: The sense of presence within virtual environments: a conceptual framework. Elsevier, Amsterdam (1993)

37. Draper, J.V., Kaber, D.B., Usher, J.M.: Telepresence. Hum. Factors **40**, 354–375 (1998)

38. Witmer, B.G., Singer, M.J.: Measuring presence in virtual environments: a presence questionnaire. Presence Teleoperators Virtual Environ. **7**, 225–240 (1998)

39. Christensen, L.: Effects of eating behavior on mood: a review of the literature. Int. J. Eat. Disord. **14**, 171–183 (1993)

40. Macht, M., Haupt, C., Ellgring, H.: The perceived function of eating is changed during examination stress: a field study. Eat. Behav. **6**, 109–112 (2005)

41. Macht, M., Simons, G.: Emotions and eating in everyday life. Appetite **31**, 65–71 (2000)

42. Macht, M.: How emotions affect eating: a five-way model. Appetite **50**, 1–11 (2008)

43. Gibson, E.L.: Emotional influences on food choice. Sensory, physiological and psychological pathways. Physiol. Behav. **89**, 53–61 (2006)

44. Kelley, A.E.: Ventral striatal control of appetitive motivation: role in ingestive behavior and reward-related learning. Neurosci. Biobehav. Rev. **27**, 765–776 (2004)

45. Meule, A., Freund, R., Skirde, A.K., Vogele, C., Kubler, A.: Heart rate variability biofeedback reduces food cravings in high food cravers. Appl. Psychophysiol. Biofeedback **37**, 241–251 (2012)
46. Teufel, M., Stephan, K., Kowalski, A., Kasberger, S., Enck, P., Zipfel, S., Giel, K.E.: Impact of biofeedback on self-efficacy and stress reduction in obesity: a randomized controlled pilot study. Appl. Psychophysiol. Biofeedback **38**, 177–184 (2013)

Embodied Space in Natural and Virtual Environments: Implications for Cognitive Neuroscience Research

Francesca Morganti[✉]

Department of Human and Social Sciences, University of Bergamo, Bergamo, Italy
francesca.morganti@unibg.it

Abstract. In the last decades, virtual reality environments are largely used in cognitive neuroscience research in order to provide participants with the possibility to navigate a space while brain activity is scanned through neuroimaging techniques such as MRI and similar. Accordingly in the field of spatial cognition research, several publications strongly assume the equivalence between exploring a not simulated and a computer-simulated environment. Albeit considering, since its first introduction in cognitive research, virtual reality simulation as an interesting possibility to study spatial knowledge organization, in the present paper I would like to address an "unrevealed question": is it reasonable to obtain the same conclusions about spatial cognition from classical neuropsychological tests and virtual reality simulations? Or are there any differences for spatial knowledge acquisition provided from the simulations' characteristics that we have to strongly consider? The main aim of this contribution is to find a possible answer to this question by introducing an embodied cognition approach to the study of wayfinding.

Keywords: Embodied cognition · Spatial orientation · Virtual reality · Enactivism

1 How the Body Contributes to Knowledge

Perceptual information, relevant to the regulation of intentional movements (that includes bodily-centered spatial patterns), changes in ways that are lawfully related to the properties of the environment and the action itself [1]. Thus, it could appear misleading to conceptualize perception and action as pure independent processes. Instead it is more parsimonious to view these two processes as opposite poles of a functional unit or action system. Moreover, the mirror neuron research developed in the last decade underlines a strong linkage between perception and action. Accordingly all the research in the field of intentional action appears to require a reshaping of the concept of "interaction".

A good description of this shift of perspective in considering interaction as situated in a specific context can be found in studies on embodied cognition [2]. Within embodied cognition, the body becomes an interface between the mind and the world allowing thought and the specific surrounding space to merge. The sensorimotor coupling of the organisms and the environment in which they live determines recurrent patterns of

© Springer International Publishing Switzerland 2016
S. Serino et al. (Eds.): MindCare 2015, CCIS 604, pp. 110–119, 2016.
DOI: 10.1007/978-3-319-32270-4_11

perception and action that allow enactive knowledge [3]. Before the enactive perspective, within the ecological psychology approach, Gibson [4] originally suggested, that an individual perceives the world not in terms of objective and abstract features but directly in terms of spaces of possible actions, or "affordances". He introduces the notion of "invariants of the physical world" to mean that during an action an agent expects that the environment will react in agreement with the basic relational laws of the body/environment interaction. In analogy with the enactive approach, the theory of affordance introduces the idea of perception-action coupling. This coupling depends on the encounter of the characteristics of the two poles of the interaction (the body and the environment) and is shaped by the overarching activity in which the agent is involved. Every human action, in fact, has to include both proprioceptive information from the agent's own body (muscles, joints, organs of balance, and so on) while it equally includes information from the "external" world (variations in the patterns of visual perception, sounds, and so on). Accordingly, in the enactive perspective, the agent's management of an action depends on the creation, on the maintenance and on the moment-by-moment reactivation of sensorimotor schemes. These schemes "guide" the agent in how to appropriately execute her movements in the specific situation in which she finds herself and what sorts of feedback to expect from the environment [5].

2 Embodied Space

Contrariwise to this research trend, the classical approach to the study of spatial cognition appears to be still mainly based on a distinctive body/environment centred approach avoiding considering humans as autonomous agents that actively generate and maintain their own coherent and meaningful patterns of activity during interaction. Instead the embodied approach on interaction has some specific implications for spatial cognition research. Orientation, in fact, is a high level cognitive ability that comprises the construction and use of a spatial representation of the context within which an action is performed. To be effective this construction requires incoming information from multiple modalities, the time by time location of the navigator, as well as the actions planning that have to be aligned and integrated with them [6]. In a more enactive sense by using affordances during an environment navigation an agent is able to construct spatial knowledge by using egocentred route maps based on regions or zones with abstract borders and landmarks and, at the same time, to localize himself by contemplating allocentred survey maps based on high-level path integration. For an explorer, in fact, the surrounding space is composed of all the affordances that are available at each moment, and his embodied representation contributes in determining what environmental dynamics are currently the most relevant, among the several available at each moment. A wayfinding may therefore be conceived of as a complex and continuously changing balance between the information available both in route and survey perspective. A recent study from Brunyé and colleagues [7] showed how the route/survey perspective flexibility could support path planning between distant origin and goal landmarks. Both route and survey perspectives are considered as a "commonplace" that allow a continuous switch and that involves translating a current ground-level egocentric perspective to a survey-based allocentric representation of environmental layout during active navigation in complex spaces. The evidence of such perspective switches suggests that they are a routine and necessary process to support successful navigation [8, 9].

Since a representation is, by definition, someone's subjective point of view, it might be argued that survey maps, even if they have a "from the above" perspective, can only be egocentric. Instead, if we consider exploration as a perception-action coupling survey maps have to be considered as allocentric representation that allow an agent to draw spatial inferences while he/she is engaged in an egocentric exploration. Survey maps, in fact, result from the pretence to be dislocated in a different position (e.g. one kilometre above the city) and watching the world from that perspective [10]. This allows to draw spatial inferences and therefore to plan in advance a path in a known as well as in a partially unknown region. Within the enactive perspective, in this case spatial plans are not allocentric representation for action sequences to be followed blindly, but they become also egocentric guides for action to be further specified in the affordance-based interaction with the environment.

Recent neuroscience studies support this allocentric/egocentric balance for spatial cognition [11], underlining the role of the retrosplenial cortex in the combination of the allocentric information (provided by the Papez circuit) with the egocentric spatial input derived from parietal areas. These data suggest that the spatial orientation is inseparable from the embodied perspective and from the specific action (affordance) performed in the surrounding environment. As stated by Gunzelmann [12], establishing correspondence between an egocentric perspective and an allocentric representation of space (such as a map) is the fundamental process assessed by orientation tasks, and we assume this process can be deeply understood by using the notion of sensorimotor coupling of the agent and its environment, as defined by enactive cognition approach.

3   Navigating the Real, Navigating the Virtual

The coupling between the egocentric embodied perception and the situated action that underlies spatial orientation is quite easy to understand when an agent is placed in a natural place, such as her house or a city square. However, this link is more difficult to understand when the agent is provided with a simulated space or when she is placed in a computer-based 3D simulation, such as virtual environments. Despite this, in the last decade, due to the progression of technology, together with paper and pencil simulation of environments (such as building plans, city maps, and so on), virtual reality simulations were widely used in neuroscience and experimental psychology to study spatial cognition [13].

In the present contribution the starting assumption is that the experiential differences between the navigation of a simulated environment and the navigation of an environment that is not simulated might have influence spatial cognition. As stated by Mellet-d'Huart [14], in fact, adopting the enactive perspective to virtual reality interaction requires reconsidering what the characteristics of the coupling between an agent and its environment are. It implies to deeply define the link that will involve reciprocal modifications between them, and to clarify the conditions for reciprocal changes. Even in a virtual reality environment, in fact, we are able to interact by choosing appropriate affordances according to our embodied perception of such environment. Moreover we gain information from this peculiar sensorimotor coupling in order to support us in creating representations of the world in terms of body-environment invariants.

Thus, according to the enactive perspective this contribution would like to speculate how this coupling can differ within two different space simulations. Meanwhile, as they are both widely used in assessing spatial cognition in clinical neuropsychology, the question remains open on how the spatial orientation obtainable from a virtual reality simulated environment (that provides the agent with an egocentric perspective) might differ from the spatial orientation obtainable from a simulation of the same environment based on a paper and pencil representation (e.g. on a sketched map) that provides the agent with an allocentric perspective. In the first type of simulation, in fact, an agent has an egocentric perspective on the environment and is able to move within it. In the second type of simulation, an agent has an allocentric perspective on the environment that requires a mental imagery effort to be translated in action. As depicted above, from literature, it could be possible to assume that both perspectives are essential for spatial orientation in a complex environment and need to be further investigated.

Accordingly, I would like to use as example the comparison between the classical paper version of the Money's Road Map test (M-RMT – [15]) and a virtual reality version of the Road Map test (VR-RMT – [16]). The M-RMT is largely used in neuropsychology for the assessment of spatial orientation ability. The M-RMT requires a mental imagery right/left turning to explore a stylized city provided to the subject in a survey perspective. The VR-MRT is a 3D version of the same environment in which participants can navigate by actively choosing right/left directions in a route perspective.

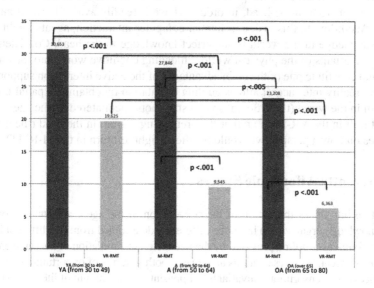

Fig. 1. Mean values and significant differences (T- test) between performances at the M-RMT and VR-RMT for age groups (Young Adults – YA; Adults – A; Old Adults OA).

In a recent research conducted with 61 healthy subjects from 30 to 80 years old (Mean age = 56.82; sd = 15.47) both the classical version of the Money's Road Map test (M-RMT) and a virtual reality version of the same test (VR-RMT) were randomly proposed. Results showed a significant difference (p < .001) for the factor Environment (M-RMT vs VR-RMT). Participants better performed the spatial task in the M-RMT (Mean = 27.10; sd = 4.6) than in the VR-MRT (Mean = 11.34; sd = 8.08). Moreover there is a significant difference in the interaction between Environment factor and age (p < .001) as depicted in Fig. 1.

By comparing the M-RMT and the VR-RMT, from these data, it was possible to understand the difference between imaging a right/left turn on a body axis (as in the M-RMT) and performing it (as in the VR-RMT). According to the embodied cognition approach, there is a difference in imaging a turn, as in the M-RMT, and performing a turn in order to obtain a spatial perspective from the simulated world. In particular in the M-RMT, an agent first look at the map, then imagine how to move on the body axis and finally obtain (and have to keep in mind) the spatial perspective derived from the turn. In the VR-RMT condition, an agent first look at the map, then physically turn on the body axis and finally perceive in the simulated world the spatial perspective derived from that turn.

These two different spatial tasks, as they provide different embodied affordances, might result in different orientation outcomes. Specifically, these differences, due to the peculiar sensorimotor coupling they provide, will be evidenced by the type of turns made by participants and the increasing complexity in their right/left turns. Moreover, the VR-MRT, by providing an external representation of the route perspective, might support perspective taking and provide better performances in spatial orientation than the M-RMT.

From the work of Gray and Fu [17], we know that, when a computer-based interface is well designed, it supports the possibility of placing knowledge in-the-world instead of retrieving it from-in-the-head, in order to have it readily available when an agent needs it. According to this vision of human-computer interaction, agents might prefer perfect knowledge in the world to imperfect knowledge in the head. Consistent with Gibson's invariants of the physical world, offloading cognitive work onto the environment could constitute one of the main advantages of the active interaction supported by the virtual reality interface: it allows guiding orientation by obtaining spatial perspectives from in the world (the different spatial snapshots encountered by the agent after a right/left turn in the VR-RMT) rather than retrieving it from in the head (the different inferences on how a perspective would be after a right/left turn in the M-RMT).

4 Differently Affordable Spaces

As enaction introduces the notion of the coevolution of the agent and its environment, spatial knowledge organization has to be differently determined from the different kind of body-environment coupling provided by the two different simulation of the same environment. This is because representations are created both in terms of opportunities for action (affordances) and sensorimotor invariants. At present a large amount of literature supports the idea that the spatial orientation in virtual reality simulation is comparable to the spatial orientation derived from direct navigation in real environments due to the "sense of presence" experienced in it [5, 18]. Nevertheless, navigating a virtual space appears to be more complex than navigating other kind of simulated space. Moreover, this difficulty seems to be directly correlated with the environment complexity. Why?

A first possible interpretation is related to the nature of the tasks. In virtual environments agents generally tried to use not simulated info to guide their movements in the virtual world and it may constitute a cognitive overload, in which subjects first processed and reached a decision about the turn using the information provided by the natural surrounding spaces and then translated this to a turn on the computerized environment. If this is true, the performing of the VR-MRT have to require both an attention switch between the environment and the screen and a reference frame switch between the allocentric perspective of the surrounding environment and the egocentric perspective of the virtual environment. However, as Schultz [19] indicated the M-RMT is solved primarily by imagining egocentric spatial transformations. Thus, in the VR-MRT, agents can reach a decision about the turn directly in front of the screen by acting the turn they considered appropriate in order to reach the subsequent turn point. In this view, the main difference between the two versions of the environments is in the imagined/perceived perspective taking. In the M-RMT, agents imagine how to move on the body axis and finally obtain (and retain) the spatial perspective derived from the turn, whereas in the VR-RMT they act the turn on the body axis and finally perceive in the simulated world the spatial perspective derived from that turn. Therefore, keeping track of each position does not require an additional cognitive effort.

Thus, independently from egocentric/allocentric strategy used, a virtual reality simulation might be more complex to perform wayfinding than a paper and pencil one. A possible explanation of this may be related to the difference between simulation and action: rotating the body on its vertical axis towards the point of reference in virtual reality is more difficult than rotating the body in a mental space. As pointed out by Tversky [20], our own body is experienced from inside, and the space around our body does not depend on the physical situation *per se*. There is also dissociation between perspective taking and mental rotation. Perspective taking involves imagining the results of changing one's egocentric frame of reference with respect to the environment. Mental rotation involves imagining the results of changing the positions of objects in the environment, while maintaining one's current orientation in the environment.

According to the pioneering research made by Hintzman and colleagues [21] we know that spatial representation mainly consists of orientation-specific perspectives, and of relational propositions. Kozhevnikov and Hegarty [22] stated that the dominant strategy used in solving items that involve a perspective change of more than 90° on a perspective-taking test was to imagine oneself reoriented with respect to the scene. For both paper and pencil and virtual simulations, following the chosen path requires agents to cognitively anticipate themselves in a particular place with a specific orientation. Under normal conditions, an agent turns on the gravitational axis while the environment remains fixed. Apparently, this embodied rotation ability created an expectation/simulation of spatial movement (defined by Gibson's affordance theory as "invariants of the physical world") that was more helpful when updating a mental world than a virtual one.

Coherently with Keehner and colleagues [23], in virtual reality agents must match the perspective that the virtual scenario is providing them to their right/left turn intentions in order to match the obtained perspective with the results of each turn, and this matching has to be tightly coupled with internal cognitive processes. The option to offload cognition onto the external visualization provided by VR-RMT (by observing the perspective resulting from a right/left turn) seems to require more effort than to base it on the embodied imaginative process (as in the M-RMT). This interpretation is consistent with the perspective proposed by Di Paolo [24] on the necessity to have an indistinguishable dialectic mechanism of monitoring and regulation poles that supports the creation of a meaning from the perspective of the organism. Accordingly here I would like to suggest that in virtual reality simulations, by perceptually offloading the turn response on the virtual scenario without involving the entire embodied information, an agent might create a meaningless experience during the environment navigation. And this failure of the sensorimotor coupling can become quite useless for spatial orientation.

Moreover, it is also necessary to consider that during the navigation of a virtual environment, any turn error causes a discrepancy between the agent's expected and actual position in the space, which might create a difficulty in subsequent turns. Thus, an error after a wrong turn in the VR-RMT could affect the results more than in the M-RMT.

5   Implications for Neuroscience Research

At present a large amount of research data are consistent with the evidence that the variability between agents involved in spatial tasks is higher in virtual than in natural spaces. By comparing exploration in natural and virtual environments, studies have concluded, in fact, that most of the abilities involved in learning in a natural world, are also needed for learning in a virtual world, but the latter presents additional demands. Consequently, the need to create an evaluation tool specific for virtual environment application is deeply felt in order to get reliable data. There is a difference between the body-environment coupling in natural and virtual environments, in fact, that can influence spatial orientation task. This difference can be partially attributed to the participant's sensation of "being there" in a simulated environment rather than in a natural one. Accordingly, in virtual reality, individuals can experience atypical patterns of sensorimotor coupling that might influence their ability to catch appropriate affordances for action in space.

In addiction it is a large shared opinion that VR interfaces can suffer from severe usability problems that can provide disorientation and inability to manipulate parts of the virtual environment and accordingly there is a need for better-designed VR systems that support perception, navigation and exploration. Up to now, in fact, VR developers don't have a coherent approach especially to interaction design, and lacked understanding of usability concepts underlying VR did not use conventional Human Computer Interaction methods or guidelines. This point could constitute one of the main issue in neuropsychology assessment because the underestimation of the cognitive efforts required from the introduction of a low level usability interface in a VR-based neuropsychological test can guide clinicians toward a misleading patient's performance evaluation and diagnostic conclusions. Accordingly, before introducing VR assessment tools in clinical research and practice, a correct usability approach have to be introduced in order to identify breakdowns and problems in interaction that can influence the cognitive performance and to provide little guidance towards a solution. Therefore, before to use in clinical assessment, there is a need to support the process of usability evaluation that addresses the new problem posed by the use of VR in a not digital native population (such as the aged one) and in particular in a cognitively impaired population (such as the neurological one) as well as linking identification of these peculiar issues to interface design guidelines.

Finally, in a more recent paper Thompson stated that cognition is a form of embodied action where cognitive processes emerge from recurrent sensorimotor patterns of perception and action [25]. This coupling between organism and environment modulates the formation of a not pre-specified and external realm but of a relational domain. Thus an agent's world is not represented internally by its brain but from the agency and the mode of coupling with the environment. This indicates that the challenge of introducing virtual reality systems in cognitive assessment is not purely technological, but also epistemic. When it comes to spatial cognition assessment, for example, beyond the contribution of technology, what ultimately matters for appropriate design of a virtual simulation is the understanding of the enaction stance that acknowledges that orientation comes from egocentric and allocentric sensorimotor invariance. Adopting this perspective means to shed a new light on this revealing how this invariance can be different from an internally and externally offloaded information, as in the classical and virtual version of the same neuropsychological test.

Hence, enaction is a good way to examine virtual reality as something more than purely a technical challenge. But how can a virtual environment be more than just a digital place that provides perceptive simulation and digital affordances for action? If an agent in a virtual simulation will be able to find spatial invariants, and progressively evolve them through the dynamics of the sensory-motor coupling, in this way he constructs a world, understands it, and feels present in it. In conclusion it is possible to state that, according to a more recent adaptive approach to enactivism [24, 26] the introduction on virtual reality in cognitive science research have to take into account how this kind of simulation more than being "realistic" has to technically support the agents' possibility to potentially distinguish the moment-by-moment different paths of encounters with the environment. Moreover, virtual reality introduces several different possibilities of sensorimotor coupling for knowledge acquisition. These are defined by the different environment simulations possibilities derived, for example, from immersive virtual reality or augmented reality systems, that can provide agents with peculiar affordances for action and different feedback information. Accordingly, in an enactive approach every one of these should be tested in order to highlights how they could provide different results for spatial cognition.

In conclusion, the integration of virtual reality with traditional evaluation methods for spatial cognition assessment may provide an interesting alternative to paper and pencil-based approaches but should be used with caution. Virtual simulations do not include the same embodied spatial information used when performing navigation in other types of environments. But it remains a great challenge for enaction research as stated by Varela [27] after his first experience with this kind of technology.

Acknowledgments. FM was funded by Department of Human and Social Sciences - MIUR grant 2014 "Embodiment, Mirroring e Intersoggettività: Implicazioni per l'apprendimento e la riabilitazione neuropsicologica".

References

1. Jeannerod, M.: The representing brain: neural correlates of motor intention and imagery. Behav. Brain Sci. **17**, 187–202 (1994)
2. Varela, F.J., Thompson, E., Rosch, E.: The embodied mind: cognitive science and human experience. MIT Press, Cambridge (1991)
3. Thompson, E., Varela, F.J.: Radical embodiment: neural dynamics and consciousness. Trends Cogn. Sci. **5**, 418–425 (2001)
4. Gibson, J.J.: The Ecological Approach to Visual Perception. Houghton Mifflin, Boston (1979)
5. Carassa, A., Morganti, F., Tirassa, M.: A situated cognition perspective on presence. In: Bara, B., Barsalou, L.W., Bucciarelli, M. (eds.) XXVII Annual Conference of the Cognitive Science Society, pp. 384–389. Sheridan Printing, Alpha, NJ (2005)
6. Gramann, K., Muller, H.J., Eick, E., Schonebeck, B.: Evidence of separable spatial representations in a virtual navigation task. J. Exp. Psychol. Hum. Percept. Perform. **31**, 1199–1223 (2005)
7. Brunyé, T.T., Gardony, A., Mahoney, C.R., Taylor, H.A.: Going to town: visualized perspectives and navigation through virtual environments. Comput. Hum. Behav. **28**, 257–266 (2012)
8. Ishikawa, T., Montello, D.R.: Spatial knowledge acquisition from direct experience in the environment: individual differences in the development of metric knowledge and the integration of separately learned places. Cogn. Psychol. **52**(2), 93–129 (2006)
9. Hartley, T., Maguire, E.A., Spiers, H.J., Burgess, N.: The well-worn route and the path less traveled: distinct neural bases of route following and wayfinding in humans. Neuron **37**, 877–888 (2003)
10. Tirassa, M., Carassa, A., Geminiani, G.: A theoretical framework for the study of spatial cognition. In: Ó Nualláin, S. (ed.) Spatial Cognition Foundations and Applications, pp. 19–31. Benjamins, Amsterdam (2000)
11. Serino, S., Cipresso, P., Morganti, F., Riva, G.: The role of egocentric and allocentric abilities in Alzheimer's disease: a systematic review. Ageing Res. Rev. **16**, 32–44 (2014)
12. Gunzelmann, G.: Strategy generalization across orientation tasks: testing a computational cognitive model. Cogn. Sci. **32**, 835–861 (2008)
13. Morganti, F.: Virtual interaction in cognitive neuropsychology. Stud. Health Technol. Inf. **99**, 55–70 (2004)
14. Mellet-d'Huart, D.: A model of (en) action to approach embodiment: a cornerstone for the design of virtual environment for learning. Virtual Reality **10**, 253–269 (2006)
15. Money, J., Alexander, D., Walker, H.T.: A Standardized Road Map Test of Direction Sense. Johns Hopkins Press, Baltimore (1967)
16. Morganti, F., Marrakchi, S., Urban, P.P., Iannoccari, G.A., Riva, G.: A virtual reality based tools for the assessment of "survey to route" spatial organization ability in elderly population: preliminary data. Cogn. Process. **10**, 257–259 (2009)

17. Gray, W.D., Fu, W.T.: Soft constraints in interactive behavior: the case of ignoring perfect knowledge in-the-world for imperfect knowledge in-the-head. Cogn. Sci. **28**, 359–382 (2004)
18. Riva, G., Waterworth, J.A., Waterworth, E.L., Mantovani, F.: From intention to action: the role of presence. New Ideas Psychol. **29**, 24–37 (2011)
19. Schultz, K.: The contribution of solution strategy to spatial performance. Can. J. Psychol. **45**, 474–491 (1991)
20. Tversky, B.: Spatial cognition: embodied and situated. In: Robbins, P., Aydede, M. (eds.) The Cambridge Handbook of Situated Cognition, pp. 201–216. Cambridge University Press, New York (2008)
21. Hintzman, D.L., O'Dell, C.S., Arndt, D.R.: Orientation in cognitive maps. Cogn. Psychol. **13**, 149–206 (1981)
22. Kozhevnikov, M., Hegarty, M.: A dissociation between object-manipulation spatial ability and spatial orientation ability. Mem. Cogn. **29**, 745–756 (2001)
23. Keehner, M., Hegarty, M., Cohen, C.A., Khooshabeh, P., Montello, D.R.: Spatial reasoning with external visualizations: what matters is what you see, not whether you interact. Cogn. Sci. **32**, 1099–1132 (2008)
24. Di Paolo, E.A.: Autopoiesis, adaptivity, teleology, agency. Phenomenol. Cogn. Sci. **4**, 429–452 (2005)
25. Thompson, E.: Sensorimotor subjectivity and the enactive approach to experience. Phenomenol. Cogn. Sci. **4**, 407–427 (2005)
26. Di Paolo, E.A.: Extended life. Topoi **1**, 9–21 (2009)
27. Varela, F.J.: Il corpo come macchina ontologica. In: Ceruti, M., Preta, F. (eds.) Che cos'è la conoscenza, pp. 43–53. Laterza, Bari (1990)

Virtual Reality Enhanced Biofeedback: Preliminary Results of a Short Protocol

Luca Morganti[✉] and Michele Cucchi

Centro Medico Santagostino, Piazza Sant'Agostino 1, 20100 Milan, Italy
luca.morganti@cmsantagostino.it

Abstract. Technology allows innovative ways to perform biofeedback: virtual reality is a promising tool to improve the sense of involvement in the activity reducing the gap between the subject and the kind of feedback given. In this manuscript we report the efficacy of 4-session short protocol of virtual reality enhanced biofeedback with patients suffering from physical symptoms related to clinical conditions marked out by high arousal, i.e. anxiety disorders and hypertension. Preliminary results suggest that biofeedback reduces both state anxiety and anxiety sensitivity. Future research should compare the short protocol with other biofeedback intervention, both virtual and traditional ones.

Keywords: Biofeedback · Virtual reality · Anxiety · Hypertension

1 Introduction

Biofeedback is a mind-body technique in which individuals gain information regarding a physiological function in order to improve the perception of control over it (Frank et al. 2010). The learning process driven by biofeedback enhances the ability to manage personal arousal helping the subject increasing the awareness about his/her physiological patterns and developing new possible ways of self-regulation.

Biofeedback has proven efficacy in many clinical conditions: specific parameters and protocols have been identified to treat different medical symptoms (Wheat and Larkin 2010). The applications of biofeedback range from clinical rehabilitation (Patla and Marteniuk 2013) to positive psychology (Serino et al. 2013) because it helps the subject improving the knowledge about specific body functions. Biofeedback can be used to improve both subject's perception of muscles' activity, for example in the rehab of a specific limb after injuries or as a consequence of a stroke, and the perception of physiological parameters, such as breath pattern or heart rate. So, the technique can be applied in contexts where the goal is to improve the efficacy of the selected biological target or skills (Beauchamp et al. 2012), both when the main cause of subjective pain is an intense psychological arousal and when it is linked to a bodily pain.

1.1 Virtual Reality

The technique of virtual reality biofeedback was firstly developed by Budzynski (1995) and clinical trials are increasing over years. It differs from common biofeedback because

© Springer International Publishing Switzerland 2016
S. Serino et al. (Eds.): MindCare 2015, CCIS 604, pp. 120–127, 2016.
DOI: 10.1007/978-3-319-32270-4_12

of the type of technological feedback shown to the user: instead of the rough pattern of the physiological signal, he/she looks at a virtual reality environment where an object is placed whose size varies according to the biological signal detected in real-time. The subject is absorbed into the virtual environment experienced through a monitor with joystick or specific glasses, enhancing the presence of the subject in the environment (Ijsselsteijn and Riva 2003). The application of virtual reality on biofeedback is promising because traditional biofeedback simply gives to patients very simple audio or video feedback information from a computer that processes their physiological data. The use of virtual environments has proven its efficacy as an affective medium so it can be used as an added value to show to the patient. The interaction with relaxing environments produces relaxation and an enhanced stronger feeling of presence in the environment allows a stronger effect on the emotional state of the patient (Riva et al. 2007).

1.2 Clinical Applications

Virtual reality is widely used for the treatment of anxiety disorders (Wiederhold and Wiederhold 2005; Gorini et al. 2010). Its efficacy for the treatment of anxiety (Repetto et al. 2013) is to get the patient in touch with the phobic situation and/or the related physiological arousal. Biofeedback has been included in virtual reality enhanced protocols (Pallavicini et al. 2009; Repetto et al. 2009), for example to help the management of psychological stress (Gaggioli et al. 2014). The efficacy of biofeedback on anxiety states has been also demonstrated among healthy subjects (Wells et al. 2012). The use of virtual reality to enhance biofeedback for the treatment of anxiety is effective, because this psychological condition may also increase the feeling of presence in virtual reality (Bouchard et al. 2008).

As regards hypertension, it has been demonstrated that devices slowing and regularizing breathing is efficacious in reducing high BP (Blood Pressure) during 2 months of self-treatment. The change in breathing pattern appears to be an important component in this reduction (Schein et al. 2001). In a review by Yucha et al. (2001), biofeedback and other active control techniques resulted in a reduction in systolic blood pressure (SBP) and diastolic blood pressure (DBP), but only biofeedback showed a significantly greater reduction in both SBP (6.7 mm Hg) and DBP (4.8 mm Hg) when compared with inactive control treatments. Nakao et al. (2003) found biofeedback to be effective in reducing blood pressure in patients with essential hypertension, being superior to sham or non-specific behavioral intervention.

More recently, Palomba et al. (2011) demonstrated that a short biofeedback training, including guided imagery of stressful events, was effective in reducing BP reactions to a psychosocial stressor: Heart rate biofeedback appears to be a suitable intervention for hypertensive patients, mostly when blood pressure increase is associated with emotional activation. A specific analysis (Yucha et al. 2005) about the kind of patients who seem to be more suitable for biofeedback identified through a regression: (1) subjects who were able to lower their systolic blood pressure 5 mmHg or more were not taking anti-hypertensive medication, (2) subjects with smallest standard deviation in daytime mean arterial pressure and (3) subjects with a low internal health locus of control.

The aim of our investigation was to evaluate the efficacy of a enhanced virtual reality biofeedback short protocol in the management of clinical disorders related to higher arousal, i.e. anxiety disorders, especially with panic attacks, and hypertension.

2   Methods

Participants. Twenty-one patients of the clinic were selected to start the biofeedback training, after having received this specific clinical suggestion by other clinician. Six of them stopped it before the end of the treatment: the reasons were fear of the Bluetooth technology and its possible effects on personal health (one person), no interest in the suggested activity if compared to pharmacological treatment (one person) and no benefits gained after the first two session (four people). A patient asking biofeedback was stopped after two meetings because his clinic situations suggested to interrupt it to focus on his general psychological issues. Further, three of them did not fill the questionnaires so they are not included in our sample.

The mean age of the final sample (N = 11) was 46.73 (SD = 11.92). The biofeedback training was suggested to them by various specialists as reported in the table below (Table 1).

Table 1. Composition of the sample

Participant	Age	Gender	Sender	
1	59	F	Cardiologist	Support to pharmacotherapy
2	27	F	Psychologist	Manage anxiety
3	51	F	Psychologist	Way to slow down daily routine
4	38	F	Psychologist	Support to face an exam
5	45	F	Neurologist	Migraine
6	58	M	Family physician	Hypochondriac symptoms
7	60	F	Psychologist	Symptoms of social phobia
8	50	M	Autonomous	Extrasystole
9	49	F	Psychologist	Nervous tics
10	36	M	Psychiatrist	Panic attacks
11	33	F	Psychologist	Manage anxiety

Using virtual biofeedback as a possible clinical intervention for different clinical conditions allowed us to think also about the role that this technique can have in a medical clinic. Even when the initial request of the patient is not about the use of this technique, biofeedback could be considered as a resource for the treatment of various symptoms. After being sent to the biofeedback specialist, all the patients attended a preliminary psychological session to be sure that the biofeedback intervention could be recommended for their clinical situation: subjects needing a deeper psychological intervention were excluded from the training. It was also possible to start both the biofeedback training and a simultaneous psychological treatment: this happened only to patient 4.

Patient 8 decided to start a psychological treatment after the biofeedback short protocol in order to investigate the type of different situations that forced her to a high arousal.

Procedure. The first meeting starts with a deep explanation of the technique both from a theoretical and a practical perspective. Our biofeedback short protocol focuses on two biological parameter (breathing frequency and heart rate): each session will involve one of the two parameters, which will be shown to the patient via a virtual reality scenario consisting of a wood with a fire in the middle of it. The size of the flame depends on the parameter: the higher it is, the bigger the flame will be on the screen. The short protocol consists in two biofeedback sessions on breathing frequency and two following sessions on heart rate. The preliminary meeting ends with the assessment of personal breathing pattern through a Thought Technology Pacer: the patient is asked to try to perform a relaxed breath and then to start practicing it during the week before the first biofeedback session. The specific personal parameters gathered via the Pacer are sent via mail together with the questionnaires to be filled via a online form. All the participants filled the same set of questionnaires again after 4 biofeedback sessions. A basic plan is hypothesized to focus on breath frequency for session 1 and 2, moving then on heart rate for sessions 3 and 4. This schema helps patients to start managing their own breathing before paying attention to the heart rate and the ways to slow it down: this structure allows the patient to be guided to a deep relaxation state by enhancing personal ways to manage the physiological arousal. It is possible to have slight variations on this plan, such as working for 1 or 2 more sessions on breath frequency: if a patient is not accustomed to manage the breathing, it is beneficial to continue focusing on it.

During the first breathing biofeedback session, the patient is given a Zephyr belt (BioHarness 3) connected via Bluetooth to a Samsung Ultra 5 laptop running NeuroVR as a software to play virtual reality scenario (Riva et al. 2011); a joystick was available if the patient need to get closer to the fire or to change the point of view. The whole workstation can be easily transferred from a room to another.

The patient is told to try to decrease the size of the virtual fire, only by knowing that working on the breath pattern is the key to change it. The second biofeedback sessions starts with a small training about specific issues related to relaxed breathing, i.e. paying attention to the length of the exhalation phase, keep care about hold-in and hold-out phase and trying to use the diaphragm during the whole process.

If no further sessions are needed to let the patient see noticeable feedbacks about the physiological arousal related to breathing, sessions 3 and 4 are performed by setting heart rate as physiological parameter for the virtual reality feedback. As already done with breathing, for the first session no specific hints is given, the patient is simply encouraged to focus on the fire knowing that the size of the flame is connected to heart rate; at the beginning of the following session, information about muscular relaxation and posture are taught in order to teach further possible ways to control the arousal shown by the virtual reality scenario.

Measures. **Stai Y-1 Scale.** State-Trait Anxiety Inventory form (STAI) (Spielberger et al. 1970; Macor et al. 1990) consists of two scales containing 20 items each that measure anxiety in adults. The STAI clearly differentiates between the temporary condition of "state anxiety" (STAI-Y1) and the more general and long-standing quality of "trait anxiety" (STAI-Y2). For the initial and the final assessment in the trial, we used the STAI Y1, that is, the state version of the STAI, which measures the anxiety in a specific moment. Each item is evaluated through 4-point Likert scales ranging from 1 (at all) to 4 (very much).

Toronto Alexithymia Scale. The 20-item version of the Toronto Alexithymia Scale (TAS-20) is a self-report measure assessing components of the alexithymia construct such as the difficulties to identify and describe feelings and an externally oriented thinking (EOT). The TAS-20 offers an alexithymia measure with well-established psychometric proprieties (Bagby et al. 1994). Each item is evaluated through 5-point Likert scales ranging from 1 (totally disagree) to 5 (total agree).

Anxiety Sensitivity Index. The ASI is a 16-item questionnaire that measures fear of arousal symptoms (Peterson and Reiss, 1987). Each item assesses concern about negative consequences of anxiety symptoms. The ASI has adequate internal consistency (Telch et al. 1989) and test-retest reliability (Mailer and Reiss 1992). ASI also seems to tap fear of anxiety symptoms as opposed to state or trait anxiety (see McNally 1994).

3   Results

All the variables were assessed over two measurement points: before the intervention (after the preliminary meeting, before any biofeedback session) and after the forth session, which corresponds to the fifth meeting. All participants filled outcome measures correctly. Pre-post intervention comparisons were conducted using paired sample t-tests at a .05 significance level. Statistical elaboration was performed using SPSS™ ver. 18.0 (Statistical Package for the Social Sciences - SPSS – for Windows, Chicago, IL).

Results show significant decrease in state anxiety ($t = 2.878$, $p < .05$) and anxiety sensitivity ($t = 2.303$, $p < .05$); the analysis of alexythimia shows no pre-post differences. Main results are reported in the table below (Table 2).

Table 2. Pre-post changes on state anxiety, anxiety sensitivity and alexithymia

Variable	Mean values (SD)		T value	Significance value
	t1	t2		
State anxiety	49.91 (10.14)	41.27 (9.2)	2.878	.016
Anxiety Sensitivity	40.82 (12.00)	37.09 (12.65)	2.303	.044
Alexithymia	47.82 (11.30)	47.45 (11.38)	.126	.902

4   Discussion

Virtual enhanced biofeedback proved its efficacy when structured in a short protocol consisting of a preliminary meeting followed by four biofeedback sessions. The results show a significant decrease both in state anxiety and anxiety sensitivity; the management of the anxious state during the biofeedback session is encouraged by the specific request to try to reduce the size of the flame. This kind of training allows the patient to improve its anxiety management skills, while strengthening in the mind the idea that anxiety is not something that goes completely over the subjective control. Adding simple but specific techniques (focus on diaphragmatic breathing, muscular relaxation) in session 2 and 4 also helps stressing the idea that there are skills that can be trained to feel more confident when anxiety rises. This kind of intervention offers bottom-up techniques that are able to improve self-efficacy about the management of anxiety states.

Real-time feedback allows the management of physiological variations: the first step is surely represented by the awareness of the way the parameter swings, then the patient becomes able to identify the more effective strategies that can be applied to reduce the arousal. The sensitivity to anxiety may decrease because biofeedback teaches to the subject that a sudden increase of the physiological activation is neither extraordinary nor overwhelming; the biofeedback training gets the patient in contact with high arousal in order not to be too much scared of anxious states anymore.

Virtual reality biofeedback may be more useful than traditional biofeedback because it shows the size of the arousal better than the mechanical trend of the parameter: it might be not so important to fully understand the inhale/exhale pattern, if compared to the possibility of focusing on the impact that the breath techniques applied by the subject may directly have on the size of the arousal. Moreover, the technique of biofeedback takes advantage of the enhanced sense of presence ensured by virtual reality to affect the emotional status of the patient.

Limitations and Future Directions. The main limitation of this preliminary study is the lack of a control condition of traditional biofeedback. Further research should investigate the efficacy of the virtual reality enhanced short protocol compared to a condition without the support of virtual reality: this could clarify whether the effects of biofeedback on anxiety and anxiety sensitivity would be significant after 4 sessions also without the advantages of virtual reality. Huang's review (Huang et al. 2006) about new ways to perform biofeedback shows the lack of RCTs as a issue that needs to be faced in order to strengthen the promising results gathered from different studies.

Early dropouts in our study - 6 people out of 21- might be related to the unwillingness to use virtual reality: a preliminary assessment about patient's perception of this type of activity would be useful to comprehend this trend and identify possible barriers to the treatment.

References

Bagby, R.M., Parker, J.D.A., Taylor, G.J.: The twenty-item Toronto Alexithymia Scale I. Item selection and cross validation of the factor structure. J. Psychosom. Res. **38**, 23–32 (1994)

Beauchamp, M.K., Harvey, R.H., Beauchamp, P.H.: An integrated biofeedback and psychological skills training program for Canada's Olympic short-track speedskating team. J. Clin. Sport Psychol. **6**(1), 67 (2012)

Bouchard, S., St-Jacques, J., Robillard, G., Renaud, P.: Anxiety increases the feeling of presence in virtual reality. Presence Teleoperators Virtual Environ. **17**(4), 376–391 (2008)

Budzynski, T.H.: Virtual reality biofeedback: a brief concept paper. Biofeedback **23**, 12–13 (1995)

Frank, D.L., Khorshid, L., Kiffer, J.F., Moravec, C.S., McKee, M.G.: Biofeedback in medicine: who, when, why and how? Mental Health Fam. Med. **7**(2), 85–91 (2010)

Gaggioli, A., Pallavicini, F., Morganti, L., Serino, S., Scaratti, C., Briguglio, M., Crifaci, G., Vetrano, N., Giulintano, A., Bernava, G., Tartarisco, G., Pioggia, G., Grassi, A., Baruffi, M., Wiederhold, B., Riva, G.: Experiential virtual scenarios with real-time monitoring (interreality) for the management of psychological stress: a block randomized controlled trial. J. Med. Internet Res. **16**(7) (2014)

Gorini, A., Pallavicini, F., Algeri, D., Repetto, C., Gaggioli, A., Riva, G.: Virtual reality in the treatment of generalized anxiety disorders. Stud. Health Technol. Inform. **154**, 39–43 (2010)

Huang, H., Wolf, S.L., He, J.: Recent developments in biofeedback for neuromotor rehabilitation. J. Neuroeng. Rehabil. **3**, 11 (2006)

Ijsselsteijn, W.A., Riva, G.: Being there: the experience of presence in mediated environments. In: Riva, G., Davide, F., Ijsselsteijn, W. (eds.) Being There: Concepts, Effects and Measurement of User Presence in Synthetic Environments. Ios Press, Amsterdam (2003)

Macor, A., Pedrabissi, L., Santinello, M.: Ansia di stato e di tratto: ulteriore contributo alla verifica della validita psicometrica e teorica dello S.T.A.I. forma Y di Spielberger. Psicologia e società **15**(1/3), 67–74 (1990)

Mailer, R.G., Reiss, S.: Anxiety sensitivity in 1984 and panic attacks in 1987. J. Anxiety Disord. **6**, 241–247 (1992)

McNally, R.J.: Panic Disorder: A Critical Analysis. Guilford Press, New York (1994)

Nakao, M., Yano, E., Nomura, S., Kuboki, T.: Blood pressure-lowering effects of biofeedback treatment in hypertension: a meta-analysis of randomized controlled trials. Hypertens. Res.: Official J. Jpn. Soc. Hypertens. **26**(1), 37–46 (2003)

Pallavicini, F., Algeri, D., Repetto, C., Gorini, A., Riva, G.: Biofeedback, virtual reality and mobile phones in the treatment of generalized anxiety disorder (GAD): a phase-2 controlled clinical trial. J. CyberTherapy Rehabil. **2**(4), 315–327 (2009). (Aprile)

Palomba, D., Ghisi, M., Scozzari, S., Sarlo, M., Bonso, E., Dorigatti, F., Palatini, P.: Biofeedback-assisted cardiovascular control in hypertensives exposed to emotional stress: a pilot study. Appl. Psychophysiol. Biofeedback **36**(3), 185–192 (2011)

Patla, A.E., Marteniuk, R.G.: Bio-feedback and principles of motor learning in the rehabilitation of movement disorders. Principles Pract. Restorative Neurol. Butterworths Int. Med. Rev. **11**, 93 (2013)

Peterson, R.A., Reiss, S.: Test Manual for the Anxiety Sensitivity Index. International Diagnostic Systems, Orland Park (1987)

Repetto, C., Gorini, A., Vigna, C., Algeri, D., Pallavicini, F., Riva, G.: The use of biofeedback in clinical virtual reality: the INTREPID project. J. Vis. Exp. JoVE (33), 128–132 (2009)

Repetto, C., Gaggioli, A., Pallavicini, F., Cipresso, P., Raspelli, S., Riva, G.: Virtual reality and mobile phones in the treatment of generalized anxiety disorders: a phase-2 clinical trial. Pers. Ubiquit. Comput. **17**(2), 253–260 (2013)

Riva, G., Mantovani, F., Capideville, C.S., Preziosa, A., Morganti, F., Villani, D., Gaggioli, A., Botella, C., Alcañiz, M.: Affective interactions using virtual reality: the link between presence and emotions. CyberPsychol. Behav. **10**(1), 45–56 (2007)

Riva, G., Gaggioli, A., Grassi, A., Raspelli, S., Cipresso, P., Pallavicini, F., Vigna, C., Gagliati, A., Gasco, S., Donvito, G.: NeuroVR 2-a free virtual reality platform for the assessment and treatment in behavioral health care. In: MMVR, pp. 493–495 (2011)

Schein, M. H., Gavish, B., Herz, M., Rosner-Kahana, D., Naveh, P., Knishkowy, B., Zlotnikov, E., Ben-Zvi, N., Melmed, R.N.: Treating hypertension with a device that slows and regularises breathing: a randomised, double-blind controlled study. J. Hum. Hypertens. **15**(4), 271–278 (2001)

Serino, S., Cipresso, P., Gaggioli, A., Riva, G.: The potential of pervasive sensors and computing for positive technology: the interreality paradigm. In: Mukhopadhyay, S.C., Postolache, O.A. (eds.) Pervasive and Mobile Sensing and Computing for Healthcare. SSMI, vol. 2, pp. 207–232. Springer, Heidelberg (2013)

Spielberger, C.D., Gorsuch, R.L., Lushene, R.E.: Manual for the State-Trait Anxiety Inventory. Consulting Psychologists Press, Palo Alto (1970)

Telch, M.J., Shermis, M.D., Lucas, J.A.: Anxiety sensitivity: unitary personality trait or domain-specific appraisals? J. Anxiety Disord. **3**, 25–32 (1989)

Yucha, C.B., Clark, L., Smith, M., Uris, P., LaFleur, B., Duval, S.: The effect of biofeedback in hypertension. Appl. Nurs. Res. **14**(1), 29–35 (2001)

Yucha, C.B., Tsai, P.S., Calderon, K.S., Tian, L.: Biofeedback-assisted relaxation training for essential hypertension: who is most likely to benefit? J. Cardiovasc. Nurs. **20**(3), 198–205 (2005)

Wells, R., Outhred, T., Heathers, J.A.J., Quintana, D.S., Kemp, A.H.: Matter over mind: a randomised-controlled trial of single-session biofeedback training on performance anxiety and heart rate variability in musicians. PLoS ONE **7**(10), e46597 (2012). doi:10.1371/journal.pone.0046597

Wheat, A.L., Larkin, K.T.: Biofeedback of heart rate variability and related physiology: a critical review. Appl. Psychophysiol. Biofeedback **35**(3), 229–242 (2010)

Wiederhold, B.K., Wiederhold, M.D.: Virtual reality therapy for anxiety disorders: advances in evaluation and treatment. American Psychological Association (2005)

M-HCI: Mental-Health-Computer Interaction

Development of Web-Based Platform for Privacy Protective Avatar Mediated Distance-Care

Yu Kobayashi[1]([✉]), Dai Hasegawa[1], Shinichi Shirakawa[2], Hiroshi Sakuta[1], and Eijun Nakayama[3]

[1] Department of Integrated Information Technology,
College of Science and Engineering, Aoyama Gakuin University, Tokyo, Japan
sweep.3092@gmail.com, {hasegawa,sakuta}@it.aoyama.ac.jp
[2] Faculty of Engineering, Information and Systems,
University of Tsukuba, Tsukuba, Japan
[3] School of Nursing, Kitasato University, Tokyo, Japan

Abstract. We propose a web-based platform for privacy-protected avatar mediated distant-care. The system can avateer an elderly person based on their articular angles acquired by a motion capture system, and render the whole body animation of the avatar on a web-browser. The avatar-mediated architecture design allow caregivers to observe the elderly persons' behavior all day long, without violating their privacy. In addition, we will show an example implementation integrating multiple sensors in the platform. By integrating multiple sensors into the platform, caregivers can observe the avatar with the elderly person's health-related status. The implemented system showed the low communication bandwidth dependency, and sufficient frame-rate for the animation to be smoothly seen.

Keywords: Avatar-Mediated Communication · Health-care · Privacy Protection · Distant-Care

1 Introduction

In recent years, with the progress of aging, our life style and family form has changed. Especially, the number of households in which an elderly person lives alone has increased, and social isolation of the elderly in such households has been acknowledged as a problem. In many cases of the socially isolated elderly people, it is difficult for someone to notice the change in their health status. Their health problems can become worse unnoticed. Additionally, daily support and mental care for the elderly, which used to be supported by the mutual aid of family members and local community, have changed to human workers involved in nursing and welfare services, offered by local governments or private sectors. This is also recognized as one of the problems of this isolation, because it inevitably leads to the increase of social welfare expense.

For the reason mentioned above, various ICT based distant-care services are provided. However, in the current state of popularization of ICT based care services, only simple and low-tech services are widely used, such as emergency call

© Springer International Publishing Switzerland 2016
S. Serino et al. (Eds.): MindCare 2015, CCIS 604, pp. 131–139, 2016.
DOI: 10.1007/978-3-319-32270-4_13

services with push button devices and locating services with wearable IC tags. On the other hand, the care services that utilize advanced ICT devices such as cameras and sensors are not widely used. One of the main reasons that the elderly and family members avoid such advanced technologies is the concern about privacy compromise, despite the fact that privacy protection technologies are now implemented in many cases. When designing distant-care systems which observe the elderly, it is desirable to observe the elderly for a long-time continuously [6]. However, it is said that privacy is the person's right to control personal information revealed to others. For this reason, to protecting one's privacy in captured video, a lot of researchers developed and used technological solutions such as filters [9] and automatic blurring, etc. But in camera-based surveillance approach, it is difficult to protect one's privacy such as personal information which can be embarrassing and/or humiliating for the elderly (e.g. nudity). Thus, in order to introduce advanced ICT technologies into distant-care/health-care services, it is important to provide a platform that can explicitly express privacy protection awareness of the system, and for the safety to be understandable for anyone.

In this paper, we propose a privacy protective avatar mediated distant-care system that can avateer an elderly person based on their articular angles acquired by a motion capture system. By avateering the elderly, the distant-care platform allows us to achieve privacy protected information delivery of the elderly person. It is easy to understand how the elderly is observed, and we believe it will help the elderly and caregivers to accept this system. We developed the system as a form of web application with an inexpensive motion capture system, Microsoft KINECT Sensor. By doing so, caregivers can observe the elderly people anytime on their mobile PCs and smart phones that have modern web browsers.

In addition, many kinds of low-cost wearable sensors have been developed for general health-care purpose lately [8]. We also show sensor integration in the proposed platform, in order to extend the platform and apply it to practical distant-care/health-care situations.

2   Related Works

In the field of ICT based distant-care system employing an animated human character, there are two types of approach: virtual human approach and avatar approach. In the former approach, the virtual human is a intelligent autonomous agent that supports users through verbal and non-verbal interaction.

For example, Rizzo et al. presented the SimCoach project that aims to develop virtual human support agents to assist military personnel and family in breaking down barriers to initiating care [1]. Devault et al. developed an virtual human interviewer, SimSensei Kiosk [2]. The virtual human, named Ellie and having a figure of an woman, engages users in 15–25 m health-care discussions. Zhou et al. created a virtual nurse agent [3]. Patients talked to the nurse agent in their hospital beds, and reported very high level satisfaction and trust in the nurse agent. The virtual human approach is promising due to the advantage of its autonomy. Human involvement is not required at all. However, these interaction technologies are still in development, and there are severe limits of domain in which those systems can work.

On the other hand, in the avatar approach, systems are only used to mediate human-human interaction. However, by using computer graphical animated representations as mediations, the system can change, reinforce, and compliment various features in human-human interaction, such as protecting privacy or anonymity, changing one's appearances, and adding unrealistic expressions, etc.

Lisetti et al. developed the multi-modal intelligent affective interfaces [4]. Their system can record the face of the patient, and render one's avatar that mirrors the emotional states of the patient to show to the health-care provider. Additionally, their system can be used to measure physiological signals such as skin temperature, ambient temperature, heat flow, and movement by using a kind of wireless wearable computer. Also, Beard et al. found a wide range of health-care activities on Second Life [10]. Matti et al. also developed the avatar-based 3D visualization system consists of a server PC, client PC, and some wearable sensors in the wireless local network [7,8]. In their system, visualize one's activity as an avatar in 3D virtual environment by using the activity recognition also they developed. However, little research developed web-based systems for avatar-mediated health-care communication, and virtually no research has developed a web-based system that can avateer one's whole body by using a contactless motion-capture system.

3   System Overview

Figure 1 shows the outline of our system. The system is composed of a three-sided client-server model: the server, the caregiver side client, and the elderly person side client. The client of the elderly person side consists of a KINECT sensor, programs for articular angle data acquisition and data processing, and a program to send the processed data to the server. The server emits the received data from the elderly person side client program to the caregiver side program.

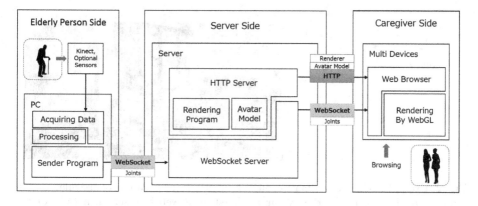

Fig. 1. System overview

The caregiver side program, which is stored in the server, is called from the web-browser in the caregiver side client, then executes the rendering program. The program receives the articular angle data from the server and applies it to the avatar model data for rendering. The frequency of data communication is approximately 15–30 times per second, so that the avatar can be animated smoothly enough.

We will describe the rendering method on the web-browser, server-client communication method, and the example of using our system below.

3.1   Avatar Animation on Web-Browser

Generally, OpenGL, DirectX and OpenGL ES (for mobiles) are used in the development of applications using 3D graphics, but one of the problems in using these APIs is that we have to develop applications for each devices and OSs used. Another problem is the applications have to be installed to the devices by users. In the rapid development of various devices of late years, it is difficult to support such devices and maintain the softwares.

So, we employed WebGL, a JavaScript API that can be run on many modern browsers such as Google Chrome, Mozilla Firefox, Safari, etc. in both PCs and mobiles. As a result, WebGL enabled to adaptation multi-platform, not depending on differences in devices and OSs, and additionally installing a software by users is reduced because such web-browsers are standard equipments in many cases.

3.2   Client-Server Communication

The sensor data is sent from the elderly person client through the server to the caregiver client. The communication requires 15–20 frequency per second. HTTP, a traditional communication protocol between a server and web-browser, needs a relatively large amount of header data for each request/response communication which leads to a significant delay for such kinds of communication. Therefore, we

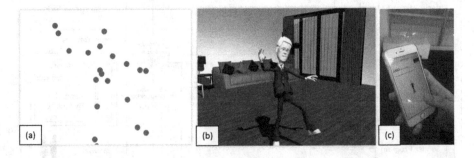

Fig. 2. Examples of avatar animation on web-browsers: (a) positions of articular angles acquired by KINECT, (b) the avatar rendered on a web browser on a PC, (c) an example of use in a mobile device.

employed WebSocket protocol for client-server communication. It is the protocol that extended HTTP, and can realize real-time two-way communication between a server and web-browser. WebSocket protocol is also supported in almost all modern web-browsers.

Figure 2 shows examples of the avatar-mediated distant-care system. KINECT can acquire twenty articular angles. The angles are represented by quaternion vector form.

4 Sensor Integration

Various types of wearable sensors have been developed in recent years, and now we can continuously monitor one's vital information such as blood pressure, heartbeat-rate, and oxygen level. The proposed avatar-mediated distant-care platform should be customized by integrating those wearable devices to adapt to a huge variety of health-care situation. In this chapter, we will show an example of sensor integration.

For this purpose, we prepared a sensing device including a temperature sensor, humidity sensor, and heartbeat-rate sensor (Fig. 3). The temperature sensor and humidity sensor are combined in one sensor module (Fig. 3(a) and (b)) shows the heartbeat-rate sensor. As described in Fig. 3(c), the sensors are connected to a micro-computer, Arduino Uno, and the micro-computer is connected to a one board computer, Raspberry Pi. The Raspberry Pi is connected to a Wi-Fi adapter and battery. The sensor data is sent from Arduino Uno to Raspberry Pi via USB cable (serial communication), then to the server via Wi-Fi. The data is processed and formatted in JSON (e.g. { "temperature": 25, "humidity": 65, "heartbeat-rate": 60}) when sent to the server. In the caregiver side, the received data is parsed and processed to render each sensor data on the web-browser.

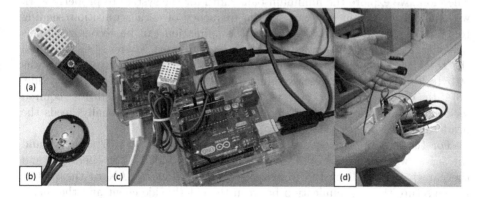

Fig. 3. Sensing devise: (a) a temperature and humidity sensor module, (b) a heartbeat-rate sensor module, (c) an overview of the sensing device, (d) a user putting on heartbeat-rate sensor.

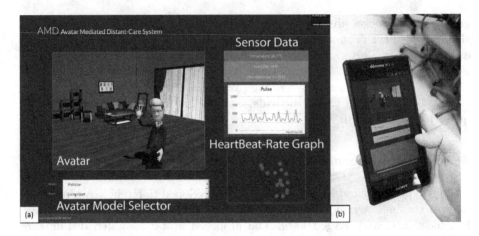

Fig. 4. Example views of avatar mediated distant-care system on the caregiver side: (a) on a PC, (b) on a smart phone.

Figure 4(a) shows a screen shot of the web-browser on the caregiver side. The temperature and humidity are shown on the top right side, and the heartbeat-rate and its animation are depicted on the middle right side. Also, Fig. 4(b) shows a user using the system (the caregiver side client) on a smart phone.

5   Experiment

The proposed system sends multiple data from the elderly side client to the server, and from the server to the caregiver client 15–30 times per second. So, if the network's communication bandwidth is below the total amount of data, it is expected that delays will occur in the animation of the caregiver client. Therefore, we explore the minimum bandwidth for the system to properly work without delays. In our test, we set the frequency of data acquisition/sending to 15 fps, which is the lower limit for the animation can be recognized one's behavior. Also, the data amount of articular angles was 6 Kbytes (48 Kbits), and the total data amount of the temperature, humidity, and heartbeat-rate was 50 bytes (0.4 Kbits) after processed into JSON format at the elderly person side. So, if the data was sent 15 times per second, 726 Kbits/s bandwidth is required for sending only the data. Usually, the communication additionally needs the header data.

For the experiment, we set up a private network, in which a router and the server was connected by a LAN cable, and the elderly side client PC and the caregiver side client PC were connected by wireless LAN to the router. In the setup, the communication between the elderly side client and the server was established with enough bandwidth. Then, we investigated the communication performance of the system by controlling the bandwidth of outbound from the server to the caregiver side PC.

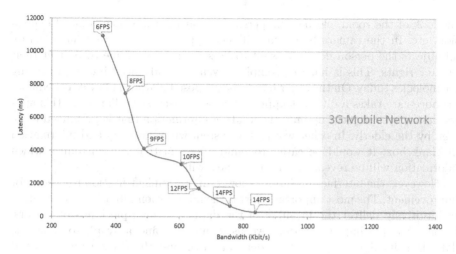

Fig. 5. Relationship between network bandwidth and animation delay and frame-rate.

We measured the performance of the system ten seconds after communication was established. To understand the performance, we used two indexes: the average frame-rate of the animation, and the average time lapse after the server sent the data until the client received the data. We measured the two indexes three times to calculate the average for each time.

Figure 5 shows the frame-rate and the time lapse when the bandwidth was controlled from 350 Kbit/s to 850 Kbit/s. The results showed that when the bandwidth was above 800 Kbit/s, the animation was rendered smoothly without delay. However, when the bandwidth was below 800 Kbit/s, a delay was seen. We measured the system performance ten seconds after the communication was established but the delay was accumulated with each passing moment.

Assuming that mobile telecommunication bandwidths of late years are not under multiple mega bit/s, caregivers can observe the animation of the avatar without delay via mobile network. And if the network bandwidth is 100 MBit/s, we can expect 140 server-client connections.

6   Discussion

It is said that privacy is the person's right to control personal information revealed to others. In the light of this point of view, when designing distant-care systems which observe the elderly for a long-time continuously, it is difficult to protect one's privacy right if the system was developed in camera-based surveillance approach. The explanation behind this is that a large amount of information about the person will be inevitably included in a picture, such as the look of the room, clothes the person is wearing, the person's facial expression, etc. In the camera-based surveillance approach, the system has to erase all objects the person does not want to be seen in every frame to protect their privacy rights. This is hard to complete even with advanced image processing technologies today. On the other hand, the proposed platform of avatar-mediated distance-care takes a different approach, sensor-based surveillance. In this approach, the system picks up only the kinds of information that is permitted to be seen by the elderly. In other words, the system will selectively add information in blank box. It would be easier to build a system that can customize which information will be revealed, reflecting one's will.

However, the interface design we showed in our implementation has room for improvement. The most important part is the information-intensive visualization to intuitively deliver the meaning of the data from multiple kinds of sensors. In our example implementation, we used numbers and a graph to show the data. But, it might be easier to understand if the visualizations were integrated with the avatar animation. For example, the room light turning red when the temperature goes up, or the avatar sweating when the heartbeat-rate goes up. We need to investigate the visualization principles and methods through user experiments.

7   Conclusions and Future Works

In this paper, we proposed a web-based platform for privacy-protected avatar mediated distant-care. Our system avateers an elderly person and animates the avatar based on their articular angles acquired by a KINECT sensor. In addition, we implemented a system integrated with a temperature sensor, humidity sensor, and heartbeat-rate sensor. The implemented system showed a low communication bandwidth dependency, and sufficient frame-rate for the animation can be recognized one's activity.

The avatar-mediated design of the system allows us to achieve continuous long-time information delivery about elderly people, without violating their privacy such as capturing video. Our system implementation and experiment results showed the possibility for applying the proposed architecture to practical distant-care situations. In our future work, we will evaluate the system's usability, the psychological burden such as how elderly react by having their behaviors tracked and showed in the form of a virtual avatar of both being the observed and the caring by introducing our system into the nursing and personal care facility. And also, additional research is needed to reveal how to detect any other particular health problems.

Acknowledgment. This research was partially supported by Strategic Information and Communications R&D Promotion Programme (SCOPE).

References

1. Rizzo, A., Buckwalter, J.G., Forbell, E., Kim, J., Sagae, K., Williams, J., Difede, J.: SimCoach: an intelligent virtual human system for providing healthcare information and support. Int. J. Disabil. Hum. Dev. **10**, 277–281 (2011)
2. DeVault, D., Artstein, R., Benn, G., Dey, T., Fast, E., Gainer, A., Georgila, K., Gratch, J., Hartholt, A., Lhommet, M., Lucas, G., Marsella, S., Morbini, F., Nazarian, A., Scherer, S., Stratou, G., Suri, A., Traum, D., Wood, R., Xu, Y., Rizzo, A., Morency, L.: SimSensei Kiosk: a virtual human interviewer for healthcare disicion support. In: Proceedings of the 2014 International Conference on Autonomous Agents and Multi-agent Systems, pp. 1061–1068. International Foundation for Autonomous Agents and Multiagent Systems, Richland (2014)
3. Zhou, S., Bickmore, T., Paasche-Orlow, M., Jack, B.: Agent-user concordance and satisfaction with a virtual hospital discharge nurse. In: Bickmore, T., Marsella, S., Sidner, C. (eds.) IVA 2014. LNCS, vol. 8637, pp. 528–541. Springer, Heidelberg (2014)
4. Lisetti, C., Nasoz, F., LeRouge, C., Ozyer, O., Alvarez, K.: Developing multimodal intelligent affective interfaces for tele-home health care. Int. J. Hum. Comput. Stud. **59**, 245–255 (2013)
5. Leonardi, C., Mennecozzi, C., Not, E., Pianesi, F., Zancanaro, M., Gennai, F., Cristoforetti, A.: Knocking on elders' door: investigating the functional and emotional geography of their domestic space. In: CHI 2009, Proceedings of the SIGCHI Conference on Human Factors in Computing Systems, pp. 1703–1712 (2009)
6. Hayes, G.R., Abowd, G.D.: Tensions in designing capture technologies for an evidence-based care community. In: CHI 2006 Proceedings of the SIGCHI Conference on Human Factors in Computing Systems, pp. 937–946 (2006)
7. Pouke, M., Hkkil, J.: Elderly healthcare monitoring using an avatar-based 3D virtual environment. Int. J. Environ. Res. Public Health **10**, 7283–7298 (2013)
8. Pouke, M.: Using 3D virtual environments to monitor elderly patient activity with low cost sensors. In: 2013 Seventh International Conference on Next Generation Mobile Apps, Services and Technologies (NGMAST), pp. 81–86 (2013)
9. Boyle, M., Edwards, C., Greenberg, S.: The effects of filtered video on awareness and privacy. In: Proceedings of the 2000 ACM Conference on Computer Supported Cooperative Work, pp. 1–10 (2000)
10. Beard, L., Wilson, K., Morra, D., Keelan, J.: A survey of health-related activities on second life. Journal of Medical Internet Research **11** (2009)

User Experiences of a Mobile Mental Well-Being Intervention Among Pregnant Women

Salla Muuraiskangas[1](✉), Elina Mattila[1], Pipsa Kyttälä[2,3], Mirva Koreasalo[2,3],
and Raimo Lappalainen[4]

[1] VTT Technical Research Centre of Finland Ltd, Digital Health, Oulu/Tampere, Finland
{salla.muuraiskangas,elina.m.mattila}@vtt.fi
[2] School of Health Sciences, University of Tampere, Tampere, Finland
{pipsa.kyttala,mirva.koreasalo}@uta.fi
[3] Department of Health, National Institute for Health and Welfare, Helsinki, Finland
[4] Department of Psychology, University of Jyväskylä, Jyväskylä, Finland
raimo.lappalainen@jyu.fi

Abstract. Postnatal depression affects 10 to 15 percent of women after child-birth. Acceptance and commitment therapy (ACT) is associated with better mental well-being and lower levels of depression. Digital ACT solutions enable providing potentially cost-effective access to interventions. This paper reports the user experiences of an ACT-based mobile mental well-being intervention among pregnant women. Twenty-nine mothers were recruited to a 6-month study. Usage rates were collected via usage logs and user experiences via questionnaires and interviews. The total usage time of the application was about 53 min per user. The application was perceived easy to use. The most common barriers of use were: content being perceived irrelevant due to the lack of tailoring for pregnancy; lack of time; and not having the application in the personal mobile phone. The application was perceived useful by women with problems and concerns with their pregnancy, a potential target group in future.

Keywords: Postnatal depression · Acceptance and commitment therapy · Intervention · mHealth · Well-being · User experience

1 Introduction

Pregnancy and childbirth are a life-altering experience, characterized by physiological, social and emotional changes. New parents are expected to be joyful, but there may also be negative feelings associated with this period. As many as 15–25 % of women experience high anxiety or depression during pregnancy, and 10–15 % of women suffer from postnatal depression [1, 2]. Antenatal depression and anxiety can have adverse effects on family functioning and the development of infants [1]. They are also significant risk factors of postnatal depression, along with stressful events, difficult labor and lack of social support during pregnancy [2].

Women are in regular contact with healthcare services during pregnancy, which provides an opportunity for identifying potential mental health problems and providing

© Springer International Publishing Switzerland 2016
S. Serino et al. (Eds.): MindCare 2015, CCIS 604, pp. 140–149, 2016.
DOI: 10.1007/978-3-319-32270-4_14

interventions. Despite the promising results on individual health and well-being interventions, there is not yet strong enough evidence to support their uptake in midwifery training or practice [1]. Prenatal care would also enable preventative well-being interventions and preparing for the changes brought on by childbirth.

Acceptance and Commitment Therapy (ACT) is a third-wave cognitive-behavioral therapy (CBT) aiming to increase psychological flexibility, which is the ability to fully contact the present moment, thoughts and feelings, and changing or persisting in behavior that serves personal values and goals [3]. Psychological flexibility has been found to be associated with psychological well-being and inversely correlate with psychological distress, including depression and anxiety [4, 5]. ACT has been proven efficient in treating depression [6–8]. To the best of the authors' knowledge, there are no publications on ACT-based interventions for improving mental well-being of pregnant women or preventing postnatal depression. However, a pilot study on mindfulness-based intervention showed promising results in decreasing anxiety and negative affect during pregnancy [9].

Introducing new interventions to prenatal care is challenging due to the already constrained resources. Therefore, ICT interventions seem promising as they do not require a lot of extra resources in the daily practice. They could, at least, be used as the first intervention that expectant mothers could be referred to if there are some concerns related to maternal mental well-being, but not severe enough problems to warrant more intensive intervention. Mobile applications delivering psychological therapy are quickly emerging with promising results [10, 11]. Also ACT-based mobile interventions have been developed. An ACT-based program, with both mobile and web components, was tested in a 4-week trial with 11 participants with no diagnosed mental disorders [12]. The trial found increases in psychological flexibility and value-based actions, but no changes in depression, anxiety, or stress [12].

This paper reports a field study with an ACT-based mobile mental well-being intervention for pregnant women. The study focused on the usage and user experience (UX) of the application. Specifically, the aim was to study the barriers of using the application and the experienced benefits of the application among pregnant women.

2 Materials and Methods

2.1 Research Questions

This study investigated the usage and user experiences of a mobile intervention for pregnant women. The research questions are: (1) how does the mobile intervention application suit the needs of pregnant women; (2) what are the potential barriers of use; and (3) what are the perceived benefits and value of the mobile intervention.

2.2 Intervention Application

The ACT intervention was delivered through a mobile intervention called Oiva, which was originally developed for stress management and mental well-being by increasing psychological flexibility [13]. Oiva aims to teach the six core skills of ACT, namely being present, *acceptance, cognitive defusion, self as context, values,* and *committed actions* [3]. It was expected that learning those skills would improve the mental well-being and increase the psychological flexibility of pregnant women, making them less susceptible to anxiety and depression during and after pregnancy.

Oiva consists of 46 ACT-based audio and text exercises, organized under four modules: (1) Aware Mind, (2) Wise Mind, (3) Values, and (4) Healthy Body (Fig. 1). Most of the exercises are short, taking only 1–3 min to complete, making it possible to perform them independent of time and location. Introductory videos present the purpose of the application and its modules. The application allows making diary notes and mark exercise into favorites. A widget on the phone main screen reminded the users when they last used the application and how many exercises they had completed so far. It also gave short aphorisms as reminders of the skills they had learned. If the user had not used Oiva for seven days, a small icon appeared in the notification bar of the phone.

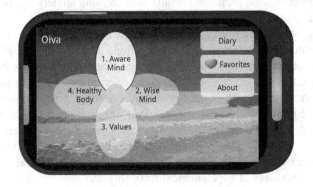

Fig. 1. Oiva home screen

Preliminary experiences among office workers showed good acceptability, usefulness and engagement [13]. A randomized controlled trial has recently been conducted to study the effectiveness of Oiva for improving the well-being of psychologically distressed overweight individuals [14].

2.3 Participants

The original study had a cluster-randomized design and included (1) a web-based nutrition intervention (N = 14) and (2) an ACT-based mobile intervention (Oiva) (N = 29), and (3) a control group with no intervention (N = 11). The interventions were provided by public health nurses (N = 52) who received training before the study started. The participating families of the control clinics received standard maternity care.

The study was conducted by public health nurses at 8 maternity clinics in the City of Vantaa, Finland. Participation in the study was offered to all families expecting their child at their standard 8 to 10 pregnancy weeks' maternity clinic visits. The exclusion criteria were age under 18 years, insufficient language skills to fill in the Finnish questionnaires and no possibility to use internet. The recruitment took place between May

2013 and August 2014. The study protocol was embedded in the standard visits at the maternity clinics until the 37–41 weeks' gestation visit. The study was approved by the Coordinating Ethics Committee of The Hospital District of Helsinki and Uusimaa. This study focuses solely on the group that received the mobile intervention through the Oiva application. In the following, the study procedures will be described for this group only.

The average age of the Oiva participants was 33, they were highly educated 74 % having Bachelor's degree or higher and 82 % were having their first child (N = 27 responding the background questionnaire).

2.4 Measures

The usage of the intervention was extracted from the usage logs collected by the application. The UX was collected via questionnaires and interviews in terms of satisfaction, intention to use, ease of use, barriers for use and usefulness.

2.5 Data Collection

Oiva was introduced to pregnant mothers through maternity clinics. Twenty-nine participants received Android mobile phones (ZTE Blade or ZTE Skate, ZTE Corporation, Shenzen, China) with the Oiva application installed around the 16th to 18th pregnancy week and they kept it until postpartum, altogether about 6 to 7 months. They were given a short introduction to the application and user instructions on paper. They were advised to use the application regularly, a few times a week.

Usage logs were collected from the study phones at the end of the study period but, due to human error in the book-keeping of mobile phones, only 21 logs of the 29 were identified to participants and analyzed. UX questionnaires were sent at the 2nd, 10th and 20th weeks after receiving the application and the number of responses was 25, 20 and 17, respectively. If the application was received after 18th pregnancy week, the UX questionnaires were sent in speeded time at weeks 2, 8 and 16 to ensure all UX questionnaires were sent before expected delivery. A subset of 8 participants was interviewed by phone around the expected date of delivery.

2.6 Data Analysis

Quantitative data included usage log files and UX questions with Likert scales. Usage log files were analyzed by first identifying the individual usage sessions of Oiva and then counting their total number and duration. UX questions were answered using 7-point Likert scale with endpoints 1 'totally disagree' and 7 'totally agree'. There was additionally 0 'cannot say' option. Zeros were excluded from the analysis and basic descriptives, such as averages and standard deviations were calculated.

Qualitative data included open-ended questions in the questionnaires and interviews. The data were analyzed using thematic analysis for barriers of use and benefits.

3 Results

3.1 Usage

The actual usage was calculated based on 21 usage logs. The median of usage days was 4 (interquartile range, IQR: 4–8.5) and the median duration of use was 52.8 min (IQR: 16.3–158). The median length of the usage period from the first log event to the last was 45 days (IQR: 12.5–153). Most of the usage was focused on the early weeks of the intervention (Fig. 2).

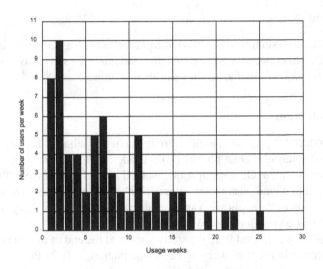

Fig. 2. Oiva users per week

The usage activity of the ones responding to the final UX questionnaire (N = 14) was somewhat higher compared to the whole group. They used Oiva on a median of 6 days (IQR: 3.8–12.5) with a median duration of 113 min (IQR: 33.6–195 min). Their median usage period was 75.5 days (IQR: 23.5–165 days).

3.2 UX

The UX items are reported in Table 1. Satisfaction was quite neutral. Intention to continue use decreased towards the end. Oiva received good ratings on usability throughout the study. Usefulness on the other hand scored lower. However, the answers had high deviations; some users rated usefulness high and some low showing differing user experiences within the group.

Table 1. User experience items, their averages and standard deviations in the brackets. Apart from the 'Grade', all items are evaluated from 1 'fully disagree' to 7 'fully disagree'.

Item	Beginning	Mid	End
Satisfaction			
Grade (1 the worst, 7 the best)	-	4.2 (1.9)	3.9 (1.9)
I would recommend Oiva to others	-	4.2 (2.2)	3.6 (2.4)
Intention to use			
I plan to continue using Oiva	5.1 (1.4)	4.7 (2.1)	2.6 (2.2)
I don't want to use Oiva	2.6 (1.7)	3.4 (1.9)	4.2 (2.2)
Usability			
It was easy to take Oiva in use/use it	6.7 (0.6)	6.2 (1.1)	6.2 (1.0)
Oiva is reliable	-	6.3 (0.9)	5.6 (1.5)
Oiva's content is understandable	5.7 (1.2)	5.0 (1.6)	5.4 (1.8)
Oiva's UI is pleasant	5.3 (1.4)	5.0 (1.8)	5.1 (1.4)
Usefulness			
Oiva fits my needs and situation in life	4.7 (1.7)	3.6 (2.1)	3.2 (2.4)
I have learnt new things with the help of Oiva	-	4.0 (2.2)	3.5 (2.4)
Content of Oiva is useful for me	-	3.9 (1.9)	3.9 (2.1)
Oiva has helped me to prepare for parenthood	-	-	2.6 (1.9)
Usage of Oiva has caused positive changes in my relationships	-	-	2.6 (1.8)
Oiva has helped me maintain and improve my well-being	-	-	2.9 (2.1)
Oiva has helped me achieve my well-being goals	-	-	2.7 (1.9)

The following analysis of the barriers is conducted for understanding the relatively low usage and benefits for realizing the future potential and efficient ways of use. Analysis is conducted with the open-ended questions in the questionnaires and interviews.

Barriers. The most prominent Oiva-related barrier of use was that the *content* of Oiva was *not perceived relevant* in terms of pregnancy. People expect information relevant to their situation and clear value from the start. The users wished Oiva's content to be *more tailored* for pregnancy, e.g. containing pregnancy or parenting related exercises. For some participants, Oiva's exercises were not nothing new since mindfulness training was already familiar. Some participants perceived the exercises as too imaginary or even "humbug". These were seen both from the questionnaires and interviews. It was also mentioned in the interviews that there were too many exercises which made the application seem harder to manage or 'complete'. Oiva was also seen a bit too problem-centered when one would have only wanted to enjoy the wonderful pregnancy.

If Oiva is meant to be targeted as a support during the pregnancy, I would have been more interested if there were more information or viewpoints related to pregnancy and parenthood. (quote from the final questionnaire).

The most prominent external barriers for use were *lack of time* and having to use a *secondary phone* which made it easy to forget Oiva. Pregnancy causes *additional activities* such as health clinic visits, job redistribution activities etc. and that is why there is even less free time than normally. When Oiva was installed in a secondary phone, often the battery was not charged at the opportune usage moment or the phone was just lying somewhere and was forgotten. Also, the interviews revealed that *pregnancy-related nausea* and *lack of energy* due to pregnancy and having extra things to do were preventing use. Many times, there was no obvious need or problem in life, which would have led to using Oiva. Also, it was reported that it is difficult to find peaceful situation to use Oiva.

> I haven't used Oiva application since the last questionnaire. I feel I don't have enough time for it and when I would, the battery is dead from the device and it must be recharged. (quote from the midterm questionnaire).

Benefits. Even though generally Oiva got rather low usefulness ratings, there was great variation between answers; there were those who did not perceive it useful at all and those who perceived it extremely useful.

The most important benefits arising from both data are *calming down* and *relaxation* benefits, *mindfulness, acceptance* and *values* which are closely related to the ACT skills Oiva was trying to teach. Other additional benefits arising from the interviews were preparing for the parenthood (in the difficult pregnancy and was related to value processing), provided good viewpoints, improved mood and self-esteem, gave peace of mind, improved stress management and relationships. It was also mentioned to offer easy access to information and was seen as a tool to process work-related worries.

> I have learnt to structure my life and things that are important to me and time which I use with them. I have learnt to loosen up and be more permissive towards myself and my feelings. These skills I have of course learnt from other sources simultaneously and even through earlier mindfulness studies. However, consolidation and repetition is still always in order! (quote from the final questionnaire).

4 Discussion

4.1 Lessons Learnt from Barriers of Use

The use and intention continue to use were low. The intention to continue use is probably connected to the low ratings and decrease in the usefulness questions, and also to the long duration of use (i.e. the intention to continue use is naturally higher in the beginning when the users have not had a lot of time to use the application). The following discussion addresses the potential reasons for the low use and ways to tackle the issues.

Find opportune moments to introduce the application. Time issues, lack of energy and not wanting to do more extra things were mentioned as barriers of use. Pregnancy itself was causing extra tasks, such as going to the maternity clinic and preparation for maternal leave, and therefore there was not much time for Oiva. Therefore, pregnancy may not be the best time to introduce a universal intervention for expecting mothers. Rather, Oiva might work better for indicated intervention, e.g. if the mother is experiencing some worries or has early signs of anxiety or low mood. A better moment could be the beginning of maternity leave as there may be more time after leaving work or right in the beginning of the pregnancy when normal life is not affected by the pregnancy too much.

Tailor the content for creating value. Some participants did not perceive Oiva's content useful and sometimes the exercises in Oiva were perceived a bit too imaginary. Therefore it is important to tailor the content for the target group, provide justification and purpose for different exercises from their point of view, and provide also down-to-earth exercises. Oiva exercises could, for example, deal with the issues that are experienced by many pregnant women, such as worries related to the well-being of the baby, feelings of guilt when doing something that is not recommended during pregnancy, or ways of mentally preparing for the labor.

Enable using primary mobile device for the intervention. Oiva was installed in a mobile phone provided by the study organizers and most users did not take it into use as their primary phone. Therefore, the Oiva phone was usually not carried along, which restricted its usage to the home environment and potentially diminished the effect of reminders. However, mobile implementation was perceived desirable as it provided mobility and choice regarding where to perform the exercises even within home. Personal mobile phone would better support usage in more varied contexts.

Enable usage in any environment. The participants reported that it was difficult to find peaceful moments for the exercises. Mobility promotes usage in any possible idle moments, for example, while riding on a bus. Therefore it is important that there are exercises that you are able to do in those less peaceful moments too, even in a crowd. There should also be search functions and filters that allow users to find them easily.

Present the content in small portions. Some participants felt Oiva contained too many exercises. Therefore, for such a long usage period, it might be a good approach to reveal the content of the application in small portions and unlock new content as the user progresses. The content could also be linked to pregnancy weeks, as suggested by one of the users.

Emphasize the benefits in the beginning. User experiences clearly reflect that many participants did not understand the purpose of Oiva and did not feel the need for using it. Probably a more extensive presentation by an ACT expert at the maternity clinic would have been needed. It has been suggested that practitioner has potential to increase the treatment credibility and treatment expectations which can influence program uptake [15]. The application should provide a clear insight of its purpose and value for the participants, or have been more engaging from the start to keep them involved long enough to gain value.

4.2 Lessons Learnt from Usefulness and Benefits

Oiva content has benefits to some, usually the ones who have needs, worries or other problems. For example, during a difficult pregnancy, Oiva was perceived extremely useful. Therefore Oiva could be provided through maternity clinics to those parents who have some worries but who are not diagnosed with mental problems.

4.3 Future Steps

Future steps should be guided to remove the revealed barriers and proper strategies to improve adherence should be included in the intervention. Also, effectiveness among the presented target group is yet to be studied.

By the time of writing this paper, a Finnish version of Oiva is already available for free for iOS and Android devices tackling one of the barriers. There is also a web version [16].

5 Conclusions

The aim of the research is to study the usage and user experiences of a mobile intervention for pregnant women and explore the barriers of use and the perceived benefits. The usage rate of Oiva was low. Most of the pregnant mothers did not perceive a need for Oiva, e.g. did not have problems or concerns related to their pregnancy. However, the persons who experienced some needs also perceived Oiva useful. It seems an application targeting psychological well-being, such as Oiva, could be especially useful for mothers who experiences problems or worries during their pregnancy. There must be some driving force, motivation, for the use. When an application is promoted to a specific user group, it should be tailored to fit their needs.

Acknowledgments. The study is supported by the Finnish Funding Agency for Innovation (TEKES) and National Institute for Health and Welfare. We express our gratitude to the parents who participated in the study. We also want to thank the public health nurses and the Social and Health Services of the City of Vantaa for good collaboration.

References

1. Alderdice, F., McNeill, J., Lynn, F.: A systematic review of systematic reviews of interventions to improve maternal mental health and well-being. Midwifery **12**, 955 (2012)
2. Robertson, E., Grace, S., Wallington, T., Stewart, D.E.: Antenatal risk factors for postpartum depression: a synthesis of recent literature. Gen. Hosp. Psychiatry **26**, 289–295 (2004)
3. Hayes, S.C., Luoma, J.B., Bond, F.W., Masuda, A., Lillis, J.: Acceptance and commitment therapy: model, processes and outcomes Behav. Res. Ther. **44**, 1–25 (2006)
4. Kashdan, T.B., Rottenberg, J.: Psychological flexibility as a fundamental aspect of health. Clin. Psychol. Rev. **30**(4), 467–480 (2010)

5. Masuda, A., Tully, E.C.: The role of mindfulness and psychological flexibility in somatization, depression, anxiety, and general psychological distress in a nonclinical college sample. J. Evid.-Based Complement. Altern. Med. **17**(1), 66–71 (2012)
6. Forman, E.M., Herbert, J.D., Moitra, E., Yeomans, P.D., Geller, P.A.: A randomized controlled effectiveness trial of acceptance and commitment therapy and cognitive therapy for anxiety and depression. Behav. Modif. **31**(6), 772–799 (2007)
7. Hofmann, S.G., Sawyer, A.T., Witt, A.A., Oh, D.: The effect of mindfulness-based therapy on anxiety and depression: a meta-analytic review. J. Consult. Clin. Psychol. **78**(2), 169 (2010)
8. Bohlmeijer, E.T., Fledderus, M., Rokx, T.A.J.J., Pieterse, M.E.: Efficacy of an early intervention based on acceptance and commitment therapy for adults with depressive symptomatology: evaluation in a randomized controlled trial. Behav. Res. Ther. **49**(1), 62–67 (2011)
9. Vieten, C., Astin, J.: Effects of a mindfulness-based intervention during pregnancy on prenatal stress and mood: results of a pilot study. Arch. Womens Ment. Health **11**(1), 67–74 (2008)
10. Morris, M.E., Kathawala, Q., Leen, T.K., Gorenstein, E.E., Guilak, F., Labhard, M., et al.: Mobile therapy: case study evaluations of a cell phone application for emotional self-awareness. J. Med. Internet Res. **12**(2), e10 (2010)
11. Harrison, V., Proudfoot, J., Wee, P.P., Parker, G., Pavlovic, D.H., Manicavasagar, V.: Mobile mental health: review of the emerging field and proof of concept study. J. Ment. Health **20**(6), 509–524 (2011)
12. Ly, K.H., Carlbring, P., Andersson, G.: Behavioral activation-based guided self-help treatment administered through a smartphone application: study protocol for a randomized controlled trial. Trials **13**, 62 (2012)
13. Ahtinen, A., Mattila, E., Välkkynen, P., Kaipainen, K., Vanhala, T., Lappalainen, R., et al.: Mobile mental wellness training for stress management: feasibility and design implications based on a one-month field study. JMIR mHealth and uHealth **1**(2), e11 (2013). doi:10.2196/mhealth.2596
14. Lappalainen, R., Sairanen, E., Järvelä, E., Rantala, S., Korpela, R., Kolehmainen, M.: The effectiveness and applicability of different lifestyle interventions for enhancing wellbeing: the study design for a randomized controlled trial for persons with metabolic syndrome risk factors and psychological distress. BMC Public Health **14**(1), 310 (2014)
15. Cavanagh, K.: Turn on, tune in and (don't) drop out: engagement, adherence, attrition and alliance with internet-based interventions. In: Bennett-Levy, J., Richards, D., Farrand, P. (eds.) Oxford Guide to Low Intensity CBT Interventions. OUP Oxford, Oxford (2010)
16. Oivamieli web site. www.oivamieli.fi. Accessed 11 June 2015

Easy Deployment of Spoken Dialogue Technology on Smartwatches for Mental Healthcare

Alexander Prange$^{(\boxtimes)}$ and Daniel Sonntag

German Research Center for Artificial Intelligence (DFKI),
Stuhlsatzenhausweg 3, 66123 Saarbrücken, Germany
{alexander.prange,daniel.sonntag}@dfki.de

Abstract. Smartwatches are becoming increasingly sophisticated and popular as several major smartphone manufacturers, including Apple, have released their new models recently. We believe that these devices can serve as smart objects for people suffering from mental disorders such as memory loss. In this paper, we describe how to utilise smartwatches to create intelligent user interfaces that can be used to provide cognitive assistance in daily life situations of dementia patients. By using automatic speech recognisers and text-to-speech synthesis, we create a dialogue application that allows patients to interact through natural language. We compare several available libraries for Android and show an example of integrating a smartwatch application into an existing healthcare infrastructure.

Keywords: Smartwatch · Speech dialogue · Text-to-speech · Automatic speech recognition · Mental health

1 Introduction

Smartwatches are becoming complex computing devices. Although these wearable computers are still relatively new, they can already compete with smartphones when it comes to processing power and hardware features. An increasing variety of devices is available today as major smartphone manufacturers, such as Samsung or Apple, joined the market and released their new models. Today's smartwatches include features such as quad-core processors, touch screens, bluetooth, wifi, GPS, sensors, cameras and many more. Mobile operating systems with rich user interfaces enabled a wide range of applications, including messengers, games, monitoring and health related apps. With the increasing availability of low-cost smartwatches we believe that they can be utilised to serve as smart objects [1] in the medical domain, and provide assistive functions for people suffering from mental disorders such as dementia.

Dementia is a general term for a decline in mental ability severe enough to interfere with daily life. Alzheimer's is the most common type of dementia. In 2014, the Alzheimer's Association documented that approximately 10–20 % of the population over 65 years of age suffer from mild cognitive impairment (MCI) [3].

© Springer International Publishing Switzerland 2016
S. Serino et al. (Eds.): MindCare 2015, CCIS 604, pp. 150–156, 2016.
DOI: 10.1007/978-3-319-32270-4_15

Memory, thinking, language, understanding, and judgement are affected. While many older adults will remain healthy and productive, overall this segment of the population is subject to cognitive impairment at higher rates than younger people [2]. Smartwatches, when used as intelligent cognitive assistance technologies, may improve the everyday life of older adults.

In this paper we propose the use of smartwatches for the development of dialogues in mental healthcare applications. In the following section we explain our choice of hardware. We compare several available automatic speech recognition (ASR) and text-to-speech (TTS) libraries for Android. We then show an example of how to integrate these smartwatch applications into our existing dialogue platform in the Kognit project.[1]

2   Smartwatches

There are many smartwatch models available from different manufacturers. Although most of them are similar considering size, price and hardware, not all of them are suitable for being used for deployment of spoken dialogue technology or for being integrated into existing healthcare environments. The vast majority of smartwatches is designed to be an accessoire accompanying a smartphone. This means that the watch cannot be used as a standalone device, but has to be connected via Bluetooth to a mobile device. Since almost all of the models have neither built-in wifi nor mobile broadband, the network connection of the smartphone is usually tethered to the smartwatch. According to our experience, these kinds of setups are prone to network errors, resulting in poor connections, address conflicts, and low utility for the target domain.

Another problem is that there are different types of mobile operating systems and not all companies grant developers access or provide a software development kit (SDK). For example, the very first smartwatch we used was running a customised version of Android 2.2 and there was neither access to the Bluetooth API nor to the microphone, although built-in applications used both features. We also tested the Samsung Gear[2] which is running on a Samsung version of the Tizen operating system. Despite the existing SDK, we were not able to implement a complex speech dialogue, because the architecture is based on the fact that the watch has to be connected to the smartphone. The applications themselves consist of a host and a wearable part, and the smartwatch is basically used as a display. Other models, such as the Pebble[3] and Apple Watch[4], have their own operating system. Fortunately, there are also devices that run on the normal Android OS and the newer Android Wear[5], which was specifically designed for smartwatches.

---

[1] http://kognit.dfki.de.

[2] http://www.samsung.com/global/microsite/gear.

[3] http://getpebble.com.

[4] http://www.apple.com/watch.

[5] http://www.android.com/wear.

Our case study for easy deployment of spoken dialogue technology uses the SimValley AW-420.RX smartwatch. In contrast to other smartwatches it comes with Android 4.2.2, wifi and even 3G network connectivity. The built-in microphone and speakers make it ideal for the implementation of speech-based dialogues. Because of the dual-core processor, the 1 GB of RAM, the built-in GPS and the camera, we conjecture a breakthrough in hardware technology for the benefit of our application development; the standard Android operating system makes it easy to deploy existing code and ensure rapid development. Considering the small screen size of smartwatches, it is quite cumbersome for elderly people to interact with the user interface using the conventional touch screen input modality. We therefore decided to use only simple touch gestures and concentrate on implementing a speech dialogue so that users can interact using natural language input.

3   Speech Libraries

There are three important technical parts of a speech dialogue: the ASR, the dialogue manager, and the TTS. In this section we describe the Android libraries for ASR and TTS that we tested and compare them to each other (dialogue management is not covered here, see, e.g., [6]).

3.1   Automatic Speech Recognition

For speech input, we tested the built-in Android API from Google, the commercially available iSpeech[6] platform and the CMU Sphinx[7] speech recognition system developed at CMU. A summary of our results can be found in Table 1; we have chosen these libraries because they work out of the box with Android and contain sample code, allowing for easy and fast development. Moreover, all of them support several different natural languages.

Google and iSpeech are both cloud-based recognisers, meaning that the voice is recorded on the mobile device and then sent to an online API for recognition. In the case of iSpeech the transaction can be done through the HTTP protocol using REST, XML or JSON format. Although the Google Voice API allows the download of offline packages for voice recognition, these can currently only be

Table 1. Comparison of Automatic Speech Recognition (ASR) libraries

	Cloud	Offline	Lang. model	Grammar	Open source	Price
Google	✓	(✓)	(✓)	-	-	Free
iSpeech	✓	-	(✓)	(✓)	(✓)	Paid
CMU Sphinx	-	✓	✓	✓	✓	Free

[6] http://www.ispeech.org.
[7] http://cmusphinx.sourceforge.net/.

used through voice typing with the keyboard. In our experience the speed of the cloud recognisers is fast enough to allow fluent speech dialogues. The recognition of the input takes places in under two seconds for most cases. When used in free-form speech mode, the recognition can however become much slower (according to the length of the input). Google's API can be used with two different language grammars, a free-form grammar and a grammar based on web search terms. The iSpeech API supports free-form models/grammars for most languages and comes with predefined models allowing the recognition of special entity formats such as numbers or addresses. There is no option to use custom grammars with the Google library and iSpeech only provides very limited support, mainly focused on new speech commands. In contrast, the CMU Sphinx speech recognition works completely offline and supports the generation of custom language models and grammars (for mental healthcare applications). We tested the PocketSphinx version, a lightweight speech recognition engine, specifically tuned for handheld and mobile devices. Results were very promising, and the continuous speech input option was particularly useful for developing speech dialogues for inexperienced users such as patients. Unlike iSpeech, which has an open source SDK but proprietary online recognisers, the PocketSphinx recogniser is fully accessible under the BSD license.

3.2   Text-to-Speech

Text-to-Speech (TTS) synthesis is a substantial part of speech dialogue systems, providing the output in natural speech. We investigate five different solutions available for the Android operating system: Google, SVOX (Pico and Classic), iSpeech and IVONA[8]. In 2009 Google included the SVOX Pico TTS into the 1.6 release of the Android platform, making it the standard TTS engine found in most Android devices. The SVOX company also released higher quality, paid versions in many different languages (SVOX Classic). Google recently made their own Text-to-Speech engine available through the play store and their online API. The previously mentioned iSpeech framework also features cloud-based speech synthesis in different languages. A relatively new system was introduced by IVONA and is currently available for free in beta testing. The features are summarised in Table 2.

Table 2. Comparison of *Text-to-Speech* (TTS) libraries

	Cloud	Offline	Quality	Price
Google	✓	✓	+	Free
SVOX Pico	-	✓	-	Free
SVOX Classic	-	✓	+	Paid ($2.99 per language)
iSpeech	✓	-	++	Paid ($0.01 per word)
IVONA	✓	✓	++	Free (Beta)

[8] http://www.ivona.com/.

Except for the iSpeech synthesiser, all TTS engines are available in offline mode. Required language models can be easily downloaded and stored on the device. Android itself has a built-in settings menu to chose from different engines and languages. The options we evaluated are easily accessible through the play store or, in case of iSpeech, through a SDK. Coding effort is minimal, and there are many sample applications available, making the implementation of speech output on Android very simple. All of the tested libraries provide many different languages and often feature both female and male voices. However, there are differences in the quality of the speech synthesis. Especially for patient-centric dialogue systems it is of great importance that the speech output sounds as natural as possible, providing best user experience. While the standard SVOX Pico voice sounds very robotic, their premium SVOX Classic series has better quality and the speaking pace is very nice. The results are similar to the Google TTS, but the voices sound even more clear and natural. Our tests suggest that sometimes words are still synthesised in a robotic voice, making the voices still sound unnatural and confusing. In our preliminary experiments in the test lab (without real patients), the most natural sounding voices are found to be iSpeech and IVONA.

4   Application Scenario

The smartwatch is used in the Kognit framework as a mobile interaction device that is always available wherever the patient goes. Patients can communicate with the smartwatch in natural language as it has a speech recognition, dialogue management, and synthesis functionality integrated. In [4] we introduced the use of NAO, a humanoid robot, as a companion to the dementia patient in order to continuously monitor his or her activities and provide cognitive assistance in daily life situations. The NAO companion could be further instrumented to keep track of real world objects (like keys or glasses) during everyday life activities. In our new scenario, we use the robot's built-in cameras together with eye-tracking technology to perform object recognition [5]. For instance in case the patient forgets where he or she has put the glasses, the smartwatch would locate them by tracing the location in the server-side memory. It would then display the location on the screen and provide audio feedback (see Fig. 1).

Since we have different components that all run on distinct operating systems, we need a reliable network communication that works well cross-platform. This is why we are using XML-RPC, a remote procedure call protocol which uses HTTP to transport XML encoded calls and works great on various devices. All components (clients) communicate through the Kognit proxy (see Fig. 2) which is running on a desktop computer. The smartwatch dialogue functionality is seamlessly integrated into the existing framework due to its networking capabilities. Currently, we are using HTTP REST requests to the cloud-based iSpeech API for speech recognition. For the Text-to-Speech synthesis, we use the offline IVONA engine. In our scenario, all data is collected in the multimodal dialogue memory from which relevant information for dialogue management can

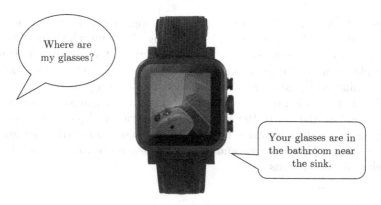

Fig. 1. Scenario example

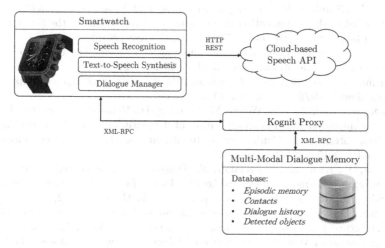

Fig. 2. Technical architecture

be retrieved. In the case of our "lost glasses" example, the NAO robot keeps track of the glasses and stored their last location in the database. During the speech dialogue, the smartwatch can be used to ask for navigation help to provide cognitive assistance to the patient.

5 Conclusions and Future Work

We discussed available smartwatch APIs for developing speech dialogues in mental healthcare applications. We described the integration of the smartwatch into our existing Kognit project, where we try to offer support through non-pharmacological treatments in daily life situations.[9] We conclude that the choice

---

[9] http://www.spry.org/pdf/cbtcoa_english.pdf.

of speech recognition and synthesis libraries is highly dependent on the application's context and provide help for choosing the right platform. Our next steps will be to use the smartwatch in conjunction with a complex multimodal dialogue platform to produce advanced context-aware multimodal dialogue applications, similar to the approaches presented in [6,7] using smartphones. Multimodal fusion and fission processes [8] are currently investigated. Future research will also evaluate the use of the smartwatch camera for object recognition and the analysis of the data provided by the built-in sensors for activity recognition. Smartwatches are highly mobile and promising devices for the rapid deployment of speech dialogue systems.

References

1. Weber, M., Schulz, C.H., Sonntag, D., Toyama, T.: Digital pens as smart objects in multimodal medical application frameworks. In: Proceedings of the Second Workshop on Interacting with Smart Objects. ACM Press (2013)
2. Pollack, M.: Intelligent technology for an aging population: The use of AI to assist elders with cognitive impairment. AI Mag. **26**(2), 9–24 (2005)
3. Alzheimer's Association, 2014 Alzheimer's Disease Facts and Figures. http://www.alz.org/downloads/facts_figures_2014.pdf
4. Prange, A., Sandrala, I.P., Weber, M., Sonntag, D.: Robot companions and smartpens for improved social communication of dementia patients. In: Proceedings of the 20th International Conference on Intelligent User Interfaces Companion (IUI Companion 2015) (2015)
5. Toyama, T., Kieninger, T., Shafait, F., Dengel, A.: Gaze guided object recognition using a head-mounted eye tracker. In: Proceedings of the Symposium on Eye Tracking Research and Applications, pp. 91–98. ACM Press (2012)
6. Sonntag, D., Schulz, C.H.: Multimodal multi-device discourse and dialogue infrastructure for collaborative decision making in medicine. In: Proceedings of the International Workshop on Spoken Dialogue Systems Technology, IWSDS12. Springer (2012)
7. Sonntag, D., Engel, R., Herzog, G., Pfalzgraf, A., Pfleger, N., Romanelli, M., Reithinger, N.: SmartWeb handheld — Multimodal interaction with ontological knowledge bases and semantic web services. In: Huang, T.S., Nijholt, A., Pantic, M., Pentland, A. (eds.) ICMI/IJCAI Workshops 2007. LNCS (LNAI), vol. 4451, pp. 272–295. Springer, Heidelberg (2007)
8. Wahlster, W.: Towards symmetric multimodality: fusion and fission of speech, gesture, and facial expression. In: Günter, A., Kruse, R., Neumann, B. (eds.) KI 2003. LNCS (LNAI), vol. 2821, pp. 1–18. Springer, Heidelberg (2003)

Higher Immersive Tendency in Male University Students with Excessive Online Gaming

Dooyoung Jung[1,2(✉)], Eun Young Kim[3], Seong Hoon Jeong[4], and Bong-Jin Hahm[1,2]

[1] Department of Neuropsychiatry, Seoul National University Hospital, Seoul, Republic of Korea
{dooyoung,hahm}@snu.ac.kr
[2] Department of Psychiatry and Behavioral Sciences,
Seoul National University College of Medicine, Seoul, Republic of Korea
[3] Mental Health Clinic, National Cancer Center, Goyang, Republic of Korea
npeunyoung@gmail.com
[4] Department of Psychiatry, Eulji University School of Medicine, Eulji University Hospital,
Daejeon, Republic of Korea
anselmjeong@gmail.com

Abstract. Although problems with online game use are gaining concerns, high-risk traits associated with excessive online gaming are not yet understood. Immersive tendency was suggested as the personality trait to behave playfully and to become involved in continuous stimuli. Because immersive tendency can be assessed through everyday activities, it may be used to find a risk group for excessive online gaming. We investigated the difference in immersive tendency, problematic online gaming, and problematic Internet use between 21 male university students with excessive online gaming and 21 matched controls. Higher immersive tendency was observed in participants with excessive online gaming. The immersive tendency can reflect an individual's susceptibility to excessive online gaming.

Keywords: Immersive tendency · Excessive online gaming · Internet gaming disorder · Problematic online gaming · Problematic internet use

1 Introduction

With the increase of impact the internet has on everyday life, problems with the Internet have become serious. Among them, excessive online gaming has gained concern as a public mental health problem in some countries, especially in older adolescent and young adult males. Due to shared properties with addictive behaviors, the American Psychiatric Association included Internet gaming disorder (IGD) in Sect. 3, 'Conditions for Further Study' of the *Diagnostic and Statistical Manual of Mental Disorders* (Fifth Edition) in 2013 [1].

Although several psychiatric conditions are known to be a risk factor in addicted gamers such as attention deficit hyperactivity disorder and depression, findings on personality trait were inconsistent. Because relations between personality and game are dependent on the motivations for the game, specific personality type does not seem to

© Springer International Publishing Switzerland 2016
S. Serino et al. (Eds.): MindCare 2015, CCIS 604, pp. 157–161, 2016.
DOI: 10.1007/978-3-319-32270-4_16

be a susceptible trait to excessive online gaming [2]. On the other hand, user experiences in a massively multiplayer online role-playing game played an important role in predicting game addiction [3]. Witmer and Singer [4] defined presence as the person's experience of being there in a mediated environment and immersive tendency as a personal trait to experience presence. Immersive tendency is the trait to behave playfully and to become involved in a continuous stream of stimuli [5]. Because the immersive tendency questionnaire rates the trait based on the experiences from everyday activities such as playing sports, watching movies, reading novels, and dreaming, it can be a valuable tool in finding risk factors prior to exposure to online games.

In a study with massively multiplayer online role-playing game players, immersive tendency showed a significant association with addiction [6]. However, there was no study on the immersive tendency in game players, in which the comorbid psychiatric conditions were investigated separately. The aim of the present study was to evaluate the difference in immersive tendency between excessive online gamers and controls without the confounding effects of psychiatric comorbidities.

2   Methods

From two high-ranking universities in Seoul, male undergraduate students aged 19–29 years were recruited for a study on the physiologic change during experimental action video game via advertisements on campus. The monetary reward was approximately 50 dollars. None of the participants was majoring in sports or related fields. In a previous study, 22 participants with excessive online gaming were matched with 22 healthy controls for sex, age, and body mass index [7]. Based on the operational criteria [8], excessive online gamers were defined as follows: maladaptive preoccupation, distress, Young's Internet Addiction Test (YIAT) score over 50 [9], at least four hour daily computer gaming, and absence of another Axis I psychiatric disorder associated with excessive computer usage. A psychiatrist interviewed the participants to screen for psychiatric disorder and rated the severity of depression using the Montgomery–Åsberg Depression Rating Scale to exclude participants with significant depression [10]. Before the participants were exposed to the experimental game, packets of self-report questionnaires were administered. In this study, we analyzed the difference between 21 excessive online gamers and 21 control participants who completed whole questionnaires.

Problematic Internet use was evaluated with YIAT which includes 20 items and ranges from 20 to 100. YIAT examines symptoms such as preoccupation with Internet use, controllability of online use and continued online use despite consequences [11]. Cronbach's α was 0.91.

Problematic Internet use was also assessed with Korea Internet Addiction Scale (KIAS) which comprises 20 items and ranges from 20 to 80 [12]. KIAS assesses psychosocial function, reality testing, addictive automatic thought, withdrawal, virtual interpersonal relationship, deviant behavior, and tolerance [13]. Cronbach's α was between 0.89 and 0.91.

Problematic online gaming was measured with Korea Internet Game Addiction Questionnaire (KIGAQ) which includes 20 items and ranges from 20 to 80 [14]. KIGAQ examines daily life, withdrawal, and pursuing a virtual relationship. Cronbach's α was 0.93.

Immersive tendency was rated with the Immersive Tendency Questionnaire (ITQ) which consists of 18 items and ranges from 0 to 108 [4]. ITQ measures the tendency towards immersion in everyday activities (e.g., "Do you easily become deeply involved in movies or TV dramas?", "How good are you at blocking out external distractions when you are involved in something?", "Do you ever have dreams that are so real that you feel disoriented when you awake?"). Cronbach's α was 0.81.

SPSS for Windows, version 21.0 (SPSS Inc., Chicago, IL, USA) was used for statistical analysis. Continuous variables were analyzed with independent samples t-test and Mann–Whitney U tests for group differences. Categorical variables were analyzed by Pearson's chi-square test and Fisher's exact test. Relationships among variables were analyzed with Pearson's correlation analysis.

3   Results

Table 1 shows participants' characteristics. There were no significant differences in age, body mass index, smoking, and alcohol consumption between excessive online gamers and controls. Excessive online gamers scored significantly higher in problematic Internet use and problematic online gaming.

Table 1. Participants' characteristics

	Excessive online gamer (n = 21)	Control (n = 21)	P-value
Age, years, mean (SD)	22.81 (2.36)	23.52 (2.52)	0.155
BMI, kg/m², mean (SD)	22.96 (2.02)	22.81 (3.18)	0.858
Smoker/non-smoker, No. of subjects	5/16	3/18	0.697
<10 cigarettes per day	1	1	
10–15 cigarettes per day	4	2	
Moderate-heavy/non-light drinker, no. of subjects	10/11	14/7	0.212
3–14 drinks per week	7	13	
>14 drinks per week	3	1	
YIAT total score, mean (SD)	70.86 (11.83)	31.48 (7.41)	<0.001
KIAS total score, mean (SD)	54.14 (10.14)	30.14 (5.43)	<0.001
KIAGQ total score, mean (SD)	43.14 (10.08)	21.86 (2.89)	<0.001

BMI, body mass index; YIAT, Young's Internet Addiction Test; KIAS, Korea Internet Addiction Scale; KIGAQ, Korea Internet Game Addiction Questionnaire.

Excessive online gamers showed a significantly higher immersive tendency, which was rated with ITQ, than controls (Table 2).

Table 2. Higher immersive tendency in excessive online gamer

	N	Df	Mean	SD	t-value calculated	P-value
Excessive online gamer	21	40	60.00	17.83	3.707	<0.001
Control	21		41.90	13.51		

Immersive tendency demonstrated significant relationships with problematic online gaming and problematic Internet use (Table 3).

Table 3. Pearson's correlation analysis of immersive tendency, problematic internet use, and problematic online gaming

	1	2	3
1. ITQ	1		
2. YIAT	0.63	1	
3. KIAS	0.69	0.94	1
4. KIAGS	0.55	0.92	0.93

ITQ, Immersive Tendency Questionnaire; YIAT, Young's Internet Addiction Test; KIAS, Korea Internet Addiction Scale; KIGAQ, Korea Internet Game Addiction Questionnaire.

All Pearson's rs are significant ($P < 0.001$).

4   Conclusion

To the best of our knowledge, this study is the first report demonstrating higher immersive tendency in excessive online gamers without comorbid psychiatric conditions. The findings are similar with the previous study of massively multiplayer online role-playing game players, in which addicted players scored higher immersive tendency than high-engaged gamers [6]. However, comorbid mental health conditions were not assessed in previous studies on immersive tendency. Because psychiatric comorbidity is very high in patients with excessive online gaming, mental health evaluation is very important. Due to the debates on IGD as a distinct disease entity, IGD was not included in non-substance-related disorders but in 'Conditions for Further Study' of the *Diagnostic and Statistical Manual of Mental Disorders* (Fifth Edition). In the current study, we recruited young adults from high-ranking universities without other psychiatric disorders to exclude other possible confounders.

In the previous study with the same participants, reduced cardiorespiratory coupling during gameplay was observed in excessive online gamers, implicating central autonomic dysregulation [7]. These differences may reflect altered central inhibitory control over the autonomic response to pleasurable stimuli. In the present analysis, excessive online gamers reported higher immersive tendency, which reflects an individual's characteristic to behave playfully and to become involved in a continuous stream of stimuli [5]. Because ITQ examines the trait through everyday activities, the immersive tendency can be used to evaluate an individual's susceptibility to IGD without gaming exposure.

With the same reasons, the immersive tendency may reflect common susceptibility regardless of gaming context and motivation.

There are some limitations to this study. The sample size is small for generalization. Further study is needed with the large population with the different gender. There is no standard diagnosis instrument for IGD. To overcome this problem, we used three different assessment tools for comparison. Although ITQ assesses personality traits through everyday activities, the immersive tendency was not examined before the gaming exposure and we cannot conclude the causal relation. Further longitudinal studies are needed to determine causality.

Acknowledgements. This study was supported by grants from the National Research Foundation of Korea (NRF-2010-0010632) and the Seoul National University Hospital (04-2013-0710).

References

1. American Psychiatric Association: Diagnostic and statistical manual of mental disorders, 5th edn. American Psychiatric Association, Arlington (2013)
2. Graham, L.T., Gosling, S.D.: Personality profiles associated with different motivations for playing World of Warcraft. Cyberpsychol. Behav. Soc. Netw. **16**, 189–193 (2013)
3. Hsu, S.H., Wen, M.-H., Wu, M.-C.: Exploring user experiences as predictors of MMORPG addiction. Comput. Educ. **53**, 990–999 (2009)
4. Witmer, B.G., Singer, M.J.: Measuring presence in virtual environments: a presence questionnaire. Presence Teleop. Virtual **7**, 225–240 (1998)
5. Wallach, H.S., Safir, M.P., Samana, R.: Personality variables and presence. Virtual Real **14**, 3–13 (2010)
6. Lehenbauer-Baum, M., Fohringer, M.: Towards classification criteria for internet gaming disorder: debunking differences between addiction and high engagement in a German sample of World of Warcraft player. Comput. Hum. Behav. **45**, 345–351 (2015)
7. Chang, J.S., Kim, E.Y., Jung, D., Jeong, S.H., Kim, Y., Roh, M.S., Ahn, Y.M., Hahm, B.J.: Altered cardiorespiratory coupling in young male adults with excessive online gaming. Biol. Psychol. **110**, 159–166 (2015)
8. Shapira, N.A., Lessig, M.C., Goldsmith, T.D., Szabo, S.T., Lazoritz, M., Gold, M.S., Stein, D.J.: Problematic internet use: proposed classification and diagnostic criteria. Depression Anxiety **17**, 207–216 (2003)
9. Young, K.S.: Caught in the Net: How to Recognize the Signs of Internet Addiction—And a Winning Strategy For Recovery. Wiley, New York (1998)
10. Montgomery, S.A., Asberg, M.: A new depression scale designed to be sensitive to change. Br. J. Psychiatry **134**, 382–389 (1979)
11. Young, K.S.: Cognitive behavior therapy with Internet addicts: treatment outcomes and implications. Cyberpsychol. Behav. **10**, 671–679 (2007)
12. Kim, D.: The follow up study of internet addiction proneness scale. Korea Agency for Digital Opportunity and Promotion, Seoul (2008)
13. Park, J.W., Park, K.H., Lee, I.J., Kwon, M., Kim, D.J.: Standardization study of internet addiction improvement motivation scale. Psychiatry Investig. **9**, 373–378 (2012)
14. Korea Agency for Digital Opportunity and Promotion: A Study of the Development of Internet Game Addiction Scale for Children and Adolescents. KADO Publisher, Seoul (2006)

Cognitive Problems and Old Age

Study of EEG Power Fluctuations Enhanced by Linguistic Stimulus for Cognitive Decline Screening

Sofia Segkouli[1,3(✉)], Ioannis Paliokas[1], Dimitrios Tzovaras[1],
Magda Tsolaki[2], and Charalampos Karagiannidis[3]

[1] Information Technologies Institute, CERTH, Thessaloniki, Greece
`{sofia,ipaliokas,dimitrios.tzovaras}@iti.gr`
[2] Greek Association of Alzheimer's Disease and Related Disorders,
Thessaloniki, Greece
`tsolakiml@ath.forthnet.gr`
[3] Department of Special Education, University of Thessaly, Volos, Greece
`karagian@uth.gr`

Abstract. Relative Electroencephalography (EEG) power can reflect cognitive decline and play a critical diagnostic role for dementia onset. The current paper investigates power changes in EEG channels on elderly people having Mild Cognitive Impairment (MCI) during a linguistic test. The main objective was to identify patterns in EEG power changes during a linguistically enriched cognitive assessment test which involved working memory abilities, selective attention and perception. Groups of MCI, demented and healthy controls were recruited to take part in an experiment. It was found that MCI and demented patients showed significantly different patterns in delta and theta frequency bands during the linguistic tasks. Results are valuable in the study of the way brain processes linguistic information in people with cognitive impairment and in screening assessment procedures.

Keywords: EEG · MCI · Dementia · Neurolinguistics · Linguistic test

1 Introduction

Increasing attention has been paid in recent years to early Mild Cognitive Impairment (MCI) detection, as well as identifying subjects with high possibility to progress to Dementia. Only a portion of MCI positives will progress to dementia· some remain stable cognitive, while others recover full function [1]. In this clinical context, existing diagnostic and prediction methods rely on neuropsychological assessment tools as the Boston Naming Test (BNT) [2], AD biomarkers [3], auditory ERP responses [4] and other approaches proposed in the literature [5].

Recently, studies on language-based assessment tests have been developed [6] and ongoing research is targeting on cerebral EEG rhythms to reflect underlying brain network activity. Moreover, most EEG-related studies conduct recordings in resting state, thereby keeping the role of language in relation to EEG monitoring degraded. The current paper targets to investigate the response of language impairments on EEG

© Springer International Publishing Switzerland 2016
S. Serino et al. (Eds.): MindCare 2015, CCIS 604, pp. 165–175, 2016.
DOI: 10.1007/978-3-319-32270-4_17

power fluctuations. An experiment was conducted to create evidence of the relation among literal components and non-literal figures of speech by MCI patients and the corresponding predictive features of EEG bands activity. The objectives can be summarized as follows:

Objective 1: Identify specific patterns of oscillations in the power of EEG frequency bands during literal expressions of language
Objective 2: Detect for significant differences in power changes between MCI, Demented and healthy elderly groups during non-literal language processing.

Previous Work on EEG signal processing has a great success in identifying demented and MCI patients [7]. Evidence-based medicine (EBM) research has pointed out that EEG power profiles are different for MCI, Demented and healthy controls at rest conditions [8]. Poil et al. [9] worked on multiple EEG biomarker models to predict progressive conversion from MCI to Dementia. This raises the question: *What can foster existing EEG features and extrude the differences between MCI/Demented and healthy control profiles?*

Some researchers study language performance in still resting states [10]. Others pay attention to specific language characteristics like syntactic and lexical features [11], or make use of various kinds of stimulus in order to enhance differences among neuro-generative diseases with promising results. Olichney et al. for example, found that category-decision tasks can actually raise differences in band waveforms [12]. Kandiah et al. [6] aimed at a linguistic MCI detection test for multilingual populations, concentrating mainly on overcoming the need of translation and cultural adaptation by using linguistic stimuli on EEG monitoring sessions.

Single frequency bands may not be the only feature affected in EEG screening tests, but relations between frequency bands may be affected as well. It has been found that the theta-to-gamma ration of relative EEG power is significantly correlated with memory decline for MCI and AD patients [13]. Theta relative power and Alpha reactivity seem to be associated with decreased performance in various cognitive domains like global cognition, language, memory and executive functioning [14].

Most of the studies exploit the potential of EEG to separate MCI patients which develop AD (Progressive MCI) from those which do not develop AD (Stable MCI) [15, 16], but not emphasizing on language assessment. This study will investigate if existing MCI screening instruments could evolve to more advanced mixed stimuli-EEG tests by taking advantage of the evidence-based abnormalities in the EEG spectrum.

2   Materials and Methods

In the proposed diagnostic model, complicated MRI or Magnetoencephalography (MEG) signal processing would not be necessary as long as determining functionality of specific localizing regions of the brain is not a priority. The main idea was not to find locations of abnormalities in human brain of MCI users, but to detect different patterns of brain activity under linguistic stimulus.

A group of elderly people were voluntarily invited to EEG monitoring sessions enhanced by linguistic stimulus. A computerized proof-of-concept testbed was created for that purpose. The stimulus consisted of verbal descriptions of everyday activities, starting from simple object naming tasks to more advanced linguistic tasks like semantic and metaphoric meaning processing.

2.1 Inclusive Criteria and Recruitment of Participants

Participants consisted of twenty one (N = 21) elderly people, ten MCI positives and three with mild Dementia based on their medical records. MCI symptoms were validated by a confirmatory MCI test given the same day (Boston Naming Test, 30-item even version). Participants were recruited from local day care organizations, while the MCI patients from the Greek Association of Alzheimer's Disease and Related Disorders. Recruitment criteria for MCI positives included typical symptoms of amnestic MCI (aMCI), but not Dementia. Participants had to be at least 60 years old, eligible and free of medication.

2.2 Used Tools

The available hardware equipment consisted of a desktop computer running the hosted application, a wearable EEG biosensor unit and a Bluetooth dongle. The sensor unit, equipped with a dry sensor, was comfortably fitted on the *Fp1* electrode scalp location, according to the international standard electrode position system '10–20' and the American Electroencephalographic Society nomenclature [17]. EEG was recorded at 512 Hz sampling rate at 12 bits ADC resolution and transmitted from the wireless wearable unit to the hosted application (~ 1 m) at a RF data rate of 250 kbit/s. Relative EEG power was analyzed after preprocessing to remove interferences from power network and adjacent 50 Hz electrical equipment (firmware filtering). Invalid datasets in which band powers appeared as null numbers (zeros) due to bad sensor-sculpt contact were removed from the samples. Timestamp annotation and the recording of user's responses were made in real time, while EEG data from in between linguistic task periods was ignored.

The software used for logging the user's activity and EEG frequency bands (developed in-house) was engineered with the SDK provided by the manufacturer of the EEG headset (NeuroSky), COM port simulation libraries to access the Bluetooth-enabled device and Delphi IDE for GUI design to deliver a windows desktop implementation.

2.3 Experimental Conditions and Procedure

The overall procedure was in line with the ethical committee of the hosted institution and it was safe and comfortable for the participants. Just before the actual testing, participants had a short introduction on the scopes of the experiment and a short demonstration of how the EEG sensor has to be properly fitted in the forehead. The test was not self-administered in order to ensure that variations in computer-driving abilities will not affect results.

2.4   Cognitive Tasks and Linguistic Stimulus

Participants were asked to perform a typical BNT test in order to monitor EEG fluctuations during object naming ability. In this study, BNT represents the simple linguistic stimulus, while the advanced one has three distinct parts concerning the literal and non-literal understanding and production ability of lexical components.

The content of the first text included sentences verbs and nouns underlined in order to be transmitted in the proper corresponding component. Sentences were semantically correlated constituting a whole paragraph with comprehending meaning. In Table 1 two examples from each part of the test are presented as a reference.

Table 1. Examples of the advanced linguistic test

Section		Statement	Fill in the blank
Part A	A1	'Every morning I enjoy my coffee in my beautiful balcony'.	_ It is a ... to drink my coffee every morning in my beautiful balcony
	A2	'There I created a green oasis to be as beautiful as possible'.	_ The ... of a green oasis was made to be as much as possible beautiful space
Part B	B1	'I avoid frying while cooking'.	_ When I cook, I avoid to ....
	B2	'After having finished all other tasks, she wiped the counter in order to be dry'.	_ The ... of clothes becomes faster in the summer sun.
Part C	C1	'The ocean of his mind was awash with new ideas'.	_ ... may be composed of water or other elements and compounds
	C2	'His mom each morning squeezes oranges to make him juice'.	_ A ... my mind but I could not find the right word to say.

The statements in part A were used as a stimulus to record the nouns derived from verbs or verb roots and reverse. Verb fluency appears, on the basis of these results, to be a possible linguistic marker for the progression from Subjective Cognitive Impairment (SCI) to MCI [18]. In this task patients had to retrieve and produce concrete nouns that derived or not from verbs' roots.

In the second section (part B) the same task was provided through sentences that have semantically different meaning. Verbs' production ability has been assessed in the absence of external stimuli [19]. Broader areas of the brain are involved in retrieving verbs [20].

In the last part (part C) semantic implicated words and semantic connotations, metaphors are used in order to detect semantic and lexical deficits. Non literal figurative language expression is affected in demented populations. In the present task, filling in and interpreting non-literal sentences seems a daunting one task for this population [21].

3 Results of EEG Analysis with Linguistic Stimuli

Because the EEG headset was quite stiff and the dry sensor mounted on it was sensitive to head movements, especially the vertical ones, very noisy recordings were removed from the pool. This resulted to twenty one (N = 21) valid recordings, eight coming from the MCI, three from demented and another ten from the healthy elderly. Due to the fact that subjects completed the test in their own times, log recordings had varying lengths. The length of the EEG data used in the log analysis was limited by the shortest sample, starting from the beginning of the EEG recordings.

3.1 Demographics

Participants were 67.10 year old in average (SD = 4.54) and fairly balanced in both sexes (57 % females, 43 % males). Half of the participants had completed high school (50 %) and almost one third were of university level (35 %). The rest 15 % stated Elementary Education completed. Demographic information is presented in Table 2 along with the results of the BNT and the advanced linguistic test.

Table 2. Demographics and linguistic test results

Parameters	Groups of participants			Total
	Healthy elderly	MCI	Mild dementia	
N	10	8	3	21
Sex M/F	6/4	4/4	2/1	12/9
Age (in years)	66.20 ± 2.89	67.38 ± 7.81	65.33 ± 3.78	66.52 ± 5.21
30BNT score	25.90 ± 1.19	23.13 ± 3.35	20.33 ± 3.78	24.05 ± 3.18
Linguistic test-total	16.08 ± 1.5	14.75 ± 2.21	12.66 ± 1.15	15.44 ± 1.85
Linguistic test-Part A	5.42 ± 0.99	5.00 ± 1.41	4.50 ± 0.71	5.22 ± 1.06
Linguistic test-Part B	5.33 ± 0.88	5.00 ± 1.41	5.00 ± 0	5.22 ± 0.94
Linguistic test-Part C	5.33 ± 0.49	4.75 ± 0.50	3.50 ± 0.71	5.00 ± 0.76

3.2 Cognition Assessment

In the most typical form, 30BNT scores include the correct answers given spontaneously without any help, those given after 30 s with semantic help and lastly the number of correct answers after another 30 s with phonemic help. For the sake of simplicity, the number of rights answers without any help (first number in BNT test result triplex) was considered the critical variable to distinct the MCI group (M = 21.00 ± 5.29) from the healthy elderly (M = 25.89 ± 1.05).

Concerning the results of the linguistic test itself, in average, healthy elderly achieved better results (M = 16.08 ± 1.5) than MCI testers (M = 14.75 ± 2.21) and demented (M = 12.66 ± 1.15). A one-way analysis of variance was calculated on testers' results (ANOVA). The analysis was marginally significant with $F(2,19) = 3.55$ (p = .05), but an interesting finding was found on the part C results. The scores of participants on the third part of the linguistic test was statistically significant with F (2,19) = 11.65 (p < .001). The processing of the metaphoric meanings of words was more demanding for MCI and demented people.

3.3 EEG Band Monitoring on BNT Test

In this section, the results of EEG band power analysis are presented (Table 3). After normality tests, the followed statistical tests reported a significant difference between cognitive groups as determined by the one-way analysis of variance (ANOVA) test with F(2,21) = 11.94 (p < .001) for Delta band and F(2,21) = 8.18 (p < .05) for Theta band.

Table 3. EEG power bands* during BNT and the proposed Linguistic test

Parameters	Healthy elderly		MCI		Mild dementia	
	BNT	Ling	BNT	Ling	BNT	Ling
AlphaLow (8–9 Hz)	32104 (±8837)	34729 (±8532)	39848 (±13040)	33951 (±13706)	23952 (±8992)	31166 (±7881)
AlphaHigh (10–12 Hz)	25606 (±7066)	28279 (±7113)	32234 (±9154)	28005 (±10514)	15933 (±786)	18465 (±6121)
BetaLow (13–17 Hz)	23033 (±6648)	25487 (±9418)	25576 (±8510)	24202 (±8810)	13984 (±1947)	16566 (±2545)
BetaHigh (18–30 Hz)	22578 (±6849)	24450 (±8456)	26625 (±8536)	24830 (±9277)	11862 (±2890)	16627 (±9735)
GamaLow (31–40 Hz)	15710 (±6992)	18262 (±7423)	19661 (±10629)	19080 (±10706)	6891 (±2916)	12519 (±9191)
GamaHigh (41–50 Hz)	7772 (±3764)	8909 (±3715)	8859 (±5092)	8303 (±3868)	3408 (±1428)	6358 (±4310)
Delta (0.1–3 Hz)	633633 (±192611)	698421 (±276600)	723693 (±149335)	624907 (±239170)	163452 (±89855)	304342 (±67961)
Theta (4–7 Hz)	137610 (±33351)	150567 (±62269)	165826 (±60226)	154284 (±61949)	46684 (±10164)	68412 (±4536)

*In ASIC EEG power units [22]

Weaker results, but still significant, were found on the high frequency bands of Alpha (F(2,19) = 5.14, p < .05) and Beta (F(2,21) = 4.47, p < .05). A Tukey post-hoc test revealed that the band power of Delta was statistically significantly lower in demented subjects (163452 ± 89855, p < .001) compared to the healthy elderly (633633 ± 192611). Delta band results of MCI testers (723693 ± 149335) did not have significant differences compared to the other two groups although their results were closer to healthy elderly.

For the Theta frequency band, for which the Homogeneity of Variances was not assumed, a Games-Howell test indicated that in demented people (46684 ± 10164) the power was significantly lower than both healthy elderly (137610 ± 33351, p < .001) and MCI testers (165826 ± 60226, p < .05).

3.4   EEG Band Monitoring with Advanced Linguistic Test

EEG power histograms were normally distributed, except Delta band which marginally failed to meet the normality condition (possibly caused by the biosensor's unit signal filtering). Its bimodality was attributed to a dual peaks feature and not platykurtosis, so finally it was not excluded from the ANOVA test which is quite robust in non-normal distributions. No correlation was found between EEG bands and age, but they were found highly correlated with each other with Pearson's correlation coefficients lying in the range [.764, .955] with average M = .861 in $p < .001$.

For EEG data from all frequency bands, which meet the homogeneity of variances assumption given by Levene's test, the Tukey HSD test was used for post-hoc to tell which specific groups differed in which EEG frequency bands. In the next step, the one-way ANOVA test was performed to determine if there are any statistically significant differences among EEG band powers in the three groups. The one-way ANOVA test was applied, having EEG power bands as dependent variables and the cognitive condition (Healthy, MCI, and Demented) as an independent categorical variable. In general, EEG strength was found lower in demented people than in MCI and healthy controls in most frequency bands.

The ANOVA results revealed statistically significant differences in Delta band power among state of cognition groups $F(2,19) = 3$, ($p < .5$). Healthy people (M = 698421 ± 27660) were not very different than MCI (M = 624907 ± 239170), but quite higher than demented (M = 621292 ± 273155). There were also only marginal differences on the Theta power band $F(2,19) = 2.6$ ($p = .09$) which show a similar to the BNT results trend, in which demented people have lower band power. A similar trend was observed in EEG data coming from demented people. Power was found weak (M = 50723 ± 7453) in comparison to the healthy elderly (M = 158524 ± 62444), but this cannot be taken into account as a valid dementia separator.

In overall, plots of EEG recordings (Fig. 1) during simple linguistic stimuli (object naming in BNT) locate MCI users on the top of other groups, while EEG activity is seriously reduced on people with mild dementia. On the other hand, the presence of advanced linguistic stimuli cause EEG power signals to correct the slope of the line and follow a downhill route from healthy cognition to Dementia.

4   Discussion

Language and cultural dependencies of this approach can be diminished by designing the task material with simplicity and focus on EEG analysis. The proposed linguistic test, provided as stimuli for EEG signal analysis and not as a screening test itself, can be easily translated to major international and local languages, without significant loss in its usefulness to distinct patterns in EEG power fluctuations. This study showed that features in EEG power band oscillations can be detected under a linguistic stimulus, either simple or advanced. The most common pattern was the decrease in power bands detected on lower frequencies and more specifically on the Delta and Theta bands (Objective 1). In some degree Alpha and Beta were affected too, but no strong patterns were found in either frequency bands.

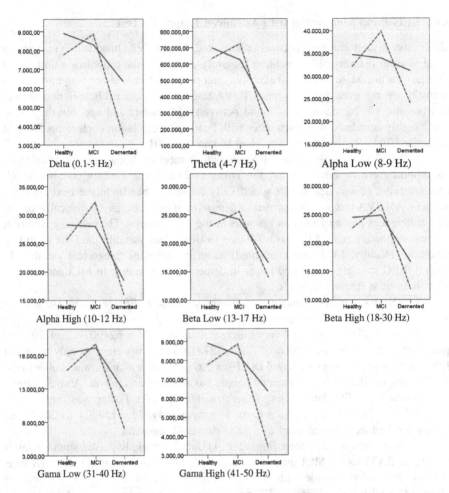

Fig. 1. Mean plots of the EEG bands power (in ASIC EEG power units [22]) of the healthy elderly, MCI positives and demented people groups during the BNT test (green dotted line) and the advanced linguistic stimuli (blue solid line) (Color figure online)

The strong linguistic stimuli showed that MCI, demented and controls actually have significant differences in EEG power fluctuations (Objective 2). Delta and Theta bands were equal or slightly higher in MCI, but clearly reduced in demented people. Also, MCI preserved the average power of EEG bands in most cases and no significant difference was found in comparison to the healthy elderly. On the contrast, demented people showed strong evidence that their EEG pattern is significantly different than others, especially in lower frequencies (Delta & Theta bands).

A systematic benchmarking on the findings may not be possible due to known difficulties in gaining access to EEG databases from MCI and AD patients and to different experimental conditions applied in various studies (scull locations, EEG frequency bands and cognitive states). Some of the most similar studies can confirm that

Beta band is stronger in controls [8], age is not affecting EEG power spectrum in any way [23] and that Delta band reveals a larger response for health controls than MCI subjects ([24].

5 Conclusion

In contrast with traditional approaches in neuropsychological tests, which tend to avoid linguistic tasks due to their language and cultural limitations, the proposed task aims to able language users to measure the inclination in cognition quantified as EEG band power. It is designed for clinical and research purposes using inexpensive EEG equipment limited to detect features in frequencies and not features of magnetic-resonance images (MRI) or other heavy and stationary machinery.

In this ERP (Event-Related Potentials) study, temporal brain patterns of activity were captured using a single frontal sensor. The source of the activity (brain-region) cannot be located with accuracy and this is a known limitation of EEG/ERP studies because the electrical potentials measured vary from time to time and from person to person as a result of the varying conductivities of the tissues involved (sculpt, brain matter, blood etc.). A broader layout with more sculpt locations might have given more data, but resulted information on brain-region activity would not be much higher. Nonetheless, the potentiality to find stronger statistical differences between groups of participants on other sculpt locations cannot be excluded.

Currently, understanding complex biological processes of the brain with EEG monitoring is not a safe approach and EEG signal analysis cannot offer diagnosis alone [25]. Having a long way to go before making accurate and valid EEG-based predictions on dementia progress, but seizing the opportunity given by the promising results derived especially from part C of the advanced linguistic stimuli test, future plans include a retest that will focus on a mixed stimuli-EEG test using figurative language processing only. The use of cliché figurative language is expected to maximize the portability of the proposed test to different language settings, but in the same cultural clusters as proposed by other studies on GLOBE societies [26].

References

1. Arevalo-Rodriguez, I., Smailagic, N., Roqué, I., et al.: Mini-mental state examination (MMSE) for the detection of Alzheimer's disease and other dementias in people with mild cognitive impairment (MCI). Cochrane Database Syst. Rev. 3 (2015)
2. Kaplan, E., Goodglass, H., Weintraub, S.: The Boston Naming Test, 2nd edn. Lea & Febiger, Philadelphia (1983)
3. Vos, S.J., van Rossum, I.A., Verhey, F., et al.: Prediction of Alzheimer disease in subjects with amnestic and nonamnestic MCI. Neurology 80(12), 1124–1132 (2013)
4. Laskaris, N.A., Tarnanas, I., Tsolaki, M.N., et al.: Improved detection of amnestic MCI by means of discriminative vector quantization of single-trial cognitive ERP responses. J. Neurosci. Methods 212(2), 344–354 (2013)

5. Ahmed, S., de Jager, C., Wilcock, G.: A comparison of screening tools for the assessment of mild cognitive impairment. Neurocase **18**, 336–351 (2012)
6. Kandiah, N., Zhang, A., Bautista, D.C., et al.: Early detection of dementia in multilingual populations: visual cognitive assessment test (VCAT). J. Neurol. Neurosurg. Psychiatry (2015, in print). doi:10.1136/jnnp-2014-309647
7. Stam, C.J., Made, Y., Pijnenburg, Y.A., Scheltens, P.: EEG synchronization in mild cognitive impairment and Alzheimer's disease. Acta Neurol. Scand. **108**(2), 90–96 (2003)
8. Baker, M., Akrofi, K., Schiffer, R., O'Boyle, M.W.: EEG patterns in mild cognitive impairment (MCI) patients. Open Neuroimag. J. **2**, 52–55 (2008)
9. Poil, S.S., (de) Haan, W., (van der) Flier, W.M., et al.: Integrative EEG biomarkers predict progression to Alzheimer's disease at the MCI stage. Aging Neurosci. **5**, 58 (2013)
10. Schiavone, G., Linkenkaer-Hansen, K., Maurits, N.M., et al.: Preliteracy signatures of poor-reading abilities in resting-state EEG. Front Hum. Neurosci. **8**, 735 (2014). doi:10.3389/fnhum.2014.00735
11. Orimaye, S.O., Wong, J.S.M., Golden, K.J.: Learning predictive linguistic features for Alzheimer's disease and related dementias using verbal utterances. In: Workshop on Computational Linguistics and Clinical Psychology, pp. 78–87 (2014)
12. Olichney, J.M., Morris, S.K., Ochoa, C., et al.: Abnormal verbal event related potentials in mild cognitive impairment and incipent Alzheimer's disease. J. Neurol. Neurosurg. Psychiatry **73**, 377–384 (2002)
13. Moretti, D.V., Fracassi, C., Pievani, M., et al.: Increase of theta/gamma ratio is associated with memory impairment. Clin. Neurophysiol. **120**(2), 295–303 (2009)
14. Hiele (van der), K., Vein, A.A., Reijntjes, R.H., et al.: EEG correlates in the spectrum of cognitive decline. Clin. Neurophysiol. **118**(9), 1931–1939 (2007)
15. Olichney, J.M., Taylor, J.R., Gatherwright, J., et al.: Patients with MCI and N400 or P600 abnormalities are at very high risk for conversion to dementia. Neurology **70**(19), 1763–1770 (2008)
16. Missonnier, P., Deiber, M.P., Gold, G., et al.: Working memory load related electroencephalographic parameters can differentiate progressive from stable mild cognitive impairment. Neuroscience **150**(2), 346–356 (2007)
17. American Electroencephalographic Society-AES: Guideline thirteen: guidelines for standard electrode position nomenclature. J. Clin. Neurophysiol. **11**, 111–113 (1994)
18. Östberg, P., Fernaeus, S.E., Hellström, Å., et al.: Impaired verb fluency: A sign of mild cognitive impairment. Brain Lang. **95**(2), 273–279 (2005)
19. Mousavi, S.Z., Mehri, A., Maroufizadeh, S., Koochak, S.E.: Comparing verb fluency with verbal fluency in patients with Alzheimer's disease. Middle East J. Rehabil. Health **1**(2), e23609 (2014)
20. Druks, J., Masterson, J., Kopelman, M., et al.: Is action naming better preserved (than object naming) in Alzheimer's disease and why should we ask? Brain Lang. **98**(3), 332–340 (2006)
21. Roncero, C., De Almeida, R.G.: The importance of being apt: metaphor comprehension in Alzheimer's disease. Front. Hum. Neurosci. **8** (2014). doi:10.3389/fnhum.2014.00973
22. Neurosky: EEG Band Power values: Units, Amplitudes, and Meaning (2014). http://support.neurosky.com/kb/development-2/eeg-band-power-values-units-amplitudes-and-meaning
23. Solís-Ortiz, S., Pérez-Luque, E., Gutiérrez-Muñoz, M.: Modulation of the COMT Val158Met polymorphism on resting-state EEG power. Front. Hum. Neurosci. **9** (2015)
24. Kurt, P., Emek-Savas, D.D., Batum, K., et al.: Patients with mild cognitive impairment display reduced auditory event-related delta oscillatory responses. Behav. Neurol. **2014** (268967), 11 (2014)

25. Tsolaki, A., Kazis, D., Kompatsiaris, I., Kosmidou, V., Tsolaki, M.: Electroencephalogram and Alzheimer's disease: clinical and research approaches. Int. J. Alzheimer's Dis. **2014**, 10 (2014)
26. Gupta, V., Hanges, P., Dorfman, P.W.: Cultural clusters: methodology and findings. J. World Bus. **37**(1), 11–15 (2002)

Age Characterization from Online Handwriting

José C. Rosales, Gabriel Marzinotto, Mounim A. El-Yacoubi[✉],
and Sonia Garcia-Salicetti

Institut Mines-Telecom, Telecom SudParis, Evry, France
{jose.rosales_nunez,gabriel.marzinotto_cos,mounim.el_yacoubi,
sonia.garcia}@telecom-sudparis.eu

Abstract. Age characterizationfrom handwriting (HW) has important applications as it may allow distinguishing normal HW evolution due to age from abnormal HW change, potentially related to a cognitive decline. We propose, in this work, an original approach for online HW style characterization based on a two-level clustering scheme. The first level allows generating writer-independent word clusters according to raw spatial-dynamic HW information. At the second level, the writer words are converted into a Bag of Prototype Words that is augmented by a measure of his/her writing stability across words. For age characterization, we harness the two-level HW style representation using unsupervised and supervised schemes, the former aiming at uncovering HW style categories and their correlation with age and the latter at predicting age groups. Our experiments on a large database show that the two level representation uncovers interesting correlations between age and HW style. The evaluation is based on entropy-based information theoretic measures to quantify the gain on age information from the proposed two-level HW style representation.

Keywords: Age · HW styles · Two-layer clustering · Supervised learning

1 Introduction

Handwriting (HW) analysis has recently been investigated in health tasks such as pathology detection [3]. In this context, age characterization from HW [12] is fundamental as it may allow distinguishing normal HW change due to age from abnormal one, potentially related to a cognitive decline. In this paper, we address the problem of age characterization from online HW. The goal is to detect HW styles and study their correlation with age, by the analysis of spatio-temporal HW parameters.

HW style classification has been widely studied for both online [1] and offline [2] HW recognition tasks, and used to design writer style-dependent recognition models. Inference of HW styles, however, is difficult as there are no rules to define or label a HW style. A clustering algorithm is thus usually required (Gaussian Mixture Models [2], K-means [5], Self-Organizing Maps [1], Agglomerative Hierarchical Clustering [4]). Previous works for clustering HW styles have tackled the problem at the stroke level [4],

© Springer International Publishing Switzerland 2016
S. Serino et al. (Eds.): MindCare 2015, CCIS 604, pp. 176–185, 2016.
DOI: 10.1007/978-3-319-32270-4_18

the character level [5], or the word level [6]. We believe, however, that style character-ization should rely not only on this raw signal information but also on high-level infor-mation associated with the variability observed across the writer words.

We propose, in this work, an original approach for HW style characterization based on a 2-level clustering scheme. The 1st level allows generating writer-independent word clusters according to raw signal information. At the 2nd level, the HW words of a person are converted into a Bag of Prototype Words (BPW) [13] by assigning each word to its closest cluster and generating the person's cluster frequency histogram. At this level, we also extract the writer stability across words, obtained by the histogram of distances between his/her word descriptions. The 2nd-level features are then given as input to the 2nd clustering for generating HW styles based on 2 kinds of information, raw spatio-temporal HW parameters, and intra writer word variability. This 2-level scheme might better characterize HW styles and their correlation with age, as the variability across words is highly informative of writer categories.

For age characterization, we harness the 2-level HW style representation using unsupervised and supervised schemes. In the former, no *a priori* knowledge on a writer's age is used. HW styles are inferred through clustering algorithms and then analyzed in terms of age distributions. In the supervised mode, writers' ages are divided into groups, used to train a classifier to characterize HW styles for each writer group. Thus, the unsupervised method aims at uncovering HW style categories and their correlation with age while the supervised approach aims at predicting age groups.

We have evaluated our approach on a large database of online HW words [7]. We propose information theoretic measures to quantify the gain on age information from the 2-level scheme. The results show that the latter uncovers interesting correlations between age and HW style. The remaining of the paper is as follows. Section 2 presents the proposed approach including spatiotemporal feature extraction, and the two-level clustering scheme. Section 3 describes the experiments and gives qualitative and quan-titative analyses of age characterization using the unsupervised and supervised schemes. Finally, Sect. 4 concludes and envisages future directions.

2 Proposed Approach

Online HW words are described as a sequence of 3 temporal functions $(x(t), y(t), p(t))$ representing the pen trajectory and pressure on a digitizer. At the 1st layer, we extract from each word 2 feature types. The 1st gathers local dynamic information, such as speed, acceleration and jerk [4], while the 2nd describes the static shape by measures such as stroke angles and curvatures [8], or inter-character spaces [6]. As dynamic parameters, we consider horizontal and vertical speed computed locally at point n as $V_x = |\Delta x / \Delta t|$ and $V_y = |\Delta y / \Delta t|$ where $\Delta x(n) = x(n+1) - x(n-1)$, $\Delta y(n) = y(n+1) - y(n-1)$ and $\Delta t(n) = t(n+1) - t(n-1)$. These values are computed along the word and quantized to build 4-bin histograms over the X and Y axes. We similarly compute local acceleration and jerk values, associated respectively with horizontal and vertical derivatives of speed and acceleration. In addition, pen pressure, its variation, and the pen-up duration ratio, computed as $PR = (Pen\text{-}up\ Duration)/(Total\ Duration)$ [12], are considered, thus obtaining 33 global dynamic features. For spatial parameters, a resampling process is first performed to ensure that consecutive word points are equidistant, so as the parameter values at each point become equally representative, regardless of speed. Local direction and curvature angles are then extracted as in [8] and used to build 2 histograms of 8 bins quantized in the 0°–180° range. We also consider the number of pen-ups, the average horizontal in-air distance, the number of strokes (defined as writing movements between 2 local minima of speed) and their average length, as well as the average length of the stroke projections on X and Y axis. This results in 22 spatial features. When combining dynamic and spatial features, a feature vector has dimension 55. At the 2nd layer, features are computed at the writer level. The writer's words are converted into a Bag of Prototype Words (*BPW*) [13] by assigning each word to its closest 1st-layer cluster and then generating the person's cluster frequency histogram. We add the histogram of intra-writer word distances by computing the Euclidean distance between the feature vectors of each possible pair of the person's words, and quantizing these distances into a 5-bin histogram.

2.1 Unsupervised Approach: Clustering

As no *a priori* knowledge on HW styles is available, HW style classification is usually performed in an unsupervised way through clustering. The styles detected depend on the static and dynamic features. These features may fluctuate across words, which is actually relevant for characterizing HW styles in terms of age [12]. Thus, we propose a novel 2-level approach: the 1st one, denoted as "1st layer", is related to raw signal information (spatial and dynamic parameters), while the 2nd or "2nd layer", is related to high-level information associated with fluctuations observed across words.

In the 1st layer, we propose to cluster all words of all persons, each word being described by a global feature vector composed of the 55 features described in Sect. 2.1. The aim here is to generate word clusters regardless of person identity. Each cluster will group words of similar global descriptors. In the 2nd layer, the clustering is performed at the writer level, using as features the person's cluster frequency histogram and the histogram of distances between his/her words. These are given as input to the 2nd layer stage for generating HW categories that take into account both spatiotemporal word similarities and similarities in HW variability between writers. Since there is no fixed number of HW styles, the number of categories in each layer is estimated using two criteria: the Silhouette [10] and the Calinski-Harabasz [11] criteria.

Clustering Validation and Visualization. To quantitatively analyze age distribution, we incorporate the entropy efficiency $\eta(x)$ measure, defined by Eq. (1). It consists of the entropy associated with the distribution of the classes considered (age groups), normalized by the maximal possible entropy of the system, $\log(n)$, where n is the number of classes. The lower the entropy efficiency, more predictable the distribution of the classes will be.

$$\eta(X) = \sum_{i=1}^{n} \frac{p(x \in X_i) \log(p(x \in X_i))}{\log(n)} \tag{1}$$

where X_i corresponds to class or age group A_i defined in Sect. 3.2. The clustering efficiency is defined as the average of the efficiencies at each cluster weighted by their sizes (Eq. (2)). This measures the change of age distribution in each cluster.

$$\eta(X) = \frac{1}{\log(n)} \sum_{j=1}^{M} \frac{|C_j|}{\left|\bigcup_{k=1}^{M} C_k\right|} \sum_{i=1}^{n} p(x \in X_i | x \in C_j) \log(p(x \in X_i | x \in C_j)) \qquad (2)$$

where C_i stands for the ith cluster obtained in either the first or the second layer. For visualizing clustering results, Principal Component Analysis (*PCA*) and Stochastic Neighbor Embedding (*SNE*) are used. *PCA* also allows computing the correlations between features and their relevance for style characterization. *SNE* [9] is a non-linear method that projects the points from a high dimensional space onto a two-dimensional space while preserving distance relations between points.

2.2 Supervised Classification for Age Prediction and Analysis

Although some features may show a large variance that heavily influences clustering, they are not necessarily useful to distinguish age categories. For this reason, we perform a Linear Discriminant Analysis (LDA) to search a new space where features that best discriminate each age group are revealed. As for the unsupervised approach, LDA is performed for the two layers. First, it is performed over the raw spatial-dynamic word description, in order to detect features that distinguish age groups. Then, a second LDA is performed on the second layer in order to search for correlations of frequency histogram and stability measures with writers' age.

3 Experiments

We use the IRONOFF database [7], which contains online samples of words in English and French, extracted using a Wacom tablet that captures the x, y positions and the pen pressure at 100 Hz. The database contains 793 writers from 11 to 77 years old (YO) that were split into 6 age groups as often done in the literature [12]:

- 23 Teenagers: 11–16 YO (A1)
- 531 Young Adults: 17–27 YO (A2)
- 120 Mid Age Adults: 28–38 YO (A3)
- 71 Mature Adults: 39–49 YO (A4)
- 37 Old Adults: 50–59 YO (A5)
- 11 Elders: 60–77 YO (A6)

An important observation is that teenagers and elders are heavily underrepresented and age groups A2 and A3 are overrepresented in the dataset. To ensure meaningful results, we balance the database in terms of age categories: we divide the set of words written by a given person into groups from 10 to 15 words, and assign each resulting group to a virtual new writer. The generated writers do not share words. Finally, we retain the same number of virtual writers for each age group; this number was set to 24 writers per group, thus generating a total of 144 writers.

3.1 Unsupervised Approach

First Clustering Layer. The optimal number of clusters found through both Silhouette and Calinski-Harabasz methods was 6. All 23.801 words of 1883 persons were clustered into 6 groups through the K-means algorithm. The obtained clusters are visualized in Fig. 1a.

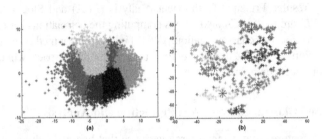

Fig. 1. (a) The 6 clusters of the first layer visualized using PCA on the two first axes. (b) The 8 clusters of the second layer visualized using *SNE*

We observe that writer-independent clusters are characterized by three main criteria. The first one is dynamic information; words are separated based on speed, acceleration and jerk (highly correlated features). The second criterion is word slant; words are clustered according to whether they are inclined to the left, to the right, or are straight. The third criterion separates words rather written in a script style from those rather written in a cursive style. Combinations of these factors characterize the six clusters, as described in Table 1, each with its corresponding color.

Table 1. Analysis of the first layer clustering results

	Associated Dynamics	Inclination	Script-Cursive
Cluster 1	Fast Velocity/Accel/Jerk	Straight Writing	Mixed Writing
Cluster 2	Slow Velocity/Accel/Jerk	Inclined to Left	Script Writing
Cluster 3	Slow Velocity/Accel/Jerk	Straight Writing	Script Writing
Cluster 4	Medium Velocity/Accel/Jerk	Straight Writing	Mixed Writing
Cluster 5	Fast Velocity/Accel/Jerk	Inclined to Right	Cursive Writing
Cluster 6	Medium Velocity/Accel/Jerk	Inclined to Right	Mixed Writing

Second Layer Clustering. In the 2nd layer, Kmeans was performed to cluster data into 8 groups, again using the number of clusters retrieved by the Silhouette and Calinski-Harabasz methods. Each point here represents a writer, described by 11 features: the distribution of his/her words into the 6 first layer clusters, plus the 5 bin histogram of his/her intra-writer word distances. As these features are highly uncorrelated and *PCA* was not effective in reducing data dimensionality, we used *SNE* to visualize clusters as shown in Fig. 1b. In the following analysis, we will refer to the clusters obtained on the second layer as categories, in order to distinguish them from the clusters in the first layer.

To interpret the second layer 8 writer categories, we introduce the diagrams shown in Fig. 2. Each category is represented by its central writer (cluster center), and is described in the left side by this writer's word distribution into first layer clusters, using the color bars C1 to C6. In the right side of the diagram (bars H1 to H5), we represent the normalized histogram of this writer's inter-word distances, used to reflect his/her HW stability. Distances assigned to bin H1 correspond to small distances between words and therefore, to a larger stability, while distances assigned to bin H5 characterize unstable handwriting.

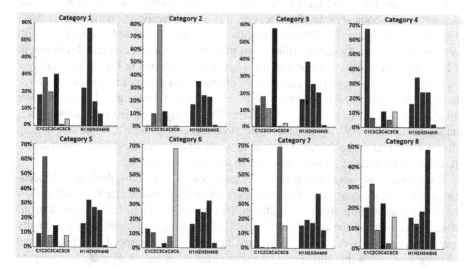

Fig. 2. Feature distribution in the 2nd layer for the central writer in each category. Left: percentage of words in each 1st-layer cluster (C1 to C6); Right: histogram of inter-word distances.

To study the correlation between age and handwriting, we analyze the age distribution of the HW categories displayed in Fig. 3. These histograms show the percentage of each age group in each category relatively to the initial balanced age distribution.

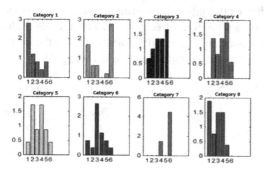

Fig. 3. Age histogram (using 6 age groups) in the 8 categories (2nd layer)

For example, if age group A5 in category 4 takes value 2, this group is twice more represented in category 4 than in the balanced dataset. The 1st and 8th categories have the largest concentration of teenagers (from 11 to 16 years old). The 1st category is the most evenly distributed in terms of the 6 clusters that emerged in the 1st layer, and shows a very homogeneous distribution among 1st layer clusters 1, 2, 3 and 4. In spite of this, we notice that persons in the 1st category achieve the greatest stability (H1 and H2 are predominant values). This can be explained by the fact that this age interval corresponds to the period of maturation of handwriting skills and of the emergence of a personal style; for this reason it contains writers that write very slowly (close to 11 years old) and others that write faster and more fluently (close to 16 years old).

On the other hand, teenagers have the greatest HW stability, as they probably still stick to the copybook style taught at school. It is also interesting to notice that persons in the first category are distributed among first layer clusters 2, 3 and 4, associated with low velocity and mostly script writing. This may be due to an incomplete development of HW skills, proper to that age. On the other hand, as shown in Fig. 3, second layer category 8 shows a large concentration of children and a high proportion of adults. However, this category has low stability, as can be seen from features H4 and H5. We can also notice that this category is represented by the styles of first layer clusters 1, 2 and 4, that involve HW styles either with slow velocity (cluster 2, 4) or fast writing (cluster 1). This is probably caused by the presence of older teenagers with more developed HW skills and that show similarities to the adult population.

Analogously, we note that second layer categories 2 and 7 have the largest concentration of elders. Category 2 is greatly represented by first layer cluster 3, related to slow and script handwriting styles. In addition, this group of elders has a good level of stability. We observe the opposite in category 7 of the second layer, which is mostly represented by first layer cluster 5, related to the highest writing speed, acceleration and jerk. We also notice that this group of elders is the most unstable class. This may be caused by the tendency of handwriting to vary when writing speed increases, and also by a trend of deterioration of handwriting capabilities for some aged people.

Entropy/Efficiency Measures. We have measured the entropy and the efficiency of clustering in terms of age distribution, on a database balanced with respect to the 6 age groups. The reduction of entropy is used as a measure of how efficient is the clustering across both layers in detecting handwriting styles that describe tendencies in age groups.

Table 2 shows that our two layered clustering significantly reduces the initial entropy. This result clearly shows the role of each layer. From Table 3 showing the entropy efficiency of each category, we observe that Category 7 has the lowest entropy which is consistent with the fact that it contains mostly elders (Fig. 3).

Table 2. Normalized entropy ($\eta(X)$) results across layers

	Initial database	First layer	Second layer
Age (6 groups)	1	0.91	0.82

Table 3. Normalized entropy ($\eta(X)$) results at the second layer for each cluster (category)

	Cat 1	Cat 2	Cat 3	Cat 4	Cat 5	Cat 6	Cat 7	Cat 8
Efficiency	0.79	0.80	0.89	0.92	0.92	0.83	0.60	0.84

3.2 Supervised Approach

In this section, we analyze the ability of each feature in discriminating between age groups. We apply LDA for retrieving the axis that best separates these groups. By studying the coefficients associated with each feature on that axis, we can determine features that are characteristic of a certain age group. This technique is also applied in a two-level scheme, for finding distinctive features not only in terms of raw signal information, but also in terms of a writer's stability across words.

LDA at the First Layer. Table 4 shows that there are age groups that are more easily classified than others using LDA (e.g. elders (A6) and teenagers (A1)). However, LDA is not able to distinguish middle age group pairs A2/A4, A3/A5, and A2/A3 as they completely overlap in the projections on the LDA axis (see Fig. 4). This reveals that HW styles of middle-aged persons might not be different enough to be distinguished whether the writer is a young adult (A2), a mid-age adult (A3), a mature adult (A4) or an old adult (A5).

Table 4. 1-vs.-all LDA classification error for the different age groups.

Classification error	A1	A2	A3	A4	A5	A6
Layer 1	11.88 %	14.49 %	14.86 %	17.24 %	14.64 %	8.84 %
Layer 2	14.28 %	16.67 %	16.67 %	17.36 %	15.97 %	9.03 %

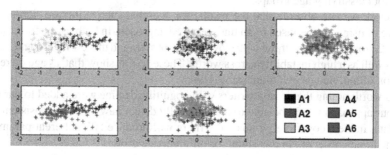

Fig. 4. LDA performance when separating the 6 age groups of persons considered

LDA at the 1st layer detects interesting features that distinguish age groups. For instance, teenagers write with more strokes than adults or elders. This larger number of strokes is actually related to not fully developed HW skills. On the other hand, middle-aged population is characterized by a low number of penups and high curvature values, which are indicators of fluent HW. Adults also show a preference for writing using long vertical lines, with the largest pressure. Elders show the largest number of penups; this could be a sign of HW degradation. Elders are also characterized by a low pen pressure that could be a symptom of weakening. Notice that teenagers are characterized by a large time on air, maybe due to not fully developed HW skills. Finally, elders and teenagers tend to write using more horizontal space; they are characterized by horizontal straight strokes as well as low curvature.

LDA at the Second Layer. At the 2nd layer, we can clearly distinguish in Fig. 5 two categories of elders: one that writes fast with cursive style tendency (represented by 1st-layer Cluster 5) and another that writes slowly with mostly a script style (represented by Cluster 3). Teenagers are represented by Cluster 2 that is related to a slow HW with mostly a right-slanted script style. Finally, we find that middle-aged groups are greatly related to first layer Cluster 1, which consists of a fast and straight handwriting style.

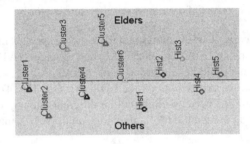

Fig. 5. Contribution of features on the second layer to classify elder writers

We note that teenagers are the most stable across words (Hist1) since they usually try to stick to copybook style. On the other hand, elders were classified as the less stable group (Hist5). Intermediate levels of stability (Hist2, Hist3, and Hist4) proved not to be useful for classifying age groups.

Overall, we can observe that the results for age characterization are similar, irrespective of using a supervised or an unsupervised approach. In both cases, for instance, we find 2 groups of elders: those with slow and script style and those with fast and cursive style as well as a high instability across words. These results show that, as age increases, a portion of individuals exhibit unstable HW.

It is worth noting that if new writers with cognitive decline were added to our database, our approach would be able to automatically detect new clusters consistent with such data. Indeed, cognitively impaired writers will produce HW different parameters w.r.t the trends observed in this study for different age groups.

4   Conclusions and Perspectives

We have proposed a novel approach for age characterization from online handwriting based on a 2-level scheme. The 1st level characterizes HW styles by raw spatial and dynamic information extracted from words, and generates writer-independent word clusters. The 2nd level extracts, by contrast, the writer's HW style variability across words. This 2-layer representation is analyzed using supervised and unsupervised learning techniques, for detecting relations between age and HW styles. Interesting correlations were uncovered: teenagers were shown to have highest HW stability, while the stability has a general tendency to decrease with aging. When we analyze low level information, we find that children and elders are characterized by a larger number of strokes and penups, respectively. This may be explained by the hesitation of children and elders, due to initial difficulties when acquiring HW skills for the former, and to possible degradation of psycho-motor abilities for the latter.

Our experiments did not show a significant difference between the 4 middle-aged groups. This confirms that HW does not vary much during this period of life. For further studies, a simplified age distribution should thus be studied, by considering only 3 age groups: children, middle aged persons and elders. As expected, our findings also confirm that not all persons in the same demographic category write in the same way. For instance, our study reveals at least 2 types of elders.

Finally, we intend to run experiments on a larger database with a more homogeneous age distribution, including elders showing cognitive or psychomotor disorders. Based on the new data, the methods proposed in this work will be further investigated to automatically characterize the HW degradations related to these disorders.

Acknowledgments. This work was partially funded by Fondation MAIF through project "Biométrie et santé sur tablette". For more information, please refer to: http://www.fondation-maif.fr/notre-action.php?rub=1&sous_rub=3&id=269.

References

1. Vuori, V.: Clustering writing styles with a self-organizing map. In: IWFHR 2002 (2002)
2. Sarkar, P., Nagy, G.: Style consistent classification of isogenous patterns. IEEE PAMI **27**(1), 88–98 (2005)
3. Teulings, H.-L., et al.: Adaptation of handwriting size under distorted visual feedback in patients with Parkinson's disease and elderly and young controls. J. Neurol. Neurosurg. Psychiatry **72**, 315–324 (2002)
4. Bharath, A., Deepu, V., Madhvanath, S.: An approach to identify unique styles in online handwriting recognition. In: ICDAR 2005 (2005)
5. Chan,S.K., Tay, Y.H., Viard-Gaudin, C.: Online text independent writer identification using character prototypes distribution. In: SPIE Electronic Imaging 2008 (2008)
6. Crettez, J.-P.: A set of handwriting families: style recognition. In: ICDAR 1995 (1995)
7. Viard-Gaudin, C., et al.: The IRONOFF dual handwriting database. In: ICDAR 1999 (1999)
8. Guyon, I., et al.: Design of a neural network character recognizer for a touch terminal. Pattern Recogn. **24**, 105–119 (1991)
9. Hinton, G., Roweis, S.: Stochastic neighbor embedding. NIPS **15**, 833–840 (2002)
10. Rousseeuw, P.: Silhouettes: a graphical aid to the interpretation and validation of cluster analysis. J. Comput. Appl. Math. **20**, 53–65 (1987)
11. Calinski, R.B., Harabasz, J.: A dendrite method for cluster analysis. Commun. Stat. Theor. Methods **41**, 2279–2280 (2012)
12. Rosenblum, S., et al.: Age-related changes in executive control and their relationships with activity performance in handwriting. Hum. Mov. Sci. **32**, 1056–1069 (2013)
13. Sivic, J.: Efficient visual search of videos cast as text retrieval. IEEE Trans. PAMI **31**(4), 591–605 (2009)

RAMCIP: Towards a Robotic Assistant to Support Elderly with Mild Cognitive Impairments at Home

Ioannis Kostavelis[✉], Dimitrios Giakoumis, Sotiris Malasiotis, and Dimitrios Tzovaras

Centre for Research and Technology Hellas, Information Technologies Institute, 6th Km Charilaou-Thermi Road, 57001 Thermi-Thessaloniki, Greece {gkostave,dgiakoum,malasiot,tzovaras}@iti.gr

Abstract. During the last decades the mild cognitive impairments (MCI) as well as the early stage of dementia comprises a societal challenge in the growing elderly population. This fact is highly related to the physical and cognitive decline of aged people, influencing the way they apprehend their environment and, thus, their daily activities. Towards this direction, the "Robotic Assistant for MCI patients at home" (RAMCIP) project, initiated by the European Union, intends to build a service robot that will operate in domestic environments with the aim to proactively and discreetly support older persons and MCI patients. The key component to achieve this goal is the design of a robot endowed with high-level cognitive functions, driven by advanced human and environment perception mechanisms, that will enable the artificial agent to autonomously decide when and how to assist. The paper in hand demonstrates the RAMCIP concept through identified user requirements and provides an overall system description. Additionally, the architecture design of the robotic system is exhibited here, firstly by providing a conceptual analysis and then by further decomposing the identified modules into functional components. The overall architecture envisaged in a user centric manner aiming to convert the real needs of the MCI patients into capabilities of the robotic assistant.

Keywords: Mild cognitive impairments · Early dementia · Robotic assistant · Domestic environment · High-level cognitive functions · Architecture design

1 Introduction

According to the Word Health Organization (WHO) [1] dementia is one of the major causes of disability and dependency among older people, whereas it is estimated that worldwide, 35.6 million people have dementia and there are 7.7 million new cases every year. Dementia is a syndrome of a chronic or progressive nature in which there is deterioration in cognitive function beyond

© Springer International Publishing Switzerland 2016
S. Serino et al. (Eds.): MindCare 2015, CCIS 604, pp. 186–195, 2016.
DOI: 10.1007/978-3-319-32270-4_19

what might be expected from normal ageing [2]. However, there is an early stage before dementia called mild cognitive impairments (MCI), which is characterized by abnormal memory performance for age but with normal general cognition and preserved normal activities of daily living [3].

Ageing is typically associated with physical and cognitive decline, altering the way an older person perceives and interacts with its environment. The thinks are getting worse at early stages of dementia, where elder people are not fully aware of their cognitive impairments and in this respect, their participation in everyday activities inherently involves significant risks. Furthermore, as soon as MCI patients recognize their tendency to forget necessary actions during daily activities, the likelihood of resigning from those activities increases. In turn, resignation from daily activities may also lead to negative emotions, reduced self-respect and potentially depression, increasing among others the probability for the person's health state aggravation and the potential for MCI to evolve into dementia. This stage is very crucial to be foreseen and anticipated prohibiting thus the impairment of the cognitive condition of the patients. In order to succeed this, the last decades persistent research endeavors in the area of service robots revealing methods that significantly assist elderly and support their independence. More precisely, the conducted research brought to the surface robots capable to autonomously move, to provide entertainment and telepresence functions, to learn and bring objects, to detect falls or even to assist the older person to move safely around the house by removing small objects and obstacles. In [4] an add-on Intelligent Wheelchair System (IWS) was developed to help older adults with cognitive impairments drive a powered wheelchair safely and effectively. On another aspect, the work described in [5] targeted the construction of a robotic wheel chair, where the entire system is part autonomous and part user-decision dependent (semi-autonomous). The ultimate goal of this work is the development of a Simultaneous Localization and Mapping (SLAM) algorithm allowing the environmental learning by a mobile robot, while its navigation is governed by electromyographic signals. Moreover, in [6], the authors presented a 2-degree of freedom robot suitable for rehabilitation of lower limbs. It utilizes neural network and genetic algorithm for the optimization of the control system. More findings in the area of assisting robotics for elder people are summarized in the objectives of past projects such as the HOBBIT [7] and the ACCOM-PANY [8]. However, major challenges still need to be addressed towards service robots of the future; ones that will be capable of assisting older persons in a wide variety of activities, discreetly and transparently, yet proactively and in tight cooperation with the human, acting at the same time as effective promoters of the patient's mental health, being solutions that will evolve along with the user, thus capable to match her/his needs as they evolve over time.

To this end, the RAMCIP project aims to research and develop a novel service robot, capable to proactively assist older persons in a wide range of daily activities, being at the same time an active promoter of the user's physical and metal health. The RAMCIP robot comprises three basic objectives which are summarized as follows:

- the development of cognitive functions based on user and home environment modelling and monitoring, allowing the robot to decide when and how to assist the user;
- the development of human robot communication interfaces, focused on empathic communication and augmented reality displays;
- the establishment of dextrous and safe robotic manipulation capabilities, which, to the best of our knowledge, applied for the first time in service robots introducing assistance activities that involve physical contact.

The rest of the paper is organized as follows: in Sect. 2 the overall concept of the RAMCIP system is described, while the basic user requirements and their mapping to the system design are outlined in Sects. 2.1 and 2.2, respectively. Moreover, an conceptual software architecture analysis is summarized in Sect. 3, while a brief discussion on the acceptability issues is exhibited in Sect. 4. In Sect. 5 conclusions about the presented work are drawn, while Fig. 1 conceptually summarizes the capacities of the RAMCIP system.

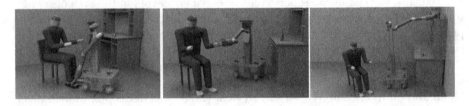

Fig. 1. The conceptual robotic platform with the manipulation hand as envisioned in the RAMCIP system.

2   The RAMCIP Concept

The RAMCIP robot is designed to assist MCI patients in their day life activities by encoding the basic needs and requirements of such people. It retains a wide range of mechanisms to observe and perceive its environment, as well as a human oriented notion to track his/her activities, while it simultaneously assess the person's cognitive and physical skills. To succeed this, the robot shall act in a safe, proactive and discreet manner employing high-level cognition with the capacity to decide when and how intervene to provide assistance. The latter will be accomplished either by initiating Human Robot communication routine or by fulfilling a robotic manipulation task, yet through an autonomous decision making mechanism.

2.1   MCI-User Requirements

The robotic assistant described in this work will be able to assist in specific occasions in the day life activities, which stem from the MCI patients' requirements. Here we append a clustering of the most indicative requirements which the RAMCIP robotic assistant is challenged to carry out during the cohabitation with an MCI patient.

1. **Taking Medication:** The robotic assistant would be responsible to facilitate the his/her medication routine. This could be accomplished either by reminding the user that is time to receive the medication or by fetching it to him/her. Additionally, the system should be able to assess the correctness of the patient's medication intake.
2. **Eating Activities:** The robot would be responsible to track the eating schedule of the patient and remind him/her for a missed meal.
3. **Dressing Activities:** The robot would be responsible to help the person to select proper clothes and identify abnormalities during dressing, e.g. to properly button his/her cloths as well as to help him/her to take off the slippers.
4. **Food Preparation:** The RAMCIP robot would be responsible to assist complementary the patient during the food preparation by fetching or lifting fallen objects, making thus the cooking task less laborious.
5. **Socialization:** The robot would help the person to be social active by reminding him/her to come in touch with family or friends or by reminding him/her about important dates.
6. **Lower-body Treatment Activities:** The robot would be responsible to carry out activities that could harm the patient's waist, while it simultaneously should be able to help the patient to put his/her feet on a footrest.
7. **Managing Home and Keep it Safe:** The robot would be responsible to continuously monitoring and prevent dangerous situations at home e.g. switch off the oven button that the patient might have forgotten.
8. **Maintaining Positive Affect:** The robot will be responsible to observe the patient's affective state by analyzing a series of observations, while it simultaneously will apply strategies to help her/him mountain positive outlooks.
9. **Exercising Cognitive and Physical Skills:** The robot will be responsible to continuously monitoring and prevent dangerous situations at home e.g. switch off the oven button that the patient might forgot.

2.2 Supporting MCI Patients Through the RAMCIP System

Towards the fulfillment of the above mentioned requirements the RAMCIP robot shall have advanced high-level cognitive functions as described in Fig. 2. These functions will be driven by thorough modelling and monitoring of the home environment and the user, allowing the robot to take optimal decisions regarding *when and how* to provide assistance, in a proactive and discreet way. Since assistance provision is deemed necessary, the robot will perform either **communication** to the user, or initiation of a **robotic manipulation task**.

Therefore, the RAMCIP platform will be specially designed in order to enclose all the aforementioned attributes. Except performance, the main concern is the safety of the user, since the RAMCIP robot will be designed for physical Human Robot Interaction applications (pHRI). Therefore, the entire robotic platform will be designed by taking into account safety issues inherent in robotic applications for human inhabited environments. Specific parameters are taken into consideration involving the inertia of the moving parts to be kept as low as possible, the compliance of the robot links as well as the robot surface to be covered with soft materials, avoiding thus human injuries in case of physical contact. From the hardware architecture point of view several sensor inputs will be utilized to perceive the environment and the human presence. RGB-D sensors will comprise the main visual input for sensing, while emphasis will be given to the depth data concealing thus sensitive and private data of the user's dailies activities. Laser range finders will be utilized for the robot safe navigation and collision avoidance within the house. RAMCIP aims to go beyond the current state of the art in safe robotic manipulation by developing a robotic manipulator of a workspace comparable to that of a human arm, overall weight of less than 10 kg and payload of 5 kg. The initial design of the robot foresees a hand mounted at the end of this arm with at least three fingers including a thumb with more than three degrees of freedom per finger ensuring dextrous grasping. Considering the communication part, human robot interaction will be established on multimodal, adaptive and empathic channels, realized through the fusion of touch-screen, voice, gestures and projective augmented reality-based interfaces. The robotic assistance tasks will be performed through either dextrous manipulation methods enabling safe object grasping, manipulation and handover, in inaccessible places including reaching of objects difficult for the user to reach (e.g. high placed objects), or through physical Human Robot Interaction during intentional and unintentional contact.

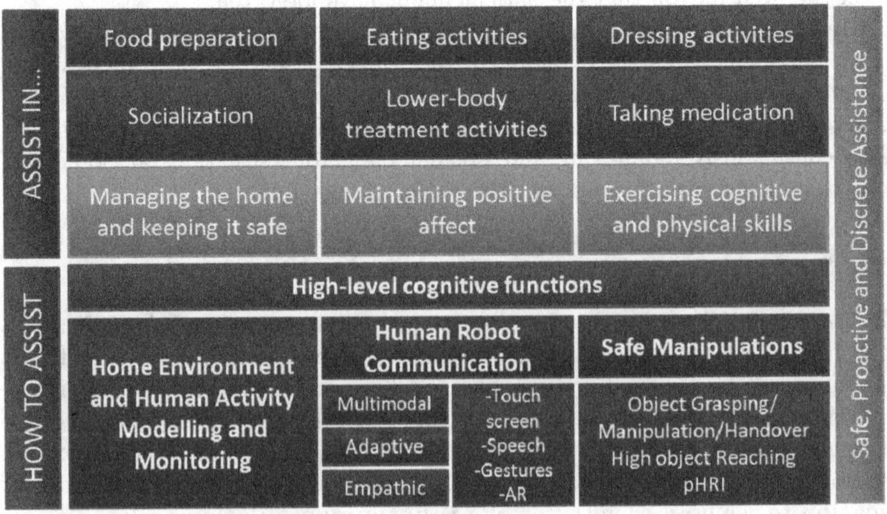

ASSIST IN...	Food preparation	Eating activities	Dressing activities	Safe, Proactive and Discrete Assistance
	Socialization	Lower-body treatment activities	Taking medication	
	Managing the home and keeping it safe	Maintaining positive affect	Exercising cognitive and physical skills	

HOW TO ASSIST	High-level cognitive functions				Safe, Proactive and Discrete Assistance
	Home Environment and Human Activity Modelling and Monitoring	Human Robot Communication		Safe Manipulations	
		Multimodal	-Touch screen	Object Grasping/ Manipulation/Handover High object Reaching pHRI	
		Adaptive	-Speech -Gestures -AR		
		Empathic			

Fig. 2. The conceptual analysis of the MCI patients needs and RAMCIP vision toward future domestic service robots for such populations

3 Conceptual Architecture of the RAMCIP System

In order to exhibit the solutions provided by the RAMCIP system, to assist the MCI patients, a conceptual software architecture will be presented here. The software to be developed within the RAMCIP scope will retain both passive perception strategies of the user and the home environment as well as active engagement solutions with the robotic platform. The RAMCIP software architecture can be decomposed into "conceptual modules", clustered "functional components", available models from the user and the environment and external data that may stem from the robot, the user or the environment. Each conceptual module comprises several algorithmic core routines which are responsible for the implementation of the subordinate functional components.

3.1 User and Home Environment Monitoring and Modelling

The user activity and behavior monitoring module, and the home environment monitoring module are the cornerstone conceptual modules of the RAMCIP system, as they connect the robot with the user and its surrounding environment. The continuously tracking of the home environment and the dynamic update of the 3D environment model, will enable the RAMCIP robot to be aware of its location in the house, its relative location to house objects and appliances, whereas moreover, it will be capable to understand also the position and state of objects and appliances.

The human activity monitoring module will be first of all responsible to identify and also recognize humans inside the house. RAMCIP shall be aware in case of multiple co-located persons, of who is its primary user, as well as persons directly related to her/him (e.g. a relative or caregiver). Upon human recognition, RAMCIP will be capable to track her/his pose, actions and complex activities. With the ultimate goal to assist MCI patients, apart from the detection of emergency situations, e.g. a sudden fall, specific emphasis will be paid to detecting cases where the user has forgotten important steps of actions e.g. the user has forgotten to turn off the oven.

Moreover, the capability of RAMCIP to recognize its user and understand her/his behavior will be based on the system's user modelling engine. This will encode both (a) generic knowledge regarding how actions compose activities and how activities compose behaviors, as well as (b) specific respective knowledge regarding its primary user (and also regarding for e.g. relatives), all encoded in the RAMCIP VUMs (Virtual User Models), which will be a virtual reflection of the user inside the RAMCIP user modelling engine.

3.2 High-Level Cognitive Functions

Toward enabling proactive and optimal assistance provision in a variety of use cases a major objective of the RAMCIP system will be to provide the robot with competent cognitive functions and reasoning. These functions will be included in the Assistance Decision Maker (ADM) module of the robot. The ADM will employ the VUM, the user and environment state to drive the robot's decisions over *when* and *how* to initiate an assistance intervention.

Consequently, the cognitive functions will ensure the development of an obedient and proactive servant undertaking difficult or forgotten tasks, to provide the robot with such a behavior that will also assist the user in exercising physical and cognitive skills, through its own behavior. This will be based on maintaining a balance between acting proactively, counteracting the user's forgetfulness by undertaking tasks that the user has forgot, and informing the user of a forgotten task, discreetly urging her/him to take a relevant action. Therefore, upon deciding that assistance provision is necessary, the robot will select through its cognitive actions to either communicate with the user or engage in a robotic manipulation task.

3.3 Human Robot Communication Module

Human robot communication will be orchestrated through the Communication Decision Maker (CDM) component, utilizing the user's VUM part encoding communication skills and preferences, as well as the user and environment monitoring system modules. The CDM will thus drive personalized and adaptive multimodal Human Robot communication based on touch-screen, voice, augmented reality and gestural modalities. The robot will be capable to automatically switch between different interaction modalities or fuse them, ensuring the provision of optimal HRI on the basis of user skills, behavior and context.

Human Robot Interaction will also be augmented through advanced empathic communication channels. On one hand, the robot should be capable to recognize the user's affective state, based on analysis of the user pose and gestures, in combination with facial expression recognition. The robot will also employ an empathic display, realized as screen-based face, capable to show facial expressions enabling human compatible communication mechanisms.

3.4 Low-Level Robot Control Module

The low-level control module of RAMCIP will be responsible to handle RAMCIP's robotic manipulations, regarding either (a) interaction with the home environment, its objects and appliances or (b) physical Human Robot Interaction with the user. Autonomous locomotion of the platform will build upon mapping and navigation methods supported from the home environment monitoring and modelling module. The low-level control module will provide RAMCIP with novel robot manipulation capabilities including advanced grasping and dexterity functions. Through these advanced manipulation capabilities, the robot will be on the one hand capable of grasping a variety of objects in the home environment ranging from very small objects to dishes, cooking utensils, etc., and on the other hand, interacting with home objects or appliances, such as doors, light switches or the oven. Therefore, a task planner will be developed to coordinate all the subordinate robotic tasks required to accomplish a specific robotic activities such as fetching objects that are placed at a height unreachable to the user. Moreover the robotic engagement in assistance activities that will involve physical contact between the robot and the user comprise an additional novel contribution of the RAMCIP system, e.g. the robot will be able to safely assist the user in lower-body treatment activities that require bending, such as changing socks or shoes, or assisting the user to place her/his feet on a footrest.

All the aforementioned conceptual modules as well as their subordinate functional components are summarized in the Fig. 3, where a flow diagram of the software architecture is illustrated.

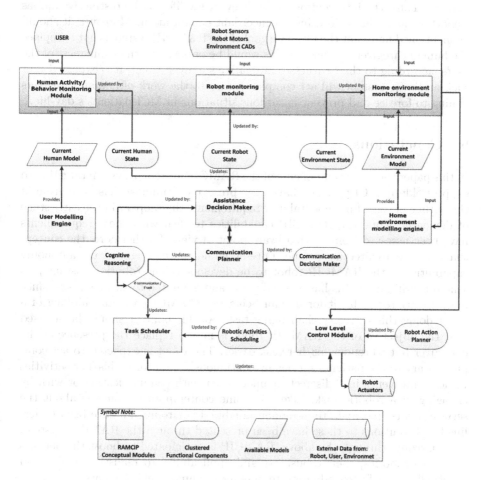

Fig. 3. The conceptual software architecture analysis of the RAMCIP system

4 Discussion

It is apparent that during the design and development of the RAMCIP system several parameters should be taken into consideration, the most important of which is the acceptability of the target users. Service robots intended for assisted living environments involve gender and ethical issues that should be paid clear attention. Gender-dependent differences are highly prone to appear in user needs and preferences, regarding either the assistance strategies or specificities in HRI, whereas privacy and ethical issues are inherently involved. Additionally, it should be stressed that the RAMCIP system would be developed so as to proactively and discreetly assist the user in his/her day-life activities by retaining autonomy and strong decision making mechanisms all developed in a human compatible manner. Thus, the intervention in user's everyday life will be distinctive and as smooth as possible, facilitating a concordant cohabitation. Moreover, it should be mentioned here that the ultimate goal of the RAMCIP system is not to replace the human caregivers services as this would be opposite to the willingness of the users, according to their witnesses in relative surveys. Albeit, it is expected that such a robotic system will act complementary to the work of human caregivers aiming to foresee and prevent hazardous situations in MCI patients's day-life.

5   Conclusions

In this paper the basic components of the RAMCIP system -a system targeting to support elderly MCI patients- have been presented. Emphasis has been given in the outline of some fundamental user requirements that appear in the early stage of dementia, while the RAMCIP capabilities to deal with these requirements have been assessed from the hardware point of view. Furthermore, the conceptual software architecture has been presented herein, highlighting the autonomy capabilities of the RAMCIP robot to be developed. The robotic assistant presented herein for MCI is has a specific role and is limited to specific tasks, since it is already too difficult for human being to help MCI patients, thinking of a robot doing this is a very challenging task. At this point it should be stressed that the objective of the RAMCIP robot is not to replace the presence of the care-giver but to render his/her task easier. The robot is expected to act complementary to the patients actions by continuously monitoring his/her activities while it intervenes in a discreet manner either with communication or with by engaging in a robotic task. Likewise, some contemporary concerns about the service robots that operate in human inhabited environments have been underlined and solutions to these have been presented through the RAMCIP system. Summarizing, through the above, RAMCIP is anticipated to boost the benefits of service robotics, their robustness and applicability to realistic settings and eventually, their future adoption to operate in human environments.

Acknowledgments. This work has been supported by the EU Horizon 2020 funded project namely: "Robotic Assistant for MCI Patients at home (RAMCIP)" under the grant agreement with no: 643433.

References

1. WHO: Word health organization (2007). http://www.who.int/mediacentre/factsheets/fs362/en/
2. Spitzer, R.L., Md, K.K., Williams, J.B.: Diagnostic and statistical manual of mental disorders. In: American Psychiatric Association, Citeseer (1980)
3. Winblad, B., Palmer, K., Kivipelto, M., Jelic, V., Fratiglioni, L., Wahlund, L.O., Nordberg, A., Bäckman, L., Albert, M., Almkvist, O., et al.: Mild cognitive impairment-beyond controversies, towards a consensus: report of the international working group on mild cognitive impairment. J. Intern. Med. **256**(3), 240–246 (2004)
4. How, T.V., Wang, R.H., Mihailidis, A.: Evaluation of an intelligent wheelchair system for older adults with cognitive impairments. J. Neuroeng. Rehabil. **10**, 1 (2013)
5. Cheein, F.A.A., Lopez, N., Soria, C.M., di Sciascio, F.A., Pereira, F.L., Carelli, R.: Slam algorithm applied to robotics assistance for navigation in unknown environments. J. Neuroengineering Rehabil. **7**(1), 10 (2010)
6. Aminiazar, W., Najafi, F., Nekoui, M.A.: Optimized intelligent control of a 2-degree of freedom robot for rehabilitation of lower limbs using neural network and genetic algorithm. J. Neuroengineering Rehabil. **10**(1), 96 (2013)
7. Hobbit:: The mutual care robot (2013). http://hobbit.acin.tuwien.ac.at
8. Accompany:: Acceptable robotics companions for ageing years (2014). http://accompanyproject.eu

Intelligent User Interfaces to Support Diagnosis and Assessment of People with Dementia: An Expert Evaluation

Anastasios Karakostas[1(✉)], Ioulietta Lazarou[1], Georgios Meditskos[1], Thanos G. Stavropoulos[1], Ioannis Kompatsiaris[1], and Magda Tsolaki[1,2]

[1] Information Technologies Institute,
Centre for Research and Technology Hellas,
Thessaloniki, Greece
{akarakos, iouliettalaz, gmeditsk,
athstavr, ikom}@iti.gr, tsolakiml@gmail.com
[2] 3rd Department of Neurology, Medical School,
Aristotle University of Thessaloniki,
Thessaloniki, Greece

Abstract. This paper presents the main user/clinician interface and the mechanisms of a sensors-based system to support clinicians' diagnosis for people suffering from Alzheimer disease and dementia. The system monitors the patient at a lab or a home environment when he/she tries to accomplish specific tasks or ordinary daily activities. The main goal of the system is to support both the clinical assessment and therapy. The system can be divided into two main parts: (a) the sensors, which monitor the patients and (b) the clinician user interface, which includes the main system operation as well as the results of the monitoring. The data between these two parts is transferred and interpreted by using knowledge-driven interpretation techniques based on Semantic Web technologies. In order to evaluate the interface satisfaction, the usefulness and the ease of use of the clinician interface both for the lab and home environments, an expert evaluation was conducted with 2 groups of professionally active psychologists with dementia expertise (14 psychologists for the lab and 10 for the home environment). The results of the questionnaire-based evaluation showed that the clinicians are quite positive about the use of the system as a supporting method to dementia assessment and therapy.

Keywords: Alzheimer · Sensors · Clinician interfaces · Semantic interpretation

1 Introduction

The frequency of dementia is rising all over the world, with considerable socio-economic impacts that are creating an imperative need for finding effective means of treatment. In current clinical practice, treatment of dementia begins with its diagnosis, which is based on behavioral assessments and cognitive tests that highlight quantitative and qualitative

S. Serino et al. (Eds.): MindCare 2015, CCIS 604, pp. 196–206, 2016.
DOI: 10.1007/978-3-319-32270-4_20

changes in cognitive functions, behaviors and activities of daily life, characteristic of the dementia syndrome and its underlying diseases. Typical questionnaire-based assessment approaches tend to introduce a high level of subjectivity, while lacking the comprehensive view of the person's life and status that only continuous monitoring can provide. This paper presents a sensor-based system that provides effective cognitive aids and supports the intervention, for example if someone's aim was to improve their sleep, the sleep sensor could be deployed to monitor sleep activity, while a sensecam together with other sensors could be used to review activity on days leading up to or following a good or bad night's sleep. The overall goal of the system is to have socio-economic benefits such as not biased and objective clinical assessment; 24/7 personalized feedback and support to patients; delay hospitalization; reduced healthcare costs; enhanced feeling of security both for patients and their families and improved cognitive and physical condition of patients.

2 Related Work

Lately, there has been a mounting interest worldwide to deploy pervasive computing technologies for advancing well-being and healthcare through remote monitoring and management services at the point of need. Within this line of research for remote healthcare, special attention has been given to the promotion of home-based continuous support and care of people with chronic conditions, to sustain their independence and eliminate the need for early hospitalization by ensuring continuous monitoring for timely intervention. Dementia, being one of the leading causes of chronic poor health and disability for the aging population, has been the subject of a number of such research works. Remote management of people with dementia involves providing tools and services that allow them to be independent. One category of such tools includes external memory aids [1] that may be calendars, diaries, alarm watches, whiteboards, notebooks, and timers. It has been shown that such devices help people with mild dementia maintain an account of their daily life [2]. Another common practice is life story work, where reminiscing activities in one's present life provides a sense of control over the past, present and future [3].

Home environment [4], which aims to promote the use of embedded technology to support a person within their own living environment and extend the period of time they can remain in their own home prior to institutionalization. Within such an environment, it is common to find sensors. Sensors are the devices, which can record information about the person or the environment. Most of the efforts described above tend to concentrate on specific aspects, such as health status monitoring, alerts and reminders based on scheduled activities (e.g. medicine taking, training activities, etc.), and not overall behaviour and daily activities modeling.

This paper presents a system, which multiple sensor outputs and interpretation through new reasoning mechanisms and knowledge structures informs clinicians with a comprehensive image of the person's ability in daily activities.

3 The Interventions

The lab intervention: The lab intervention involves short-term testing (between 1 to 1 1/2 h) in the Alzheimer day care center at lab conditions. These interventions consists of monitoring persons with dementia using the system's technology in order to provide a brief overview of their health status during consultation (cognition, behaviours and function), and to correlate the system data with the data collected using typical dementia care assessment tools. The monitoring is accomplished using a range of sensors, including wearable, physiological, activity-based, and location-based. Each participant starts with a regular consultation with a general practitioner, and then undergoes the ecological assessment, which is followed by a neuropsychological assessment. During the consultations, demographical and medical characteristics are gathered by means of widely used and generally recognized assessment tools. The lab assessment is divided into two steps conducted in an experimental setting equipped with daily objects and ambient technology. The home intervention: Our system performs functional assessment of adults with memory and functional problems in their everyday environments. This type of automated assessment also provides a mechanism for evaluating the effectiveness of alternative physical and psychological health interventions. This system is valuable for providing automated health monitoring and assistance in an individual's environments. Via examination of individual's specified problems we can adjust intervention not only for providing quality of life, suggesting helpful programs and mentioning their daily mistakes and problems, but also enhance prospective memory and everyday functionality.

Both lab and home interventions are based on clinical assessments tasks. Typical clinical everyday assessments are based on patient's perception. Our system provides crucial, reliable and validated information to the clinicians about the condition of a patient. Moreover, based on specific system outputs, the clinician is able to design and provide a series of interventions to the patient in order to enhance his/her cognitive, social and physical status.

4 The Proposed System

The system requires not only efficient user interfaces, but also a flexible and robust underlying infrastructure to support data and functions presented to the user. In the field of Ambient Intelligence (AmI), and especially Ambient Assisted Living (AAL), this requirement for flexibility on the application layer is resolved by the Service-Oriented Architecture (SOA). For the clinical intervention, we designed and developed such a service-oriented system, based on the Web Service technology. Overall, the system architecture involves three layers: the hardware, middleware and application layer. Although, the first prototype of the system has been presented in [5], this paper introduces much more extended integration and especially the inclusion of real-time sensors for energy and object movement detection.

The sensors supported by the system provide a variety of data formats and are ambient, non-intrusive, and wearable. For example, an ambient depth camera is placed to survey the whole room, collecting both image and depth data. One of the main technical obstacles in concurrent AAL systems, is to unify and timely coordinate sensor data retrieval, synchronicity and homogeneity. Indeed, the sensors used in our intervention present various data forms and especially both real-time and asynchronous data transfer. A dedicated module interfaces with each sensor, complying with its own API and platform dependencies.

After data has been either streamed online to the system (i.e. camera and audio recordings, plug consumption data and motion detection events) or transferred offline (i.e. wristwatch accelerometer values), they must be further analyzed and stored. The purpose of raw sensor data analysis is to extract higher-level, more meaningful observations, by means of aggregation or even machine learning techniques. In detail, camera depth data is used by Complex Activity Recognition (CAR) [6] algorithms to provide location based events e.g. the participant is in the zone for tea. Image data from the same camera is used by another set of techniques, namely Human Activity Recognition (HAR) [7], which perform learning to detect high-level activities such as preparing tea. The energy consumption data stream is processed in real-time and based on certain per-device thresholds, pushes detected activities i.e. KettleOn and RadioOn. Similarly, analyzing the stream of tag sensor events results in the detection of object movement events, such as KettleMoved, CupMoved etc. Audio data is similarly processed by Offline Speech Analysis (OSA) algorithms [8], to provide clustering for the patients as either healthy, MCI or Alzheimer's Disease. Raw accelerometer readings from the wristwatch are aggregated into a single numerical measurement, which signifies the participant's per minute moving intensity.

The analysis layer hosts two additional, software-based modules: Knowledge Base Manager (KBM) and Semantic Interpretation (SI). The former module is able to parse detected activities and measurements under a common exchange model and map them into rdf-triple format for storage in a common Knowledge Base (KB). This process allows for the SI module to reason upon and combine existing observations in order to extract higher-level activities. All analysis modules are exposed through universal WSDL endpoints. A controller module, implemented as the application backend, is responsible to timely invoke analysis and functions and guide data flow for storage in the KB. E.g. for audio analysis, the controller invokes microphone recordings, invokes OSA, stores results through KBM and invokes SI when the lab session is complete. Semantic Web technologies and in particular RDF/OWL ontologies, have been gaining increasing attention as a means for modelling and reasoning over contextual information and human activities in particular [9]. Formally founded in Description Logics [10], their expressiveness and level of formality make them well-suited for the open nature of context-aware computing [11–13]. For example, in OWL one can effectively model and reason over taxonomic knowledge. This is a desirable feature in pervasive applications where the need to model information at different levels of granularity and abstraction, so as to drive the derivation of successively further detailed contexts is particularly evident. Similarly, OWL supports consistency checking - another useful feature when dealing with imperfect context information coming from multiple sources, property domain/range restrictions, instance class memberships, property relationships, e.g. transitive, inverse, etc. (see [10] for the complete list of semantics). In addition to the native reasoning services, ontologies are usually combined with rules

[14, 15], allowing to express richer semantic relations, e.g. temporal relations. Under this context, low-level information acquired from detectors, such as video cameras and contact sensors, is mapped to ontology class and property assertions, while high-level interpretations are inferred through the combination of ontology semantics and rules. This is essential for sensor-driven systems where the derivation of high-level knowledge from low-level sensor data requires complex relational structures that capture the interrelation of various pieces of information in terms of time, location, actors and resources. The knowledge-driven interpretation services in our system consist of a hybrid reasoning architecture that combines the OWL reasoning paradigm and the execution of SPARQL queries. More specifically, the native semantics of OWL is used to formally represent and integrate activity-related information originated from different data sources, whereas SPARQL queries further aggregate activities, describing the contextual conditions and the temporal relations that drive the derivation of complex activities, e.g. the complex activities of the protocol. In addition, SPARQL assessment queries validate the underlying activity models, detecting abnormal behaviors, such as missed protocol activities or activities with long duration, assisting clinicians in assessment.

The Clinician Interface. We designed and developed the clinician interface based on the following main principles and goals based on the requirements provided by three clinicians with dementia expertise: -They system should be easily operated from a novice computer user -The clinicians should be always informed about the current phase of the protocol and the relevant instructions in the lab environment -The clinicians should easily operate the sensors. Moreover, they should be aware if there is a problem with a specific sensor -The clinicians should be informed about the results of each patient in a comprehensive way after the completion of the protocol. In order the human computer interaction being efficient, the tasks, the procedures and the methods that the clinician may perform with the system need to be structured in a logical and consistent manner. This means that the interface should be intuitive and the system should address the clinician's goal and objectives. Moreover, the number of actions that a user has to perform in accomplishing a task (even for technological complex tasks like the operations of the sensors) should be minimized.

Following the above goals and principles, the lab clinician interface contains 3 main areas:

The insert/edit user area. In this area the clinician is able to insert a new patient into the system and begin the assessment.

The assessment area. When the clinician enters the assessment area, he/she has to initialize the sensors (Fig. 1: B). In each phase of the protocol, the clinician is informed about the title and the guidelines of the phase (Fig. 1: A) or its order (Fig. 1: D). He/she can start and stop (or skip) the sensors' recording for this part of the protocol (Fig. 1: B). Finally, the user is informed about the sensors activation (Fig. 1: E). For example in Fig. 3, in the motion sensors section we can see that the patient has just moved the phone.

The results area (Fig. 2). After the completion of the protocol, the clinician is able to see the results for the specific patient. The "timeline" shows the order, the time and the success of all the attempts (Fig. 2: C).

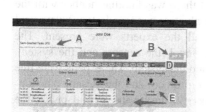

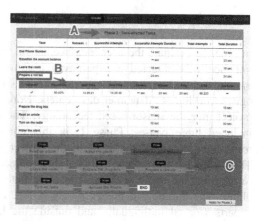

Fig. 1. Assessment area: specific protocol phase

Fig. 2. Results area: semi-directed activities

The home clinician interface allows the clinicians to see various results and data correlations from the recordings. In Fig. 3, the clinical is able to choose the input from multiple sensors and see their relation during specific time period. In such way, he/she is able to identify improvements or changes in the patient's daily performance. In Fig. 4, the clinician is able to see the patient's activities during the day, and relative patterns.

Through the system UI, the clinician is able to see among other measurements, if the patient has completed successfully or not an activity, the total efforts for each activity and the sequence of activities that he/she followed. Furthermore, in the home environment the clinician is able to see correlations between sensors (e.g. sleep duration based on the sleep sensor and physical activity based on motion sensor) in order to assess more accurately and provide the proper and personalized interventions.

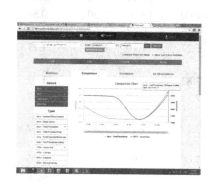

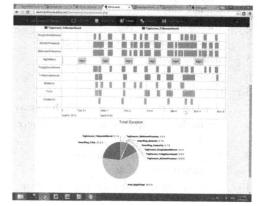

Fig. 3. Sensors' input comparisons

Fig. 4. Patient's daily activities in Home environment

5 The Expert Evaluation Method

In order to evaluate the user interface satisfaction and the usefulness of the clinician interface, we conducted an expert evaluation with 14 (for the lab interface) and 10 (for the home interface) domain experts. These experts are professionally active psychologists working at Alzheimer day centers. None of them was familiar neither with the project, nor the sensor-based technology. The evaluation process lasted 2 days and included three phases: Phase 1: in this phase all the experts were present. The researchers presented the goals of the project, protocol, the sensors and the system. There was also a live presentation of the protocol and the system. The experts were free to interrupt and make questions regarding both the protocol and the system functionalities. The duration of this section was 1 h. Phase 2: during the second phase, the experts worked individually and outside the lab. They on their own were able to operate with the system through a demo online environment and to explore all the system's functions. There was no time limit for this phase. The experts were free to interact as much as they like. Phase 3: in the last phase the experts had to answer an online questionnaire. The questionnaire consisted of two sections. The first one included the QUIS-short version, a standardized questionnaire for user interface satisfaction [17] and the second one included the PUEU questionnaire regarding the perceived usefulness and ease of use [18]. Both of these questionnaires are well known, valid and reliable (Table 1).

Table 1. Expert evaluation results

#	Questions (min: 0, max: 9)	Mean n = 14 lab	SD	Mean n = 10 home	SD
QUIS					
Overall reaction to the system					
1	terrible-wonderful	7.00	1.00	8.00	0.89
2	difficult-easy	6.82	1.40	8.17	0.75
3	frustrating-satisfying	7.09	1.14	8.33	0.82
4	inadequate power-adequate power	7.00	1.26	8.50	0.84
5	dull-stimulating	7.36	0.92	7.67	1.86
6	rigid-flexible	6.27	1.10	8.17	1.17
Screen					
7	Reading characters on the screen: hard-easy	7.82	0.98	7.50	1.52
8	Highlighting simplifies task: not at all-very much	7.36	1.29	8.17	1.17
9	Organization of the information: confusing-very clear	7.27	1.19	6.83	2.32
10	Sequence of screens: confusing-very clear	7.09	1.04	7.17	2.56

(*Continued*)

Table 1. (*Continued*)

#	Questions (min: 0, max: 9)	Mean n = 14 lab	SD	Mean n = 10 home	SD
Terminology and system information					
11	Use of terms throughout system: inconsistent-consistent	7.64	0.92	8.17	0.75
12	Terminology related to task: never-always	7.64	0.81	8.83	0.41
13	Position of messages on screen: inconsistent-consistent	7.73	1.01	7.33	1.63
14	Prompts for input: confusing-clear	7.27	0.90	7.50	1.52
15	Computer informs about its progress: never-always	8.09	0.70	7.83	0.98
16	Error messages: unhelpful-helpful	8.27	0.79	7.67	0.52
Learning					
17	Learning to operate the system: difficult-easy	7.36	1.21	7.50	1.76
18	Exploring new features by trial and error: difficult-easy	7.64	0.92	7.67	1.21
19	Remembering names and use of commands: difficult-easy	7.55	1.13	8.67	0.82
20	Performing tasks is straightforward: never-always	7.73	0.79	8.33	0.82
21	Help messages on the screen: unhelpful-helpful	7.91	0.94	7.83	0.75
22	Supplemental reference materials: confusing-clear	7.64	0.67	7.67	1.37
System capabilities					
23	System speed: too slow-fast enough	7.91	0.83	7.83	0.75
24	System reliability: unreliable-reliable	7.91	0.94	7.83	1.17
25	System tends to be: noisy-quiet	8.18	1.17	7.83	0.75
26	Correcting your mistakes: difficult-easy	7.00	1.34	7.50	2.26
27	Designed for all levels of users: never-always	6.73	0.90	8.50	0.84
PUEU					
Usefulness					
28	Using the system in my job would enable me to accomplish tasks more quickly: unlikely-likely	6.36	1.29	8.50	0.55
29	Using the system would improve my job performance: unlikely-likely	6.27	1.19	8.33	0.82
30	Using the system in my job would increase my productivity: unlikely-likely	6.00	1.00	8.00	1.10
31	Using the system would enhance my effectiveness on the job: unlikely-likely	6.64	1.03	8.33	0.52

(*Continued*)

Table 1. (*Continued*)

#	Questions (min: 0, max: 9)	Mean n = 14 lab	SD	Mean n = 10 home	SD
32	Using the system would make it easier to do my job: unlikely-likely	6.18	1.17	8.33	0.82
33	I would find the system useful in my job: unlikely-likely	6.55	1.04	8.33	0.52
Ease of use					
34	Learning to operate the system would be easy for me: unlikely-likely	8.00	1.26	8.33	0.82
35	I would find it easy to get the system to do what I want it to do: unlikely-likely	7.73	1.35	8.50	0.55
36	My interaction with the system would be clear and understandable: unlikely-likely	7.91	1.14	8.33	0.52
37	I would find the system to be flexible to interact with: unlikely-likely	7.82	0.98	8.67	0.52
38	It would be easy for me to become skillful at using the system: unlikely-likely	8.00	1.10	8.33	0.52
39	I would find the system easy to use: unlikely-likely	7.91	1.04	8.83	0.41

Moreover, there were some positive comments regarding the systems' functionality as: "innovative and flexible", "it is quite simple", "easy to use", "easily evaluation of specific patient's daily operations", "effortlessly monitor the patient's skill at real time" and "Clear and easy to follow". On the other hand there was one negative comment: "Choice of colors for messages and buttons could be problematic for someone with color-blindness."

6 Conclusions

This paper presented a sensors-based system that aims to help clinicians to diagnose and support more efficiently people suffering from Alzheimer disease and dementia. The end-user interface helps the clinician (a) to operate the system and (b) to see the results for each patient, which derived from semantic interpretation analysis. The psychologists' overall reaction to the system was very positive. The usability testing of our system by the psychologists showed that our system responded to their needs, was efficient in support of diagnose a patient and was easy to learn to use. Overall we can say that it was very much appreciated by the psychologists. Though these outcomes seem rather promising, we need to verify these results in a future evaluation study by including more clinicians working with the system. However, regarding the usefulness of the system of the lab environment we see that the means are between 6.00 and 6.64. Although, this indicate positive attitude, these values are not high as the values of interface satisfaction answers. In our opinion, this can be explained by the limited time that the psychologists interacted with the system. We believe that only after consistent use the users will fully identify the benefits. Finally, with respect to the ease of use, the psychologists seem to have rather positive attitude. Especially, they believe that it would be easy for them to learn to operate the system and to become skillful at using the system. This result indicates that the psychologists feel confident and ambitious to use the system even though they are not familiar with relevant systems and interfaces.

Overall, this study confirmed what we already expected; that carefully designed clinician interfaces would be positively accepted by professionally active psychologists as a supporting material for their clinical assessment. The future plan of this work includes more experiments with patients and the enrichment of the UI with more advanced techniques. Finally, patients' acceptance of the system is going to be evaluated.

Acknowledgment. This work has been supported by the EU FP7 project Dem@Care: Dementia Ambient Care – Multi-Sensing Monitoring for Intelligent Remote Management and Decision Support under contract No. 288199.

References

1. Lee, M.L., Dey, A.K.: Capturing and reviewing context in memory aids. In: Workshop on Designing Technology for People with Cognitive Impairments Human-Computer Interaction Institute, Carnegie Mellon University, Pittsburgh, PA (2006)
2. Kapur, N., Glisky, E.L., Wilson, B.A.: External memory aids and computers in memory rehabilitation. In: The Hand-book of Memory Disorders, 2nd edn., pp. 757–784 (2002)
3. Housden, S.: Reminiscence and lifelong learning. Int. J. Comput. Healthcare **2007**, 161–176 (2007)
4. Augusto, J.C., Nugent, C.D.: Smart homes can be smarter. In: Augusto, J.C., Nugent, C.D. (eds.) Designing Smart Homes. LNCS (LNAI), vol. 4008, pp. 1–15. Springer, Heidelberg (2006)
5. Stavropoulos, T.G., Meditskos, G., Kontopoulos, E., Kompatsiaris, I.: Multi-sensing monitoring and knowledge-driven analysis for dementia assessment. Int. J. E-Health Med. Commun. (IJEHMC) **6**(4), 77–92 (2015)
6. Romdhane, R., Crispim, C.F., Bremond, F., Thonnat, M.: Activity recognition and uncertain knowledge in video scenes. In: 2013 10th IEEE International Conference on Advanced Video and Signal Based Surveillance (AVSS), pp. 377–382 (2013)
7. Avgerinakis, K., Briassouli, A., Kompatsiaris, I.: Recognition of activities of daily living for smart home environments. In: 2013 9th International Conference on Intelligent Environments (IE), pp. 173–180 (2013)
8. Satt, A., Sorin, A., Toledo-Ronen, O., Barkan, O., Kompatsiaris, I., Kokonozi, A., Tsolaki, M.: Evaluation of speech-based protocol for detection of early-stage dementia. In: INTERSPEECH, pp. 1692–1696 (2013)
9. Tiberghien, T., Mokhtari, M., Aloulou, H., Biswas, J.: Semantic reasoning in context-aware assistive environments to support ageing with dementia. In: Cudré-Mauroux, P., Heflin, J., et al. (eds.) ISWC 2012, Part II. LNCS, vol. 7650, pp. 212–227. Springer, Heidelberg (2012)
10. Baader, F.: The Description Logic Handbook: Theory, Implementation, and Applications. Cambridge University Press, Cambridge (2003)

11. Riboni, D., Bettini, C.: COSAR: hybrid reasoning for context-aware activity recognition. Pers. Ubiquit. Comput. **15**(3), 271–289 (2011)
12. Chen, L., Nugent, C.: Ontology-based activity recognition in intelligent pervasive environments. Int. J. Web Inf. Syst. **5**(4), 410–430 (2009)
13. Okeyo, G., Chen, L., Wang, H., Sterritt, R.: Dynamic sensor data segmentation for real-time knowledge-driven activity recognition. Pervasive Mob. Comput. **10**, 155–172 (2012)
14. Okeyo, G., Chen, L., Wang, H., Sterritt, R.: A hybrid ontological and temporal approach for composite activity modelling. In: Trust, Security and Privacy in Computing and Communications (TrustCom 2012), pp. 1763–1770 (2012)
15. Wessel, M., Luther, M., Wagner, M.: The difference a day makes–recognizing important events in daily context logs. In: Contexts and Ontologies Representation and Reasoning (2007)
16. Shaw, R., Troncy, R., Hardman, L.: LODE: linking open descriptions of events. In: Gómez-Pérez, A., Yu, Y., Ding, Y. (eds.) ASWC 2009. LNCS, vol. 5926, pp. 153–167. Springer, Heidelberg (2009)
17. Chin, J.P., Diehl, V.A., Norman, K.L.: Development of an instrument measuring user satisfaction of the human-computer interface. In: Proceedings of CHI 1988 ACM, pp. 213–218 (1998)
18. Davis, F.D.: Perceived usefulness, perceived ease of use, and user acceptance of information technology. MIS Q. **13**, 319–340 (1989)

Stay Positive and Well

A Positive Technology System for the Promotion of Well-Being: From the Lab to the Hospital Setting

Macarena Espinoza[1(✉)], Ernestina Etchemendy[2], Luis Farfallini[1],
Cristina Botella[1,3], and Rosa María Baños[2,3,4]

[1] Universitat Jaume I, Castellón de la Plana, Spain
macaespinoza@gmail.com, lfarfallini@gmail.com, botella@uji.es
[2] Ciber, Fisiopatología Obesidad y Nutrición, Instituto Salud Carlos III, Madrid, Spain
ernestina.etchemendy@gmail.com, banos@uv.es
[3] Red de Excelencia PROMOSAM (PSI2014-56303-REDT), MINECO, Madrid, Spain
[4] Universitat de Valencia, Valencia, Spain

Abstract. There is growing evidence of the effectiveness of Positive Psychology Interventions (PPIs) to enhance subjective and psychological well-being in different populations, and the Information and Communication Technologies (ICTs) are becoming into a key help to increase the efficiency of this type of interventions. Recently, the use of technology to foster well-being and personal growth has been named as *Positive Technology*. The aim of this paper is to describe and to present data about a positive technology example (EARTH of Well-being system) and to examine its usefulness in different populations and settings. Data of four studies are presented: two with non-clinical population (university students) and two with clinical population (cancer patients). Outcomes show that this system is capable of promoting subjective well-being in both populations. Also, its efficacy was proved in different settings (laboratory and hospital contexts). Limitations and future research are discussed.

Keywords: Positive technology · Well-being · Efficacy · Non-clinical population · Clinical population

1 Introduction

A positive psychology intervention (PPI) has been defined as a "treatment method, strategy or intentional activity that aim to cultivate positive feelings, behavior, or cognition" [1]. Currently, there is evidence that shows the effectiveness of PPIs to enhance the subjective and psychological well-being and to reduce depressive symptoms in both general and clinical populations (e.g. anxiety, depression) [1–3]. PPIs are mainly brief and simple exercises or activities that can be implemented as part of one's daily routine, and where commitment and daily practice become essential elements of their efficacy [4].

The literature suggests that PPIs can be used in conjunction with preventive interventions and traditional treatments with the aim to strengthen personal psychological resources. In addition, the majority of PPIs is delivered in a self-help format, as evidenced in the meta-analysis conducted by Bolier et al. [2], where this format obtained

© Springer International Publishing Switzerland 2016
S. Serino et al. (Eds.): MindCare 2015, CCIS 604, pp. 209–219, 2016.
DOI: 10.1007/978-3-319-32270-4_21

small but significant effects. From a cost-effective perspective, self-help interventions can be effective and appropriate tools in mental health field, although it is necessary to enhance their efficacy [2].

The Information and Communication Technologies (ICTs) are becoming into a key help to enhance the efficacy and efficiency of psychological interventions [5–9]. The connectivity, the speed and the availability of ICTs are redefining our daily life, and also have an impact on Psychology and other behavioral sciences [10]. ICTs are presented as effective and sustainable solutions to public health demands that allow reaching a large number of people with a high quality and low costs. All these advantages are being already used in the PPIs [eg., 11, 12].

Taking into account the growing relationships between ICTs and PPIs, and the increasing literature of PPIs delivered through technologies, is not strange the appearance of different terms to name this intersection. For example, Ritterband et al. [13] has proposed "Online Positive Psychological Interventions" to define those interventions offered by the Internet and focused on behavioral aspects, designed to modify and establish certain behaviours and the subsequent improvement in symptomatology. Mohr et al. [14] proposed "Technological Behavioral Interventions" to refer to technological apps (e.g., smartphones, computers, virtual reality, videogames, social networks, etc.) specifically designed to intervene on behavioral, cognitive and emotional aspects, in order to improve physical and psychological health and well-being. In addition, Botella et al. [15] and Riva et al. [16] have suggested the term "Positive Technologies" to refer to the scientific and applied approach focused on the study of the use of technology to improve the quality of personal experiences. It is a perspective that seeks to promote the use of technology to foster personal growth and the development of human virtues and strengths, thus contributing to social and cultural development.

The term proposed by Botella et al. [15] and Riva et al. [16] is the only one that establishes a classification of technologies based on conceptualizations of subjective, psychological and social well-being [15, 16]. According to Botella et al. [15], each of these levels has critical variables (hedonic level: emotion regulation; eudaimonic level: flow and presence; and social level: collective intentions and social connections) that can be used to guide the design of technological applications that seek to influence different aspects of well-being. Examples of hedonic PTs would be those that induce a positive and enjoyable experience, such as a virtual reality environment of joy induction. Eudaimonic PTs include technologies that help people to achieve experiences focused on the search for a full and meaningful life. Social PTs include technologies that support and enhance communication among individuals, groups and organizations.

Until now, the efforts have been put mainly into the assessment of the efficacy of PTs to improve well-being. Given the strengths and benefits of these tools [11, 17] the issue of its transference to other settings than the Lab should be now a priority. It is possible to translate the PTs developed so far to natural settings, like schools, organizations or hospitals?, Its positive outcomes obtained with general populations in controlled environments remained significant when they are implemented with other populations and contexts?.

Taking into account the previous, this paper aims to describe and to present data about `EARTH of Well-being´ (Emotional Activities Related to Health) system, a technology based on the PT approach proposed by Botella et al. [15] and Riva et al. [16] and developed as a system designed to generate hedonic and eudaimonic experiences through self-applied PPIs. Its usefulness in two different populations and two settings will be examined. Therefore, the purpose is double: to analyze its benefits and also to explore the viability of implement this type of systems in other environments than the Lab.

2 EARTH of Well-Being System

The EARTH system is a self-guided platform initially developed for the Mars-500 project [18] with the purpose of promote positive experiences in a closed and controlled environment (a simulated Mars mission). Subsequently, it was adapted for the other population with the aim of promote different aspects of positive affect and hedonic and eudaimonic well-being for a variety of people.

This system includes several strategies structured in three modules. Two of the modules are positive Mood Induction Procedures (MIPs), and the third one includes narrative exercises of reminiscence and future projection. All the strategies included in EARTH are based on theories of well-being, regarding positive emotions [e.g., 19] optimal functioning and psychological health [e.g., 20]. EARTH system offers several techniques and tasks, since some authors have suggested that the use of different positive intervention techniques could be useful for the maintenance and enlargement of their effects [17, 21].

MIPs are experimental strategies designed to produce, in a controlled manner, specific transient emotional states similar to those experienced in natural situations [22]. In EARTH system, the specific emotions targeted are joy and relaxation, because there is evidence about their undoing effects on negative emotions [23–26] and their impact on other positive emotions, by creating the appropriate conditions for experience them [23].

To promote these positive emotional states, Virtual Reality (VR) environments were used as a frame to apply several MIPs in a structured and interactive way, overcoming some of the limitations of the traditional MIPs [27, 28].

EARTH's narrative exercises include the recall of positive life event memories and also the generation of specific plans for the future. Writing activities were included given their beneficial effects on mental health [29–31], and the reminiscence activity was considered given its potential to generate positive emotions through past memories [32, 33]. Besides, several studies have shown the effectiveness of exercises focused on the development of positive future plans for well-being, for example the 'Best Possible Self', [4, 34, 35] or the 'Life Summary' of Seligman et al. [36].

To work on these narrative exercises, EARTH includes several multimedia resources (music, pictures, videos, writing) with the purpose of expand the possibilities to represent and express personal experiences and emotions in a more dynamic way [37, 38]. In this sense, to include personal material (like photos, letters, music) is also available, as a way of enriching the meaningfulness of the activity and facilitating the "positive mental time travel" [39].

2.1 Modules Description

Park of Well-Being. This module includes two virtual environments aimed to induce joy or relaxation (MIP-VR). Both simulate a park in a city, and the colors, sounds and content of the exercises were adapted to the specific target emotion. In this setting several exercises are included: self-statements, choosing pictures, listening to music while interacting with the surroundings, watching movie scenes, and recalling an autobiographical emotional experience. Before and after each exercise, users can walk throughout the park and listen a specific music depending on the target emotion. The music used was 'EineKleineNachmusik' for joy and 'Heavenly Theme' for relaxing. Both songs were validated in previous studies [28, 40]. Five self-statements (e.g. 'I feel happy and cheerful') [41] were included in each VR environment (5 for relaxation and 5 for joy). In the exercise, each self-statement was accompanied by four emotional pictures (IAPS) [42] and users had to choose the image that best represented each statement. Next, users were invited to watch a movie scene in an outdoor cinema. The movies included were: 'Singing in the Rain' for joy and 'Out of Africa' for relaxation [43]. Finally, users had to remember moments of their own lives that could produce a specific emotion (joy or relaxation, respectively) [44].

Well-Being Through Nature. This module includes two virtual environments where users can learn some techniques to generate positive emotions (joy and relaxation) (MIP-VR). Both environments simulate a natural landscape, and welcome narratives, colors and sounds were chosen to generate the target emotions (joy or relaxation) [45, 46]. Three psychological techniques were also included: positive reminiscence, savoring and slow breathing. Users can choose in which order to perform each exercise.

The Book of Life. This module consists of a personal diary designed to help users to recall positive and meaningful moments of their lives, and write about positive and significant future plans. This diary is composed by 16 chapters, each targeting different psychological resources. Eleven chapters are directed to recall positive past experiences (happiest moment, the best place, significant people, achievement and effort, giving to others, enjoying social relationships, beauty, enthusiasm and passion, gratitude, courage, optimism). The other five exercises involve defining objectives and significant future plans regarding different areas of their lives (oneself, work, family, friends, or general life). Each exercise contains a general statement that explains the goal of the exercise, and a series of questions to guide the writing (to avoid negative, impersonal or nonspecific contents). Users can use different multimedia resources besides writing (music, pictures and videos) to represent their memories and plans, and develop each chapter of the book. Participants can use their own multimedia elements or use the ones available in the EARTH system.

3   EARTH of Well-Being Outcomes

Some of the exercises included in this platform have been validated in different populations: people with adjustment disorders [47] or elderly [48]. Below, data about the usefulness of the EARTH system in two samples (general population and cancer patients), will be presented.

3.1 EARTH System in General Population

Two studies have been focused on the examination of the system in non-clinical population (university students). The first one [18] assessed users' acceptance and perceived usefulness of the system, as well as preliminary data about its efficacy in the promotion of well-being. The second one explored the efficacy of the system compared to a control activity [49].

Study 1. In this first study [18], 38 university students (mean age 24.6 years, range 18–41 years old) used the application along 6 sessions distributed over 2weeks (3 sessions per week). Each week they received one session of the MIP-VR module (sessions 1 and 4), one session of the Book of Life (sessions 2 and 5) and one free-choice session (sessions 3 and 6). After each session, participants indicated their mood change in a 7 point Likert scale (1 = much worse; 7 = much better). Participants came to the lab to complete each session on a computer.

Regarding preferences, most of participants choose MIP-VR modules in the two free-choice session (Session 3: 89.47 % vs. 10.53 %; Session 6: 78.95 % vs. 21.05 %). However, both modules (MIP-VR and Book of Life) were considered highly useful by the participants (above 92 % of coded responses) and an important proportion of agreement (above 78 %) was found regarding the possibility to have access to the system in their own homes ('If it were possible, would you like to have the system available in your home?'). Taking into account mood changes, an improvement was found after all sessions (mean scores were from 4.95 to 5.37) [18].

Study 2. In the second study [49], 95 university students (mean age 24.9 years, range 18–47 years old) were randomly assigned to two conditions: experimental (EG) and control group (CG). Participants included in the EG used the system at the lab 3 times a week along 1 month (12 sessions). Participants of the CG did not perform any guided activity during 1 month. Both groups were evaluated at the same times (Baseline, pre-intervention, post intervention, and follow up at 1 and 3 months). Besides, EG participants rated their emotional state before and after each session, using visual analog scales to assess 10 emotions (joy, surprise, relax, vigor, sadness, anger, anxiety, boredom, stress, loneliness) using a 7 point Likert scale. They also indicated their mood change after sessions, like in the previous study. Results showed that participants who used EARTH of Wellbeing system increased their mood and positive emotions and decreased negative emotions, both in a significantly way (joy: $F = 52.83, p<.001, \eta2 = 0.50$; relax: $F = 49.35; p<.001, \eta2 = 0.48$; sadness: $F = 12.49, p = .001, \eta2 = 0.19$; anger: $F = 35.93, p<.001, \eta2 = 0.40$; anxiety: $F = 61.01, p<.001, \eta2 = 0.54$; stress: $F = 61.95, p<.001, \eta2 = 0.54$; loneliness: $F = 9.20, p = .004, \eta2 = 0.15$). This outcome was also observed in participants with high scores in depression and anxiety [49].

3.2   EARTH System in Cancer Population

Given that the EARTH system was initially designed as a PT for non clinical populations, the next step was to analyze the possible implementation of this system in other groups or settings, and therefore assess also its transferability.

Following this aim, two studies have been carried out to assess the feasibility of this system in cancer population, specifically in hospitalized patients, which implied to take into account new variables such as participants' physical discomfort, and also a complex setting for implementing the intervention (a hospital).

A previous adaptation of contents and functioning was made, specially on the Park of Well-being, with the purpose of simplify the interaction (e.g. self-statements words order by themselves) and adjust some contents to the vital situation of these participants (e.g. instead of the phrase: 'I feel happy and cheerful' it was included the sentence: 'There are things that make me happy').

Study 1. In a pilot study, the feasibility and benefits of the two VR modules of EARTH in oncology inpatients with metastatic cancer were assessed [50]. The sample was composed by 19 patients (mean age 60.9 years; range 29-85 years old). The most frequent diagnoses were breast (26.3 %) and lung cancer (15.8 %). Intervention was delivered in patients' room along 4 sessions and they had the possibility of interact with the 4 VR environments. The first and third sessions were oriented to joy and the second and fourth to relaxation induction. After each session, participants experienced higher positive emotions intensity as well as lower negative emotions intensity (2nd session: general mood [$t = -4.616, p<.001, \eta2 = 0.62$], relaxation [$t = -2.110, p<.05, \eta2 = 0.26$], sadness [$t = 3.580, p<.003, \eta2 = 0.50$]; 4th session: joy [$t = -3.202, p<.009, \eta2 = 0.51$]). Besides, participants commented that the main perceived benefits were distraction, entertainment, and relaxation [50]. Its brevity, low cost and easiness of use (keyboard and a mouse as interaction devices) helped to implement this system in the hospital routine with encouraging results.

Study 2. Subsequently, the entire system was tested with hospitalized cancer patients in different stages of the disease. The Book of Life module was also included. As in the first pilot study with the VR modules, some modifications were made. Specifically, work was focused on the positive reminiscence exercises, selecting 6 life moments from the 11 available in the system, and the exercises oriented to future planning were excluded. This study had two phases:

Pilot study. In a first exploratory study [51], 16 patients (mean age 62.5, range 44–75 years old) with different diagnoses (lung 33.3 %, digestive 20 %, colon-rectum 20 %) were included. They received one or more sessions (up to 4) and their response and disposition in front of the Book of Life module was assessed. Participants could choose the module to work with, in each session (Book of Life or VR environments). Outcomes shown the acceptability of reminiscence exercises (most of patients who did both modules, preferred the reminiscence one [71.4 % vs 28.6 %] as well as its positive effect on subjective well-being (it was found a higher proportion of cases with better perceived mood after sessions in the reminiscence module) [51].

Protocol Study. Taking into account the outcomes obtained in the pilot study, it was carried out a second study in which participants received two sessions of Book of Life and two sessions of the VR modules [52]. The group of participants was composed by 11 inpatients (mean age 58.7 [range 38–82 years old] with different diagnoses (27.3 % other, 18.2 % lung cancer). Most of the participants had metastatic cancer (63.6 %). Data suggest the usefulness of the system to promote higher positive emotional states after each session (there were statistically significant changes in positive mood, well-being and calmness after 1st and 3rd session (S1 = positive mood, $Z = -2{,}333$, $p = .020$, $d = -0.68$; well-being, $Z = -1.890$, $p = .059$, $d = -0.67$) (n = 11) (S3 = positive mood, $Z = -2.121$, $p = .034$, $d = -1.20$; well-being, $Z = -2.060$, $p = .039$, $d = -1.63$; calmness, $Z = -2.121$, $p = .034$, $d = -1.44$) (n = 8). Besides, no patient stated being "worse" of mood after the sessions, and in all of them more than 60 % of the participants commented feeling "better" of mood after the activities. In addition, participants' response was positive in terms of acceptance and satisfaction with the procedure [52].

4 Discussion

Four studies have been done with the purpose of explore the feasibility and preliminary usefulness of EARTH of Well-being system in the promotion of positive experiences. Outcomes suggest that this system is able of promoting subjective well-being not only in nonclinical population in a controlled setting [49] but also in participants with a medical condition in natural settings (e.g. hospital) [50]. These findings are quite relevant taking into account that PTs try to improve the quality of the personal experiences, and therefore, must be accessible and easy to use in different context and daily conditions.

In this sense, it is of relevance to consider the fact that both populations included in this paper (students and cancer population) had very different age range (x=25 vs x=60 years) and educational level (superior vs basic level) which suggests the viability of this PT system for different types of population.

Beyond testing the usefulness of this system for different groups of people, is also interesting to analyze the particularities that could arise when different populations use the system. Regarding this, it seems that for both groups the use of VR environments was quite attractive, and although for all participants both modules of the system (VR and Book of Life) were useful, data suggest that for cancer patients the book of life was a relevant component of the intervention. It would be of interest to continue exploring the specific weight of each component of the system to better understand its possibilities and limits.

Another aspect to take into account when analyzing PT is the role of expertise with technologies. As this could be a serious limitation, PTs usually try to include simple interaction devices and brief instructions. However, it seems that even more important than the experience per se, is the proneness to technologies the key gap to overtake. In the case of the populations included in this paper, university students usually are prone to technologies' use. However, this is not the case of cancer participants: they were no very familiar with technologies (some of them had no experience at all) and some were even reluctant. However, they were able of use the system and obtained psychological benefits from it, just like the university students did. Possibly, to introduce the system as a tool designed to help them to achieve a better mood state, and as a "working together" exercise (participant plus researcher) may have been of help to approximate these technologies to this population.

It should be noted that one limitation of the studies with nonclinical population is that they were composed by University students, who are not representative of general population, and the generalizability of our findings is limited. Despite this, data obtained so far are encouraging, and invite us to continue exploring the possibilities of this system with more heterogeneous populations. Future studies with bigger and more diverse samples will allow us to identify in a better way the particular needs and benefits obtained by each type of population who use EARTH system.

Another limitation is the absence of control group in the studies with oncology patients. It will be necessary to include a comparison group to confirm the preliminary data obtained so far with this population. Besides, it is important to notice the short-term of the benefits obtained with EARTH system in the populations assessed. In the case of cancer patients there were improvements after sessions but no follow-ups were included. In the case of university students, no differences were found between EG and CG in the evaluations post intervention, and therefore, is not possible to state the maintenance of the benefits obtained post sessions. Future studies should investigate the efficacy of EARTH in protocols that includes a longer intervention time, given that previous research have indicated the hedonic adaptation as an important obstacle in the efficacy of PIs [53]. To explore this aspect in natural settings could also generate valuable information regarding the feasibility of implement these systems in daily life environments, and its capacity to maintain the benefits even in variable conditions.

Finally, another relevant line to explore is the cost-effectiveness of EARTH in particular, and PTs in general. Previous studies have suggested the importance of economic evaluations and the absence of studies which addressed this issue [54]. To continue exploring the advantages and disadvantages of these technologies in terms of efficacy, efficiency, usability and costs is vital to add more solid evidence to support the health professional's decisions.

References

1. Sin, N.L., Lyubomirsky, S.: Enhancing well-being and alleviating depressive symptoms with positive psychology interventions: a practice-friendly meta-analysis. J. Clin. Psychol. **65**, 467–487 (2009)
2. Bolier, L., Haverman, M., Westerhof, G.J., Riper, H., Smit, F., Bohlmeijer, E.: Positive psychology interventions: a meta-analysis of randomized controlled studies. BMC Public Health **13**, 119 (2013)
3. Seligman, M.E.P., Steen, T., Park, N., Peterson, C.: Positive psychology progress: empirical validation of interventions. Am. Psychol. **60**, 410–421 (2005)
4. Sheldon, K.M., Lyubomirsky, S.: How to increase and sustain positive emotion: the effects of expressing gratitude and visualizing best possible selves. J. Posit. Psychol. **1**, 73–82 (2006)
5. Cavanagh, K., Shapiro, D.: Computer treatment for common mental health problems. J. Clin. Psychol. **60**, 239–251 (2004)

6. Layard, R., Clark, D., Knapp, M., Mayraz, G.: Cost-benefit analysis of psychological therapy. Natl. I. Econ. Rev. **202**, 90–98 (2007)
7. Opris, D., Pintea, S., García-Palacios, A., Botella, C., Szamosközi, S., David, D.: Virtual reality exposure therapy in anxiety disorders: a quantitative meta-analysis. Depress. Anxiety **29**, 85–93 (2012)
8. Powers, M., Emmelkamp, P.: Virtual reality exposure therapy for anxiety disorders: a meta-analysis. J. Anxiety Disord. **22**, 561–569 (2008)
9. Roy-Byrne, P., Craske, M.G., Sullivan, G., Rose, R.D., Edlund, M.J., Lang, A.J., Bystritsky, A., Welch, S.S., Chavira, D.A., Golinelli, D., Campbell-Sills, L., Sherbourne, C.D., Stein, M.B.: Delivery of evidence-based treatment for multiple anxiety disorders in primary care: a randomized controlled trial. JAMA **303**, 1921–1928 (2010)
10. Miller, G.: The smartphone psychology manifesto. Perspect. Psychol. Sci. **7**, 221–237 (2012)
11. Bolier, L., Haverman, M., Kramer, J., Westerhof, G.J., Riper, H., Walburg, J.A., Boon, B., Bohlmeijer, E.: An Internet-based intervention to promote mental fitness for mildly depressed adults: randomized controlled trial. J. Med. Internet Res. **15**, e200 (2013)
12. Drozd, F., Mork, L., Nielsen, B., Raeder, S., Bjørkli, C.A.: Better days. A randomized controlled trial of an internet-based positive psychology intervention. J. Posit. Psychol. **9**, 377–388 (2014)
13. Ritterband, L.M., Gonder-Frederick, L.A., Cox, D.J., Clifton, A.D., West, R.W., Borowitz, S.M.: Internet interventions: In review, in use, and into the future. Prof. Psychol. **34**, 527–534 (2003)
14. Mohr, D.C., Burns, M.N., Schueller, S.M., Clarke, G., Klinkman, M.: Behavioral intervention technologies: evidence review and recommendations for future research in mental health. Gen. Hosp. Psychiat. **35**, 332–338 (2013)
15. Botella, C., Riva, G., Gaggioli, A., Wiederhold, B.K., Alcaniz, M., Baños, R.M.: The present and future of positive technologies. Cyberpsychol. Behav. **15**, 78–84 (2012)
16. Riva, G., Baños, R.M., Botella, C., Wiederhold, B.K., Gaggioli, A.: Positive technology: using interactive technologies to promote positive functioning. Cyberpsychol. Behav. **15**, 69–77 (2012)
17. Parks, A.C., Della Porta, M.D., Pierce, R.S., Zilca, R., Lyubomirsky, S.: Pursuing happiness in everyday life: the characteristics and behaviors of online happiness seekers. Emotion **12**, 1222–1234 (2012)
18. Baños, R., Etchemendy, E., Farfallini, L., García-Palacios, A., Quero, S., Botella, C.: EARTH of Well-Being system: a pilot study of an information and communication technology-based positive psychology intervention. J. Posit. Psychol. **9**, 482–488 (2014)
19. Diener, E.: Subjective well-being. Psychol. Bull. **95**, 542–575 (1984)
20. Ryff, C.: Happiness is everything, or is it? explorations on the meaning of psychological well-being. J. Pers. Soc. Psychol. **57**, 1069–1081 (1989)
21. Layous, K., Lyubomirsky, S.: The how, who, what, when, and why of happiness: Mechanisms underlying the success of positive interventions. In: Gruber, J., Moscowitz, J. (eds.) The Light and Dark Side of Positive Emotions. Oxford University Press, New York (2012)
22. García-Palacios, A., Baños, R.: Eficacia de dos procedimientos de inducción del estado de ánimo e influencia de variables moduladoras. Rev. Psicopatología y Psicol. Clínica **4**, 15–26 (1999)
23. Fredrickson, B.L.: Cultivating positive emotions to optimize health and well-being. Prev. Treat. 3 (2000)
24. Fredrickson, B.L.: Positive emotions broaden and build. In: Plant, E.A., Devine, P.G. (eds.) Advances on Experimental Social Psychology, vol. 47, pp. 1–53. Academic Press, Burlington (2013)

25. Fredrickson, B., Levenson, R.: Positive emotions speed recovery from the cardiovascular sequelae of negative emotions. Cogn. Emotion **12**, 191–220 (1998)
26. Fredrickson, B., Mancuso, R., Branigan, C., Tugade, M.: The undoing effect of positive emotions. Motiv. Emotion. **24**(4), 237–258 (2000)
27. Baños, R.M., Botella, B., Alcañiz, M., Liaño, V., Guerrero, B., Rey, B.: Immersion and Emotion: The impact on the sense of presence. Cyberpsychol. Behav. **7**, 734–741 (2004)
28. Baños, R.M., Liaño, V., Botella, C., Alcañiz, M., Guerrero, B., Rey, B.: Changing induced moods via virtual reality. In: IJsselsteijn, W.A., de Kort, Y.A., Midden, C., Eggen, B., van den Hoven, E. (eds.) PERSUASIVE 2006. LNCS, vol. 3962, pp. 7–15. Springer, Heidelberg (2006)
29. Burton, C.M., King, L.: The health benefits of writing about intensely positive experiences. J. Res. Pers. **38**, 150–163 (2004)
30. Burton, C.M., King, L.: The health benefits of writing about positive experiences: the role of broadened cognition. Psychol. Health. **24**, 867–879 (2009)
31. Pennebaker, J., Seagal, J.: Forming a story: the health benefits of narrative. J. Clin. Psychol. **55**, 1243–1254 (1999)
32. Haight, B.K., Webster, J.D.: The Art and Science of Reminiscing: Theory, Research, Methods, and Applications. Taylor & Francis Ltd., London (1995)
33. Serrano, J.P., Latorre, J.M., Ros, L., Navarro, B., Aguilar, M.J., Nieto, M., Ricarte, J., Gatz, M.: Life review therapy using autobiographical retrieval practice for older adults with clinical depression. Psicothema **24**, 224–229 (2012)
34. King, L.A.: The health benefits of writing about life goals. Pers. Soc. Psychol B. **27**, 798–807 (2001)
35. Peters, M.L., Flink, I.K., Boersma, K., Linton, S.J.: Manipulating optimism: can imagining a best possible self be used to increase positive future expectancies? J. Posit. Psychol. **5**, 204–211 (2010)
36. Seligman, M., Rashid, T., Parks, A.: Positive Psychotherapy. Am. Psychol. **61**, 774–788 (2006)
37. Abbott, J., Klein, B., Ciechomski, L.: Best practices in online therapy. J. Technol. Hum. Serv. **26**, 360–375 (2008)
38. Barak, A., Klein, B., Proudfoot, J.G.: Defining internet-supported therapeutic interventions. Ann. Behav. Med. **38**, 4–17 (2009)
39. Fredrickson, B.: Positivity. Crown Publishers, New York (2009)
40. Sutherland, G., Newman, B., Rachman, S.: Experimental investigations of the relations between mood and intrusive unwanted cognitions. Brit. J. Med. Psychol. **55**, 127–138 (1982)
41. Velten, E.: A laboratory task for induction of mood states. Behav. Res. Ther. **6**, 473–482 (1968)
42. Lang, P.J., Bradley, M.M., Cuthbert, B.N.: International affective picture system (IAPS): Technical manual and affective ratings. NIMH Center for the Study of Emotion and Attention, Gainesville: University of Florida (1995)
43. Gross, J.J., Levenson, R.W.: Emotion elicitation using films. Cogn. Emot. **9**, 87–108 (1995)
44. Brewer, D., Doughtie, E.B.: Induction of mood and mood shift. J. Clin. Psychol. **36**, 215–226 (1980)
45. Gabrielsson, A., Lindström, E.: The influence of musical structure on emotional expression. In: Juslin, P., Sloboda, J.A. (eds.) Music and Emotion: Theory and Research, pp. 223–248. Oxford University Press, Oxford (2001)
46. Guilford, J.P., Smith, P.C.: A system of color preferences. Am. J. Psychol. **72**, 487–502 (1959)

47. Andreu-Mateu, S., Botella, C., Quero, S., Guillén, V., Baños, R.: La utilización de la realidad virtual y estrategias de psicología positiva en el tratamiento de los trastornos adaptativos. Psicol. Conduct. **20**, 323–348 (2012)
48. Baños, R.M., Etchemendy, E., Castilla, D., García-Palacios, A., Quero, S., Botella, C.: Positive mood induction procedures for virtual environments designed for elderly people. Interact. Comput. **24**, 131–138 (2012)
49. Farfallini, L.: Validación de una intervención positiva auto-aplicada orientada al bienestar: EARTH of Well-being. Tesis doctoral. Unpublished manuscript (2014)
50. Baños, R.M., Espinoza, M., García-Palacios, A., Cervera, J.M., Esquerdo, G., Barrajón, E., Botella, C.: A positive psychological intervention using virtual reality for patients with advanced cancer in a hospital setting: A pilot study to assess feasibility. Support. Care Cancer **21**, 263–270 (2013)
51. Espinoza, M., Baños, R.M., García-Palacios, A., Botella, C., Cervera, J., Esquerdo, G., Barrajón, E.: Preferences and usefulness of a brief psychological intervention that uses information and communication technologies (ICT) to promote well-being in adult oncology inpatients. In: Poster Presented at Third World Congress on Positive Psychology, IPPA, Amsterdam, Holland, June 2013
52. Espinoza, M., Baños, R.M., García-Palacios, A., Botella, C.: La Realidad Virtual en las Intervenciones Psicológicas con Pacientes Oncológicos. Psicooncología **10**, 247–261 (2013)
53. Lyubomirsky, S.: Hedonic adaptation to positive and negative experiences. In: Folkman, S. (ed.) The Oxford Handbook of Stress Health and Coping, pp. 100–124. Oxford University Press, Oxford (2011)
54. Bolier, L., Majo, C., Smit, F., Westerhof, G.J., Haverman, M., Walburg, J.A., Riper, H., Bohlmeijer, E.: Cost-effectiveness of online positive psychology: Randomized controlled trial. J. Posit. Psychol. **9**, 460–471 (2014)

Maintain and Improve Mental Health by Smart Virtual Reality Serious Games

András Sárkány[1], Zoltán Tősér[1], Anita L. Verő[1], András Lőrincz[1(✉)], Takumi Toyama[2], Ehsan N. Toosi[2], and Daniel Sonntag[2]

[1] Faculty of Informatics, Eötvös Loránd University, Pázmány Péter Sétány 1/C, Budapest 1117, Hungary
lorincz@inf.elte.hu
[2] German Research Center for Artificial Intelligence, Trippstadter Strasse 122, 67663 Kaiserslautern, Germany

Abstract. Serious games for mental health is seen as the groundwork for assistive technology to maintain and improve mental health. We present a technical system layout we partly implemented for demonstration purposes and highlight vision-based perception and manipulation capabilities. These include physical interactions employing artificial general intelligence in virtual reality applications. We employ hand gesture tracking, as well as an Oculus Rift integrated gaze and eye tracking system. The resulting serious games should eventually cover daily life activities, which we additionally monitor. The dynamic and contextual modelling of obstacles are central issues, and capabilities required for serious games include knowledge about the 3D world. Such knowledge include gaze and hand sensors interpretations for multimedia information extraction in causal relationships. Towards this goal, we envision to make use of virtual reality with a physics engine (rigid and soft body dynamics including collision detection) for the observed objects. We also exploit semantic networks to enable the machine to filter information and infer ongoing complex events including hidden BDI (beliefs, desires, intentions) variables. We see this combination of employed technology as the relevant groundwork for reaching human-level general intelligence and to enable real-world applications. Future applications and user groups we target on include dementia patients.

1 Introduction

Recognition of ongoing activities and prediction of intentions of players in serious games environments is a big challenge as so many context factors have to be taken into account. On the other hand, it provides considerable advantages in behavioral understanding and thus, in the evolution of the capabilities of serious games: (1) the efficient harmonization and synchronization of behaviors of multiple players and the AI engine, (2) the disambiguation of speech-based input, and (3) the potential compression of user input information to be communicated or monitored.

A. Lőrincz—This research was supported by EIT Digital in the *CPS for Smart Factories* activity and Kognit, http://kognit.dfki.de.

© Springer International Publishing Switzerland 2016
S. Serino et al. (Eds.): MindCare 2015, CCIS 604, pp. 220–229, 2016.
DOI: 10.1007/978-3-319-32270-4_22

Our main application is the provision of novel methods of treatment of dementia, the modelling of the cognitive impairments in particular. It is increasingly recognised that pharmacological treatments for dementia should be used as a second-line approach and that non-pharmacological options should, in best practice, be pursued first [7]. People with dementia and their caregivers are often advised that 'mental exercise' (in the form of a serious game in virtual reality (VR)) may be helpful in slowing down the decline in memory and thinking experienced by many affected individuals. [26]

We concern ourselves with daily life situations of the patient in VR, where we use robust detectors of hands and gaze, and embed observed objects into VR having a physics engine. Our game example shows that we can interpret ongoing events as well as intentions. The development of such serious games is additionally supported by a number of clinical research and related works about memories of daily life activities, a design case study for Alzheimer's disease [5], reality orientation for geriatric patients [23], using validation techniques with people living with dementia [3], and computer based technology and caring for older adults [22]. Recent studies investigate whether a VR cognitive training application, e.g., a virtual supermarket (VSM), can be used as a screening tool for mild cognitive impairment [29]. We try to classify and work against such impairment for serious games in daily life activities.

For everyday life activities, motion detection based on vision or sound, and motion prediction is of great importance. We learn models of the three dimensional world and a naïve model of physics at a very young age. Today, one can embed such knowledge into artificial intelligence applications when observations are properly transferred to VR environments together with the computer models of the virtual world. As a result, dynamical properties of flexibility, rigidness, properties of solids, liquids gases can be simulated. In turn, potential interactions between objects (e.g., when a glass falls down, then it might break) become part of the model based approach. Other potential events, e.g., that a sharp knife can cut the skin, are conveyed by different additional information sources for common sense reasoning, including large databases, books, scientific literature, and the semantic web—knowledge bases constructed via crowdsourcing have become broadly available.

We argue that complementing symbolic knowledge with a physics engine improves machine interpretation capabilities for serious games for mental health to a great extent. Machine intelligence needs additional information about intention, which is hidden from direct observations, but is needed for interaction, e.g., for knowing if the game player is missing some information, or his or her capabilities are limited and help is needed for efficient cooperation, for competing task, or for general task completion. Information about individual BDIs may improve assistive technologies to a great extent even in very small tasks. In daily life activities, examples of task completion include to successfully pour coffee into a cup or to spread butter on a toast. Such knowledge about task performance and completion may be extracted from gaze orientation and gestures (including facial expressions) and from general and individual behavioural regularities.

The purpose of the serious games would be to stimulate the memory and thinking process of dementia patients while they perform everyday activities in VR, which can be supervised by the system we describe to the extent of giving appropriate hints via simple text-based communication. For example, the user has to perform spreading butter on the bread which requires searching for the applicable tool (knife) in its everyday location (kitchen) and executing proper actions with her hand.

In this paper, we provide two illustrative task examples for dementia related tasks as serious games, and disambiguate their task execution for a better understanding and monitoring. We show by an exemplary technical evaluation that the interpretation and prediction of such ongoing events have become feasible (Sect. 2). Then, we argue that monitoring of daily task events in serious games for mental health may involve only little additional effort that can be delivered by sensing and data processing. Last, but not least, we discuss the general relevance of such VR serious games and conclude in Sect. 3. As a test system based on qualitative judgements, the argumentation is based on observations or indications rather than rigorous or scientific analysis. Researchers may use our scenario and findings for suggesting new hypotheses for mental health applications.

2 Illustrative Examples

First, we showcase our concept in a VR human-computer interaction scenario that can infer the goals of gestures towards intention recognition by means of gaze tracking. In our illustrative example, object recognition can also disambiguate the situation. Although we present a very simple case, the combined information of recognized objects and gaze information tells more about the targeted motion pattern than the object recognition (and tracking) alone. This example is followed by the description of a more complex scenario that should exploit predictive models, symbolic knowledge, as well as cost and risk considerations. Assisting technologies can be implemented in both cases.

2.1 Activity and Intention

The VR scenario includes the perception of human intentions (conveyed by state-of-the-art sensors) and visual feedback provided by a VR headworn display, i.e., the *Oculus Rift*. We attached a LeapMotion tool to the front of the Oculus Rift to detect hand poses in real-time and the *SMI gaze and eye tracking system*, which is built into the Oculus Rift[1], is used to recognize the gaze patterns.

In this way VR and its attached physics engine can mirror and model the environmental manipulations. We also include *ConceptNet* [14,21], a semantic network collected by crowdsourcing. We use it for inferring information about tools and human activities.

---

[1] http://www.smivision.com/en/gaze-and-eye-tracking-systems/products/eye-tracking-hmd-upgrade.html.

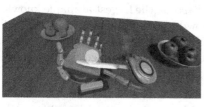
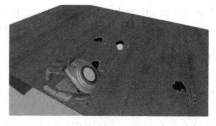

(a) spread butter   (b) wipe table

Fig. 1. Two activities, (a): *"butter spreading"* and (b): *"wiping the table"*. Yellow disk: target of gaze. Hand gestures are very similar, while gaze reflects both attention (buttering and wiping) and intention (clean next dirty spot, also shown) (Color figure online).

We present two illustrative scenarios, *"butter spreading"* and *"wiping the table"*; we try to distinguish and interpret these activities. We use compressed, low-dimensional VR features being useful when building semantic representations of spoken or written speech [28] from multimodal input, event annotation [1], or question answering scenarios [13]. The high level sensors eliminate noise and we have (i) a pure 3D skeleton model of the hand and (ii) the target of gaze in 3D. One can extract and recognize what the hand is holding and what the user is looking at. In our example, hand gestures (grabbing combined with periodic motion) are similar and data in a short time frame can be misleading. This low-dimensional information may be sufficient, e.g., if it is known that the user is resting, has nothing in his or her hand, or has got tremor. In this scenario, the frequency of the periodic motion is low and the periodicity is irregular are sufficient for eliminating tremor as an option. If there is no object manipulated then the quasi-periodic motion may be related to communication (e.g., waving.) Gaze is an additional source of information that can detect if the user is waving to somebody. Gaze alone may provide additional information, e.g., when the user is searching for something. In fact, we may detect what the user is looking for (see, e.g., [2]) based on episodic information [24].

Gaze direction may differ in the two scenarios. Spreading the butter may need attention (if the butter is even or not) and then the bread is the target of the gaze. Wiping may require less attention (if the dirt disappeared or not) and the gaze can search for the next spot to be removed (Fig. 1). Assume now that the objects used and thus the engaging activities are recognized. Assume further that monitoring in the past shows that focus of attention is needed for butter spreading, but not needed for cleaning a spot on the table. If the system detects different behaviors in these scenarios, then this comes unexpected and the causes can be guessed. In either case, speech-based interaction is possible, e.g., when the activity is about to finish.

Considerable knowledge about human needs and material properties is required. Background knowledge about objects that are manipulated or gazed at, including bread, butter, knife, and sponge is available on the Internet.

The question is how to query such knowledge from the individual knowledge source. Below, we show examples based on *Wikipedia*, the largest available knowledge base at the moment, *ConceptNet*, a crowdsourced semantic network, and the probabilistic language model of *Google Ngram*. These are samples of crowdsourced knowledge bases (Wikipedia and ConceptNet) combined with machine learning models (Google Ngram) in a broader sense.

Wikipedia. Cleaning the table, having breakfast and cleaning the table again make a natural order of episodes and could be part of the daily routine. Similar routines are typical in our daily life activities in many different dimensions [20] and the temporal order enables efficient predictions about the ongoing event. So, if the breakfast has been finished and the typical practice is cleaning, then sensory information about hand motion may be sufficient to properly infer what is happening. We can also use Wikipedia for context based filtering. Explicit Semantic Analysis [8] (ESA) is a good example. Roughly speaking, this method (i) takes a word and its textual environment, (ii) measures the relative frequency of that word on all Wikipedia pages, and (iii) uses the pages with highest relative frequency for semantic restrictions. It restricts potential interpretations very efficiently. Special methods demonstrate that noisy automatic character recognition input can be interpreted by means of ESA [18,19].

ConceptNet. While Wikipedia can restrict the domain interpretation, it can't provide information about the ongoing events, e.g., if the conditions of the expected event are satisfied, if it is being performed successfully, and when it may be finished. Crowdsourcing has been directed towards collecting such information and this is one of the goals of ConceptNet. ConceptNet collects common-sense information about what for example a household article is *UsedFor*, is *CapableOf* and if it *HasPrerequisite*. One can use ConceptNet and Wikipedia for inferring about ongoing event within spatio-temporal contexts.

N-Grams. Neither Wikipedia nor ConceptNet knowledge snippets facilitate dialogue management directly. One can however use a simple and inexpensive method for generating sentences, although only with moderate success. It serves illustration purposes well and it has been applied in augmentative and alternative communication [25] as a statistics based method that exploits n-grams collected from texts. The method exploits the order of the words and can put forth the next word ordered by the probabilities that it followed the previous words in written texts. The method is related to data compression. It has already been used in some early applications in this domain [4].

2.2   Architecture that Combines the Methods

The architecture that combines the methods is sketched in Fig. 2. The first part (in blue) evaluates ongoing gaze and hand motions. This portion of the information restricts observations about the tools and objects present to the tools

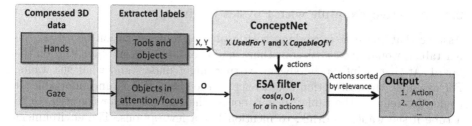

Fig. 2. Method of evaluation of potential activities. For more information, see text (Color figure online).

and objects attended and to those that are subject of the ongoing manipulation (in green). Part of the returned information is relevant for the situation that can be inferred from spatial and temporal constraints and past episodes and practices. The tool for the contextual information is ESA based on Wikipedia (grey), whereas the tool for inferring about the ongoing event is ConceptNet (pink). The resulting assistive system would–in principle–sort the interactions, including non-actions, according to relevance. If communication is needed, then the probabilistic language model can be used.

2.3 ConceptNet in the Example

We experimented with ConceptNet for the above example on 'knife' in hand with context 'bread+butter' and 'bread' with context 'knife+butter' (Fig. 3(a)) on 'sponge' in hand with context 'dirt' (Fig. 3(b)). We ranked the offered solutions according to their ESA ranks cummulated in the ESA vectors of the word and their contexts, respectively. The resulting ordered list ranks more relevant activities higher. However, for both cases we found sensible gaps between relevant and irrelevant words (Fig. 3). In Fig. 3 red line shows the position of the gap with some examples included.

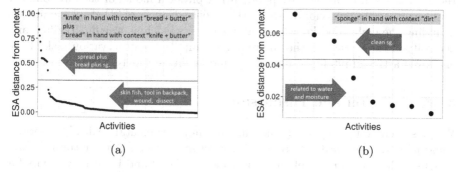

(a)   (b)

Fig. 3. Semantic similarity between concepts derived from ConceptNet from the objects held in the hand(s) and the 'context', i.e., the objects gazed. Red line: gap threshold for relevant and irrelevant activities (Color figure online).

2.4   Assistive Example with Physics Engine

Assume that the user is working with a picture communication board [12] on her tablet, would like to ask something, and chooses the symbol for 'tilt' on the board. At that point, an intelligent partner might understand what she wants. For example, the instruction could refer to the chair, if it is uncomfortable. It could also refer to the tablet, if it is not at the right angle for the user, or to a tube if she wants to drink, to mention but a few options. The environment and the ongoing events can disambiguate what she wants. For example, if she is wearing smart clothes then it can be inferred that she is sitting comfortably. If the tablet is on the table facing her at the right angle, but the tube is out of reach at that moment, then she might want to drink. Episodic understanding and prediction may change this belief. Assume that the tablet is on the table, but it started to flip towards the edge, so that it may/will fall. In this case, she most probably wants the table tilted and the instruction may concern either the intelligent wheelchair or the accompanying robot to make this happen. However, falling is not a feature of the tablet. Nonetheless, if the assistive robot is using 3D VR models which exploit physics and have a 3D model of the room, then ongoing dynamical processes can be identified, computed, and *predicted* immediately. In turn, the accompanying assistive robot or 3D model would be able to figure out that the moving *object* may/will fall and the short instruction 'tilt' should refer to the table holding the tablet.

The critical features are as follows: (i) The assistive robot or 3D VR engine should observe that something is moving. (Motion detection has been solved in the community to a large degree.) (ii) It should identify that the moving object is the tablet. This detection is much more difficult when the object is occluded. Occlusion can be tackled by using 3D models that can track objects and their features, and thus 'know' about the occluded parts: they can complete the pattern of the object from a few features in 3D. 3D model is the solution to many partially observed problems, including the walls or obstacles behind the moving wheelchair or the robot. If the robot or the wheelchair are missing parts of necessary information, then they should either (re-)identify those, or, the accuracy can be arbitrarily poor. (iii) A physical model of the environment enables pro-active behavior. In short, the recent advances of 3D graphical models including the embedded knowledge about physics, such as weight, fragility, and elasticity of the objects in the environment simplify the observation task of the employed artificial intelligence modules and facilitate timely interactions.

3   Conclusion and Discussion

We presented system layout to maintain and improve mental health by a serious game in VR. The hardware tools of our setup allow for very natural control actions such as movement of the head to look around and hand movements for manipulation of the 3D world, thus we expect fast acceptance even by older adults. The game includes a model of the observable part of the physical world. Such information alleviates interpretation and prediction since laws of physics are deterministic. We added the models of sensed information about the user, including the objects held in the hands and the objects gazed at. We exemplified how common sense and language resources can be connected to the potential actions occurring in the physical world, and that these sources can be exploited to select the best options by means of semantic similarities. We also discussed certain aspects of intentions, which are needed for efficient assistance.

When identifying an event, each sensory modality can add more information. On the other hand, many information sources can be abandoned if the activity is identified and a deterministic 3D dynamical model is matched. We illustrated both of these by utilizing sensory information processed by high tech devices and collected textual databases. Our illustration utilizes VR with 3D physics engine, high level sensors, symbolic components such as Wikipedia and ConceptNet, and sub-symbolic components, such as gaze. High-level inference was implemented via methods operating on the symbolic level.

When the sensory information is insufficient for disambiguation and interpretation, then information about what has just happened could be of value. Furthermore, episodic information collected over longer times can be exploited, too, since longer term individual behavioral patterns have low entropy [20]. Once the situation is disambiguated, and an activity contained in the knowledge base recognised, the activity model can be used to predict potential outcomes enabling pro-active interaction with the ongoing event.

Crowdsourcing efforts [10] that exploit human intelligence are booming and improving [6] and may guide artificial intelligence to human level understanding if complemented with high-level sensors and 3D physics [15]. There are a few directions worth mentioning here:

Special AI Methods: Recent advances in deep learning methods have passed human performance in a number of classification task. The same technology shows strengths in goal-oriented behavior even when only low-level visual information is available [16]. Expectations are high in this respect and we might see considerable breakthrough in the coming years.

Emotions: The prerequisites of emotionally sensitive assistive responses include (i) emotion detection and (ii) personalized reactions. The former may take advantage of facial expression estimation [11], gaze direction measurements [27], gesture [17], and prosody estimations [9] among others in this fast developing field.

Personalization and forecasting: Web 3.0 technology and IoT scenarios can lead to precise monitoring, spatio-temporal regularity extraction, and inference about ongoing events given collected data about past events of the individual and also from many other people, including individuals with similar personalities and problems. This direction belongs to the cross section of collaborative filtering, big data, data mining, and recommender systems, all undergoing fast evolution recently.

Beliefs, desires, intentions: Emotions, personalization and forecasting are linked to BDIs; i.e., to motivations, fears, explicit and implicit goals. Longer-term goals (on the order of hours or so) are to be matched to shorter term activities.

228 A. Sárkány et al.

Machine learning should serve a person with dementia very well: activities towards longer-term goals can be achieved if their prerequisites are satisfied and that can be tracked by IoT.

Interestingly, the successful implementation of further dementia-related VR games includes the knowledge about the 3D world, i.e., knowledge of material properties described by physics and chemistry. Knowledge at the level of a child is sufficient in many respects. We have argued about the power of virtual reality in this context. Further investigations should include high tech tools to collect sensory information as partly illustrated by our examples to be connected to a fully-integrated smart virtual reality serious games platform.

References

1. Antol, S., Zitnick, C.L., Parikh, D.: Zero-shot learning via visual abstraction. In: Fleet, D., Pajdla, T., Schiele, B., Tuytelaars, T. (eds.) ECCV 2014, Part IV. LNCS, vol. 8692, pp. 401–416. Springer, Heidelberg (2014)
2. Borji, A., Lennartz, A., Pomplun, M.: What do eyes reveal about the mind?: algorithmic inference of search targets from fixations. Neurocomputing **149**, 788–799 (2015)
3. Cirillo, A.: Using validation techniques with people living with dementia, June 2013. http://assistedliving.about.com/od/familycaregivercommunication/a/Using-Validation-Techniques-With-People-Living-With-Dementia.htm
4. Cleary, J.G., Witten, I.H.: Data compression using adaptive coding and partial string matching. IEEE Trans. Commun. **32**(4), 396–402 (1984)
5. Cohene, T., Baecker, R., Marziali, E., Mindy, S.: Memories of a life: a design case study for alzheimer's disease. In: Lazar, J. (ed.) Universal Usability, pp. 357–387. Wiley, Chichester (2007)
6. Dai, P., Lin, C.H., Weld, D.S., et al.: Pomdp-based control of workflows for crowd-sourcing. Artif. Intell. **202**, 52–85 (2013)
7. Douglas, S., James, I., Ballard, C.: Non-pharmacological interventions in dementia. Adv. Psychiatr. Treat. **10**(3), 171–177 (2004)
8. Gabrilovich, E., Markovitch, S.: Computing semantic relatedness using wikipedia-based explicit semantic analysis. In: IJCAI, vol. 7, pp. 1606–1611 (2007)
9. Gharsellaoui, S., Selouani, S.A., Dahmane, A.O.: Automatic emotion recognition using auditory and prosodic indicative features. In: 2015 IEEE 28th Canadian Conference on Electrical and Computer Engineering (CCECE), pp. 1265–1270. IEEE (2015)
10. Howe, J.: The rise of crowdsourcing. Wired Mag. **14**(6), 1–4 (2006)
11. Jeni, L.A., Lőrincz, A., Szabó, Z., Cohn, J.F., Kanade, T.: Spatio-temporal event classification using time-series kernel based structured sparsity. In: Fleet, D., Pajdla, T., Schiele, B., Tuytelaars, T. (eds.) ECCV 2014, Part IV. LNCS, vol. 8692, pp. 135–150. Springer, Heidelberg (2014)
12. Jonson, R.: Picture Communication Symbols. Mayer-Johnson, Solana Beach (1985)
13. Lin, X., Parikh, D.: Don't just listen, use your imagination: leveraging visual common sense for non-visual tasks. arXiv preprint arXiv:1502.06108 (2015)
14. Liu, H., Singh, P.: Conceptnet – a practical commonsense reasoning tool-kit. BT Technol. J. **22**(4), 211–226 (2004)

15. Lőrincz, A.: Revolution in health and wellbeing. KI-Künstliche Intelligenz **29**(2), 219–222 (2015)
16. Mnih, V., Kavukcuoglu, K., Silver, D., Rusu, A.A., Veness, J., Bellemare, M.G., Graves, A., Riedmiller, M., Fidjeland, A.K., Ostrovski, G., et al.: Human-level control through deep reinforcement learning. Nature **518**(7540), 529–533 (2015)
17. Oberweger, M., Wohlhart, P., Lepetit, V.: Hands deep in deep learning for hand pose estimation. arXiv preprint arXiv:1502.06807 (2015)
18. Pintér, B., Vörös, G., Palotai, Z., Szabó, Z., Lőrincz, A.: Determining unintelligible words from their textual contexts. Procedia Soc. Behav. Sci. **73**, 101–108 (2013)
19. Pintér, B., Vörös, G., Szabó, Z., Lőrincz, A.: Wikifying novel words to mixtures of wikipedia senses by structured sparse coding. In: Fred, A., De Marsico, M. (eds.) Pattern Recogn. Appl. Methods, pp. 241–255. Springer, Heidelberg (2015)
20. Song, C., Qu, Z., Blumm, N., Barabási, A.L.: Limits of predictability in human mobility. Science **327**(5968), 1018–1021 (2010)
21. Speer, R., Havasi, C.: Representing general relational knowledge in conceptnet 5. In: LREC, pp. 3679–3686 (2012)
22. Foundation, S.: Computer based technology and caring for older adults (2003). http://www.spry.org/pdf/cbtcoa_english.pdf
23. Taulbee, L.R., Folsom, J.C.: Reality orientation for geriatric patients. Psychiatr. Serv. **17**(5), 133–135 (1966)
24. Toyama, T., Sonntag, D.: Towards episodic memory support for dementia patients by recognizing objects, faces and text in eye gaze. In: Hölldobler, S., Krötzsch, M., Peñaloza, R., Rudolph, S. (eds.) KI 2015. LNCS, vol. 9324, pp. 316–323. Springer, Heidelberg (2015). doi:10.1007/978-3-319-24489-1_29
25. Vörös, G., Verő, A., Pintér, B., Miksztai-Réthey, B., Toyama, T., Lőrincz, A., Sonntag, D.: Towards a smart wearable tool to enable people with SSPI to communicate by sentence fragments. In: Cipresso, P., Matic, A., Lopez, G. (eds.) MindCare 2014. LNICST, vol. 100, pp. 90–99. Springer, Heidelberg (2014)
26. Woods, B., Aguirre, E., Spector, A.E., Orrell, M.: Cognitive stimulation to improve cognitive functioning in people with dementia. Cochrane Database Syst Rev 2 (2012)
27. Zhang, X., Sugano, Y., Fritz, M., Bulling, A.: Appearance-based gaze estimation in the wild. In: 2015 IEEE Conference on Computer Vision and Pattern Recognition. IEEE Computer Society (2015)
28. Zitnick, C.L., Parikh, D., Tech, V.: Bringing semantics into focus using visual abstraction. In: 2013 IEEE Conference on Computer Vision and Pattern Recognition (CVPR). IEEE (2013)
29. Zygouris, S., Giakoumis, D., Votis, K., Doumpoulakis, S., Ntovas, K., Segkouli, S., Karagiannidis, C., Tzovaras, D., Tsolaki, M.: Can a virtual reality cognitive training application fulfill a dual role? Using the virtual supermarket cognitive training application as a screening tool for mild cognitive impairment. J. Alzheimers Dis. **40**, 1–10 (2014)

Internet-Based Intervention for Secondary and Tertiary Prevention of Depressive Symptoms

Adriana Mira[1(✉)], Juana Bretón-López[1,3], Azucena García-Palacios[1,3], Rosa Baños[2,3], and Cristina Botella[1,3]

[1] Universitat Jaume I, Castellón de la Plana, Spain
{miraa,breton,azucena,botella}@uji.es
[2] Universitat de València, Valencia, Spain
banos@uv.es
[3] CIBER Fisiopatología de la Obesidad y Nutrición (CB06/03), Instituto de Salud Carlos III, Santiago de Compostela, Spain

Abstract. Depression is one of the most disabling psychological disorders worldwide. A very important challenge today consists on addressing the issue of depression from a preventive perspective. A growing body of research supports the efficacy of Internet-based treatments. We have developed an Internet-based program (*Smiling is Fun*) with the objective of helping people in prevention of depression and anxiety symptoms. It is based on classical cognitive behavioral techniques, such as behavioural activation, and also includes other positive psychological strategies to improve coping ability and positive mood. We applied this intervention program in people who had to cope at least with one stressor in their life producing interference (secondary prevention) and also in people who had to cope at least a stressor and met the diagnosis of an emotional disorder (ED) (tertiary prevention). All participants had minimal to moderate depressive symptoms. The principal objective of the present work is to present the data about the efficacy of this Internet-based intervention as a secondary and tertiary prevention tool comparing both groups.

Keywords: Prevention · Depression · Internet-based intervention

1 Introduction

Depression is one of the most disabling psychological disorders worldwide [1]. It results in a reduced quality of life because it damages family and friend networks and therefore it markedly impacts at the societal level [2] affecting about 350 million people of all ages, income and nationalities [3]. It is known that 25 % of all human beings will suffer from depression at any moment over their lives and it will become one of the three leading causes of disability in 2030 [4]. There are many arguments that suggest that prevention and treatment of depression should be a health priority strategy. The prevention of depression has been proposed as one of the central points in the European Pact for Mental Health and Wellbeing (2008). Therefore, a very important challenge today consists on addressing the issue of depression from a preventive perspective [5]

© Springer International Publishing Switzerland 2016
S. Serino et al. (Eds.): MindCare 2015, CCIS 604, pp. 230–239, 2016.
DOI: 10.1007/978-3-319-32270-4_23

operating in each of its three levels: *primary prevention*, to reduce its incidence, *secondary prevention*, for people who have some risk factor or those who show subclinical symptoms, and *tertiary prevention*, to minimize the limitations caused by an already established disorder [5]. As Cuijpers et al. [6] point out, it is important to develop better strategies and tools to identify individuals at risk and design prevention programs. We have evidence based psychological interventions for depression [7] and, although less, there are also interventions focusing on its prevention [5]. However, they have an important limitation: the provision of mental health services is generally less than adequate in terms of accessibility and quality [8]. Thus, although psychological treatments have advanced significantly they keep forgetting the central goal to reduce costs (personal, social, and economic) associated to mental health problems. Individual psychotherapy and the dominant model in the provision of services are not likely to achieve these needs [9]. The use of the Internet to support the implementation of the interventions (treatment or prevention), have proven to be a powerful means for its effective deployment in general mental healthcare provision. It has been demonstrated to be a feasible solution to accessibility problems, helping to deliver interventions focused on promoting healthy lifestyle and behaviours [8]. A growing body of research supports the efficacy of Internet-based treatments [10].

The principal objective of the present work is to present data about **the efficacy of an Internet-based intervention as a secondary and tertiary prevention tool.** We have developed an Internet-based program (Smiling is Fun) with the objective of helping people in prevention of depression and anxiety symptoms, and in promoting emotion regulation. It is based on classical CBT techniques, such as behavioural activation, and also includes other positive psychological strategies to improve coping ability and positive mood (Riva et al. 2012). We applied this intervention program in people who had to cope at least with one stressor in their life that produces interference (**secondary prevention**) and also in people who had to cope at least a stressor and met the diagnosis of an ED (**tertiary prevention**) comparing these two groups of participants. All participants had minimal to moderate depressive symptoms. We present the results until the 6 month follow up.

2 Method

2.1 Sampling Procedure and Participants Characteristics

Participants were recruited via announcements to the university community and advertisements on the media (Internet and newspapers) and posters. The advertisements described the research as a study of an Internet-based intervention for the prevention of depression and an opportunity for personal growth and to acquire psychological resources. The advertisements also stated that prospective participants would receive 15 Euros to cover travel expenses any time they had to come to the lab. People who were interested contacted us either by phone or e-mail. Eligibility and exclusion criteria were as follows: Inclusion criteria included to be aged between 18–65 years old; be willing to participate in the study; be able to use a computer and having an Internet connection at home; be able to understand and read Spanish; to have minimal, mild, or moderate depression (score not more than 28 in the BDI-II) and, to be experiencing, at least, one stressful event in their lives that provoked them an interference. Exclusion criteria included to be receiving psychological treatment or to have received another psychological treatment in the past year, to suffer a severe mental disorder on Axis I: abuse or dependence of alcohol or other substances, psychotic disorder or dementia and, the presence of suicidal ideation or plan (Evaluated by item 9 of the Beck Depression Inventory; BDI-II).

Demographic Characteristics. The final study sample (N =80) was composed mostly by women (65 %). Regarding marital status, 53.8 % of the participants were single, 38.8 % married or with a partner and 7.5 % separated or divorced. Regarding the study level most of the participants had higher education (68.8 %), 26.3 % had mid-level studies and the rest were basic studies (5 %). The age range was between 20 and 59 with a media of 35.13 and a standard deviation of 9.45.

Diagnostics. Regarding diagnosis, following the DSM-IV-TR criteria (APA, 2002), 24 participants met the criteria for one or more anxiety or mood disorders. The number and percentage of each diagnosis at baseline are presented in Table 1. As shown in the table, 13 cases fulfilled depression criteria and 1 dysthymia.

Table 1. Number of each of the diagnoses present at pre-treatment

Diagnostic	N pre-treatment
Depression	8
GAD	5
A without PD	4
SP	1
Dysthymia	1
Cases of comorbidity	
Case 1	Depression + GAD
Case 2	Depression + GAD
Case 3	Depression + GAD
Case 4	Depression + GAD + PTSD
Case 5	Depression + GAD + SP + A without PD+OCD

Note. N pre treatment = Number of each of the diagnoses in the pre-treatment; GAD = Generalized Anxiety Disorder; A without PD = Agoraphobia without Panic Disorder; SP = Social Phobia; PTSD = Post-Traumatic Stress Disorder; OCD = Obsessive Compulsive Disorder.

Stressful Events. As shown in Table 2, all participants were experiencing one or more stressful events in their lives.

Table 2. Number of each stressor present in the lives of the participants at pre-treatment.

Stressful event	N
Unemployment	48
Other unemployed relatives	35
Debts	27
Disease (own or other relatives)	45
Conflicts (work / family)	30
Other	20

Note. N = Number of each stressor at pre-treatment.

2.2 Intervention

Smiling is Fun is an Internet-based, multimedia (video, image, etc.), interactive program for the prevention and treatment of depression, which allows the individual to learn and practice adaptive ways to cope with depressive and anxiety symptoms and daily problems. It is designed for optimal use on a PC, but it can also be used on a tablet. The program includes a *Home module, Welcome module* and 8 treatment interactive modules with the following main therapeutic components: motivational, educational, cognitive, behavioural activation, and positive psychology. Smiling is Fun uses three complementary transversal tools that accompany the user throughout the implementation of the program: (1) *Activity report* for self-monitoring, which provides feedback to users, showing that their mood is related to the activities performed, and the benefits of being active. (2) The *calendar* which allows users to know at what step they are throughout the program and provides information regarding homework and tasks already achieved, reminding the user of those still outstanding. (3) *'How am I?'* which offers a set of graphs and feedbacks to chart the user's progress. It shows the evolution of: activity level, emotional distress (anxiety and sadness), positive emotionality (active, enthusiastic, energetic, etc.) and negative emotionality (angry, fearful, stressed, tense, moody, etc.).

2.3 Measures

Mini-International Neuropsychiatric Interview (MINI) [11]. This is a short structured diagnostic psychiatric interview that yields key DSM-IV and ICD-10 diagnoses.

Beck Depression Inventory II [12].This is one of the most widely questionnaires used to evaluate severity of depression in pharmacological and psychotherapy trials. The instrument has good internal consistency (Cronbach's alpha of 0.76 to 0.95) and test-retest reliability of around 0.8 [12]. The Spanish version of this instrument has also shown a high internal consistency (Cronbach's alpha of 0.87) for both the general [13] and the clinical population (Cronbach's alpha of 0.89).

Overall Anxiety Severity and Impairment Scale [14]. OASIS consists of 5 items that measure the frequency and severity of anxiety, as well as the level of avoidance, work/

school/home interference, and social interference associated to anxiety. A psychometric analysis of the OASIS scale found good internal consistency (Cronbach's alpha = 0.80) [14].

Overall Depression Severity and Impairment Scale [15]. ODSIS is a self-report measure which consists of 5 items, evaluating experiences related to depression. ODSIS measures the frequency and severity of depression, as well as the level of avoidance, work/school/home interference, and social interference associated to depression. A psychometric analysis of the ODSIS scale found good internal consistency (Cronbach's alpha = .92) [15].

Positive and Negative Affect Scale [16, 17]. PANAS consists of 20 items that evaluate two independent dimensions: *positive affect* (PA) and *negative affect* (NA). The range for each scale (10 items on each) is 10 to 50. The Spanish version has demonstrated high internal consistency (0.89 to 0.91 for PA and NA in women and 0.87 for AP and 0.89 for AN in men) in college students [17]. This is consistent with the findings in the literature [16].

Perceived Stress Scale [18]. The PSS is a 14-item self-report questionnaire that assesses the degree to which recent life situations are appraised as stressful. Spanish validation of this scale has an internal consistency of 0.86 [19]. We used the 4-item version of this scale. It is composed by the items 2, 6, 7 and 14, which correlate more strongly with the 14-item scale.

2.4 Procedure

People who were interested in the study contacted us either by phone or e-mail. We pre-screened possible participants by phone to filter some crucial criteria: age, to be receiving psychological treatment or to have received another psychological treatment in the past year, to be able to use a computer and having an Internet connection at home and to be able to understand and read Spanish. Participants who passed the pre-screening by phone were given a date for an initial face-to-face interview (screening) in our laboratory, where a research team member explained the study, asked for demographic information, evaluated the presence of depression or other ED by the MINI, and the severity of depressive symptoms by the BDI-II. Furthermore, the investigator evaluated the presence of a stressful life event and its interference. Participants interested in participating signed an informed consent form. Selected participants became part of the study (N=80). Then, the participants were given access to the program. They had to wait 24 h until being able to start with the first module of the program. Once they finished the 8 treatment modules, they performed the post-treatment evaluation also integrated into the web system (same self-report questionnaires that in the pre-treatment assessment).

3   Results

3.1   Baseline Data

The Chi-square tests indicated that there were no significant differences between the two groups before treatment on any of these variables: sex ($\chi^2(1)= 0.813; p = 0.666$); marital status ($\chi^2(2)= 2.351; p = 0.671$); educational level ($\chi^2(2)= 2.526; p = 0.640$); and age ($t=-1.349$; g.l=78; $p=0.181$).The one-way ANOVA analysis showed that the participants who where living a difficult life situation and met the diagnostic criteria of a ED, were significantly worse in the pre-treatment in all clinical variables (see Table 3).

Table 3. Clinical characteristics of Participants at Pre-Assessment

DV	Clinical Status	M	SD	F	p
OASIS	Stressor	3.34	3.32	14.032	<0.001
	Stressor + Diag.	6.42	3.46		
	Total	4.26	3.63		
ODSIS	Stressor	1.95	2.80	20.836	<0.001
	Stressor+ Diag.	5.29	3.43		
	Total	2.95	3.36		
BDI-II	Stressor	7.84	6.20	23.255	<0.001
	Stressor+ Diag.	15.42	6.97		
	Total	10.11	7.29		
PANAS +	Stressor	30.79	6.77	20.691	<0.001
	Stressor+ Diag.	23.08	7.32		
	Total	28.48	7.76		
PANAS -	Stressor	17.27	5.88	13.823	<0.001
	Stressor+ Diag.	22.63	5.95		
	Total	18.88	6.37		
PSS	Stressor	5.11	2.75	25.225	<0.001
	Stressor+ Diag.	8.33	2.33		
	Total	6.08	3.01		

Note. M = Medium; SD = ssStandard Deviation; BDI II = Beck Depression Inventory II; Stressor = group of participants who were living a stressful event (n = 56); Stressor + Diag. = group of participants who were living a stressful event and met a clinical diagnostic (n = 24); OASIS = Overall Anxiety Severity and Impairment Scale; ODSIS = Overall Depression Severity and Impairment Scale; PANAS+ = Positive Affect Scale; PANAS- = Negative Affect Scale; PSS = Perceived Stress Scale.

3.2   Difference Between the Group with Stressors and the Group with Stressors Plus Clinical Diagnostic: Pre-post-Follow up

Means, standard deviations for all outcome measures of the participants who were living a stressful event and for the participants who had also met diagnostic criteria for an ED are displayed in Table 4. The ANOVA results showed that both the time effect and the effect group were significant in all variables. Regarding the interaction effect it was significant in the variables: ODSIS ($F_{(3, 234)} =4.72$, $p=.010$), BDI-II ($F_{(3, 234)} =5.19$, $p=.005$) and PSS ($F_{(3, 234)} =3.00$, $p=0.413$). In these variables with interaction effect, the Sidak's post-hoc tests indicated that in the case of ODSIS, the participants with an ED improved significantly from pre to post ($p < .001$), in comparison with the group with only a difficult situation ($p = .079$). The improvements obtained at post-treatment remained until 3 the month follow up but not until the 6 month follow up. The same pattern was observed in the case of perceived stress (PSS): the participants with an ED improved significantly from pre to post ($p = .001$), in comparison with the group with only a difficult situation ($p = .090$). In these cases, the improvements remained at 3 and 6 month follow-up. Regarding the BDI-II the two groups improved significantly from pre to post-treatment. Nevertheless, as we can see in Table 4 and the effect size presented below, the participants with clinical diagnostic benefit more from the intervention program than the participants with only stressors. The improvements were maintained at 3 and 6 month follow up.

Table 4. - Means and Standard Deviations of the clinical variables: pre – post and follow ups.

DV	Clinical Status	PRE-TRAT		POST-TRAT		3 F-UP		6 F-UP	
		M	SD	M	SD	M	SD	M	SD
OASIS	Stressor	3.34	3.32	1.25	2.24	1.66	2.36	1.84	2.42
	Stressor + Diag.	6.42	3.46	3.00	2.62	3.25	2.88	4.29	3.34
	Total	4.26	3.63	1.78	2.48	2.14	2.61	2.58	2.94
ODSIS	Stressor	1.95	2.80	0.82	1.95	1.09	2.07	1.05	2.20
	Stressor+ Diag.	5.29	3.43	2.00	2.69	2.29	3.34	3.50	3.34
	Total	2.95	3.36	1.18	2.24	1.45	2.56	1.79	2.80
BDI-II	Stressor	7.84	6.20	4.68	4.85	4.82	5.21	4.70	5.24
	Stressor+ Diag.	15.42	6.97	7.92	7.24	8.08	7.78	9.96	8.41
	Total	10.11	7.29	5.65	5.82	5.80	6.22	6.28	6.76
PANAS +	Stressor	30.79	6.77	32.57	8.13	32.82	8.09	32.59	7.84
	Stressor+ Diag.	23.08	7.32	28.92	11.01	29.63	11.14	28.67	9.25
	Total	28.48	7.76	31.48	9.18	31.86	9.16	31.41	8.43
PANAS -	Stressor	17.27	5.88	12.75	3.15	13.80	4.04	13.91	3.97
	Stressor+ Diag.	22.63	5.95	16.88	5.03	17.67	5.56	19.29	6.10
	Total	18.88	6.37	13.99	4.23	14.96	4.86	15.53	5.28
PSS	Stressor	5.11	2.75	4.23	2.71	4.34	2.70	4.05	2.69
	Stressor+ Diag.	8.33	2.33	6.21	3.27	6.03	3.37	6.25	3.26
	Total	6.08	3.01	4.83	3.01	4.85	3.00	4.71	3.03

Note. M = Medium; SD = Standard Deviation; BDI II = Beck Depression Inventory II; Stressor = group of participants who were living a stressful event (n = 56); Stressor + Diag. = group of participants who were living a stressful event and met a clinical diagnostic (n = 24); OASIS = Overall Anxiety Severity and Impairment Scale; ODSIS = Overall Depression Severity and Impairment Scale; PANAS+ =Positive Affect Scale; PANAS- = Negative Affect Scale; PSS = Perceived Stress Scale.

3.3 Effect Sizes (Cohen's *D*) Pre-post Intervention

In the group of participants who were only experiencing a stressor, a medium effect size in the variables was obtained: OASIS ($d = .71$), ODSIS ($d=.45$) and BDI-II ($d=.55$). In the PANAS + and PSS a small effect size was obtained ($d=.23$ and .31 respectively). In the case of the PANAS –a big effect size was obtained ($d=.93$).

Regarding the participants with ED a big effect size in the variables was obtained: OASIS (d=1.03), ODSIS (d=.99), BDI-II (d=.98) and PANAS – (d=.96). Medium effect size on positive affect and PSS was found (d=.58 and d=.69 respectively).

3.4 Treatment Adherence

The adherence was high in both groups: 82.1 % participants of Stressor group completed all treatment modules and 75 % of Stressor + Diagnostic group.

4 Discussion

This work pretended to analyze the utility of the self-applied intervention program through the Internet as a secondary preventive strategy (aimed to people without any disorder symptoms, but with some risk factors or subclinical symptomatology) and tertiary (aimed to reducing disability arising from an existing disorder). In order to do that, two groups were selected (Stressor versus Stressor + diagnosis). 56 participants living one or more stressful events that caused interference in their lives took part as they were in a risky situation (secondary prevention) and 24 participants who were also living one stressor fulfilled the diagnostic criteria of an ED (tertiary prevention). In order to address such objective, different analysis were carried out. First of all, some analysis were carried out in order to determine whether there were differences in the improvement of the different clinical variables assessed according to whether, in addition to be suffering and adverse event, participants met diagnostic criteria of an ED. Participants with a diagnosis of an ED were significantly worse in all clinical variables. However, at post-treatment and follow ups, both subsamples improved significantly at OASIS and PANAS (positive and negative). Results found were relevant, as, although both groups had started with significantly different scores, the intervention was equally effective in both subsamples in improving both anxiety symptoms as negative and positive affect. This result is relevant, as it indicates that the program protects those people in a risky situation, although it does not fulfill depression criteria neither another ED (secondary prevention), improving its symptomatology. And also those already showing an ED (tertiary prevention). However, we should remember that it was not like this with ODSIS and PSS, as in these variables, the participants fulfilling diagnostic criteria of an ED significantly improved, compared to those participants who only showed one or several stressors in their lives, who did not. Furthermore, although at BDI-II both subsamples improved significantly from pre to post-treatment, those participants suffering from an ED benefited more. We have to add to this that, in all variables, the effect size found was bigger with the subsample of the participants fulfilling diagnostic criteria of an ED than with the subsamples of those participants who were just going through a difficult vital situation (with the exception of the negative affect, where a big size effect was found in both subsamples). These are interesting results, as they may suggest that, in our study, the more severe the participant was, the more was benefited. Results indicate that the self-applied intervention program has also worked as a tool to reduce the disability and discomfort showed by the sample who apart from going through a difficult vital situation, fulfilled the diagnostic criteria for an ED (tertiary prevention). On the other hand, data should read results carefully, as so far, we just have data for the 6 month follow up. Similar studies, with self-applied preventive programs through the Internet, have also showed being successful in reducing depressive and anxiety symptoms [20]. More recently, our group, within the frame of the European project OPTIMI (Online Predictive Tools for Intervention in Mental Illness) [21] has tested the efficacy of the very same program used in this study, but with a specific population that consisted of long-term unemployed men who were considered at risk, and the results are encouraging [22]. Even though, the studies focusing on prevention with self-applied programs through the Internet are quite limited. Therefore, this study is relevant to this topic. It is possible to conclude that the results show that the program would be useful as a secondary and tertiary prevention strategy. That is, it would protect those participants at risk (those suffering from a stressor interfering in their lives), but who do not fulfill diagnostic criteria of any disorder at pre-treatment (secondary prevention). Furthermore, taking into account those participants who did fulfill diagnostic criteria of an ED at pre-treatment, the disability arising from it might moderate, even going to disappear (tertiary prevention). A basic objective of this study is therefore accomplished, that is to say, to make people acquire coping resources which enable them to properly handle those difficult situations in their daily lives. To sum up, we can state that the self-applied treatment protocol through the Internet has shown to be efficient when improving the clinical state of those people who took it. Also, the improvement has been kept in time with most of the assessed clinical variables (at least, during the 6 months after the intervention).

The study has limitations: It doesn't have control group. For this reason, it is possible that the symptoms improved because often, overtime, symptoms decrease. Furthermore, it is possible that differences found between the two groups can be explained by that diagnosed group has higher scores. In any case, in view of the results, we consider the present study has contributed to improve the knowledge related to the psychological treatments which could be self-applied through the Internet, adding data that demonstrate their effectiveness.

References

1. Haro, J.M., Ayuso-Mateos, J.L., Bitter, I., Demotes-Mainard, J., Leboyer, M., Lewis, S.W., Linszen, D., Walker-Tilley, T.: ROAMER: Roadmap for mental health research in Europe. Int. J. Methods Psychiatr. Res. **23**, 1–14 (2014)
2. Merikangas, K.R., Kalaydjian, A.: Magnitude and impact of comorbidity of mental disorders from epidemiologic surveys. Curr. Opin. Psychiatry **20**, 353–358 (2007)
3. World Health Organization.: Iniciative depression in mental health. Geneva, World Health Organization (2010)
4. Mathers, C.D., Loncar, D.: Projections of global mortality and burden of disease from 2002 to 2030. PLoS Med. **3**, e442 (2006)
5. Muñoz, R.F., Cuijpers, P., Smit, F., Barrera, A., Leykin, Y.: Prevention on major depression. Ann. Rev. Clin. Psychol. **6**, 181–212 (2010)
6. Cuijpers, P., Beekman, A.T.F., Reynolds, C.F.: Preventing depression: A global priority. JAMA **307**, 1033–1034 (2012)

7. Nathan, P.E., Gorman, J.M.: A guide to treatments that work. Oxford University Press, New York, NY, US (2007)
8. Kazdin, A.E., Blase, S.L.: Rebooting psychotherapy research and practice to reduce the burden of mental illness. Perspect. Psychol. Sci. **6**, 21–37 (2011)
9. Kazdin, A.E., Rabbitt, S.M.: Novel models for delivering mental health services and reducing the burdens of mental illness. Clin. Psychol. Sci. **1**(2), 170–191 (2013)
10. Richards, D., Richardson, T.: Computer-based psychological treatments for depression: A systematic review and meta-analysis. Clin. Psychol. Rev. **32**, 329–342 (2012)
11. Lecrubier, Y., Sheehan, D., Weiller, E., Amorim, P., Bonora, I., Sheehan, K., Dunbar, G.: The Mini International Neuropsychiatric Interview (M.I.N.I.), a short diagnostic interview: Reliability and validity according to the CIDI. Eur. Psychiatry. **12**, 232–241 (1997)
12. Beck, A.T., Steer, R.A., Brown, G.K.: Manual for the Beck Depression Inventory-II. Psychological Corp, San Antonio, TX (1996)
13. Sanz, J., Navarro, M.E., Vázquez, C.: Adaptación española del Inventario para la Depresión de Beck-II (BDI-II): Propiedades psicométricas en estudiantes universitarios. Análisis y Modificación de Conducta **29**, 239–288 (2003)
14. Norman, S.B., Cissell, S.H., Means-Christensen, A.J., Stein, M.B.: Development and validation of an overall anxiety severity and impairment scale (OASIS). Depres Anxiety **23**, 245–249 (2006)
15. Bentley, K.H., Gallagher, M.W., Carl, J.R., Barlow, D.H.: Development and validation of the Overall Depression Severity and Impairment Scale. Psycholol. Assess. **26**(3), 815–830 (2014)
16. Watson, D., Clark, L., Tellegen, A.: Development and validation of brief measures of positive and negative affect: The PANAS scales. J. Pers. Soc. Psychol. **54**, 1063–1070 (1988)
17. Sandín, B., Chorot, P., Lostao, L., Joiner, T.E., Santed, M.A., Valiente, R.M.: Escalas panas de afecto positivo y negativo: Validación factorial y transcultural. Psicothema **11**, 37–51 (1999)
18. Cohen, S., Kamarck, T., Mermelstein, R.: A global measure of perceived stress. J. Health Soc. Behav. **24**, 386–396 (1983)
19. Campo, A., Bustos, G., Romero, A.: Consistencia interna y dimensionalidad de la Escala de Estrés Percibido (EEP-10 y EEP-14) en una muestra de universitarias de Bogotá, Colombia. Aquichán. 9 (2009)
20. Lintvedt, O.K., Griffiths, K.M., Sørensen, K., Østvik, A.R., Wang, C.E., Eisemann, M.Y., Waterloo, K.: Evaluating the effectiveness and efficacy of unguided internet-based self-help intervention for the prevention of depression: A randomized controlled trial. Clin. Psychol. Psychother. **20**, 10–27 (2013)
21. Botella, C., Moragrega, I., Baños, R.Y., García-Palacios, A.: Online predictive tools for intervention in mental illness: The Optimi project. In: Westwood, J.D. et al (eds) Stud Health Technol Inform, vol. 164, pp. 86–94 (2011)
22. Mira, A., Botella, C., García-Palacios, A., Riera López del Amo, A., Quero, S., Alcañiz, M.Y., Baños, R.M.: An Internet-based program to cope with regulating stress and emotion: An example of positive technology. J. Cyber. Ther. Rehabil. **2**(1), 22–23 (2012)

An Innovative Online Positive Psychology Training Addressed to Pregnant Youth

Giulia Corno[1](✉), Guadalupe Molinari[2], Macarena Espinoza[2], Rocio Herrero[2],
Ernestina Etchemendy[3], Alba Carrillo Vega[1], and Rosa M. Baños[1]

[1] Universitat de Valencia, Valencia, Spain
giulia.me.corno@gmail.com
[2] Universitat Jaume I, Castellón de La Plana, Spain
[3] Ciber. Fisiopatología Obesidad y Nutrición. (CIBERObn) Instituto de Salud Carlos III,
Madrid, Spain

Abstract. Pregnancy involves important changes for women of all ages. Specifically, young pregnant are faced with the difficult task of continuing their physical, emotional, and identity development while preparing for their role as parents. The aim of this work is to present the protocol of an innovative self-applied online positive psychology intervention addressed to pregnant youth. The purpose of this intervention is to enhance well-being, to help these women get through pregnancy in the best possible way. The intervention will be composed by four modules, for a total length of five weeks. Each module will be dedicated to the promotion of one positive dimension through the use of validated positive psychology exercises. We hypothesize that participants will report a significant higher level of happiness at post-test, and follow-up. Secondly, we hypothesize that participants will report a significant increase in positive affect, optimism, life satisfaction, social support, self-compassion, and psychological well-being, and a reduction in depression, anxiety, and negative affect at post-test and follow-up. Tertiary study objective is to examine if particular subgroups (in term of ages, different week of pregnancy, relationship status, unwanted/wanted pregnancy, and different personality profile) will benefit differently than others from the training .

Keywords: Positive psychology intervention · Pregnancy · Youth · Online intervention

1 Introduction

Pregnancy and childbirth are major life events. Pregnancy is a time of changes: it represents the start of a new role for women of all ages. Pregnancy is also a period during which women are exposed to the risk to develop some psychological disorders as depression [1], anxiety disorders (i.e. panic attack, obsessive-compulsive disorder, and general anxiety disorder) [2–5], and eating disorder [6]. The most common psychological disorder linked with pregnancy is depression. Risks to develop depression are associated with previous personal history of depressive episodes, family history, but also to

© Springer International Publishing Switzerland 2016
S. Serino et al. (Eds.): MindCare 2015, CCIS 604, pp. 240–246, 2016.
DOI: 10.1007/978-3-319-32270-4_24

some psychosocial factors, as the lack of social support, negative attitude towards the pregnancy, and negative relationship with the beloved [7, 8].

Specifically, regarding young future mothers, they are faced with the difficult task of continuing their physical, emotional, and identity development while preparing for their role as parents [9]. Comparing to older women, young future mothers have higher probability to develop some psychosocial problems linked to young pregnancy including school interruption, persistent poverty, limited vocational opportunities, separation from the child's father, divorce, and repeat pregnancy [10]. Moreover, young pregnant women experience feelings of anxiety, depression, loneliness, and confusion because they do not know what to expect from motherhood [11, 12]. They have to start to look to their lives in another way [13].

Youth pregnancy still represents a social and health concern, either in developing and industrialized countries. Each year, approximately 900.000 teenagers become pregnant in the United States [14], and more than 4 in 10 adolescent girls have been pregnant at least once before 20 years of age [14]. The majority of these pregnancies are among older teenagers (i.e. 18 or 19 years of age) [14, 15]. Specifically, Hispanic adolescents have had the highest overall birth rates and smallest decreases in recent years [16]. Considering the adolescent fertility rate (births per 1,000 women ages 15–19), for every 1.000 females 15 to 19 years of age, between 2010–2014, 55 in Argentina, 14 in Canada, 55 in Chile, 63 in Mexico, 101 in Nicaragua, 11 in Spain, 26 in UK, and 31 in USA gave birth [17]. The United States teenage birth rate of 52.1 is the highest in the developed world– and about four times the European Union average. The United Kingdom has the highest teenage birth rate in Europe. In Spain, it has been noticed an increased number of pregnant women who are living in a relational and economic difficult situation. Specifically, the 34 % of pregnant women are between 16 and 25 years old and they report several issues related to the absence of support from the family, the partner, and the social community. Giving birth while still a teenager is strongly associated with disadvantage in later life. On average across 13 countries of the European Union, women who gave birth as teenagers are twice as likely to be living in poverty [17].

Some models of adolescent pregnancy-prevention programs exist [14, 18–20]. Nevertheless, most of them are focused on abstinence promotion and contraception information, contraceptive availability, sexuality education, school-completion strategies, and job training. The aim of these program is to prevent a second pregnancy, and prevent the abuse of drugs among adolescent mothers. None of these programs is dedicated to the promotion of the well-being, and to the enhancement of the strengths already present in the participants. Thus, starting from this lack, we have developed an Internet-based positive psychology training, "Positive Pregnancy" (http://pospre.wix.com/home) aimed to the promotion of the overall well-being of the future young mothers. We think that focusing on the well-being enhancement will promote and contribute to increasing the personal and social strengths of the participants, preventing the risks to develop psychosocial problems, as school interruption, limited vocational opportunities, depression, anxiety and loneliness.

The aim of this work is to present the protocol of this innovative self-applied online positive psychology intervention addressed to pregnant youth.

Below, in order to better understand the training, we included some reflections about positive psychology interventions and the relevance of online interventions in the contemporary society.

2   Positive Psychology and Positive Psychology Interventions (PPIs)

One goal of positive psychology is to increase well-being, and research suggests that this is possible through brief exercises termed "positive interventions" (PPI) [21–23]. According to Lyubomirsky [24], positive psychology interventions are programs "aimed at increasing positive feelings, positive behaviors, or positive cognitions as opposed to ameliorating pathology or fixing negative thoughts of maladaptive behavior patterns" (p. 469). Recent meta-analyses confirm that on average, these techniques lead to reliable and sustainable boosts in well-being [25–28]. Moreover, increased positive well-being is a significant protective factor from the occurrence of future episodes of major depression [29].

In the last decades, many experimental researches based on online trials has been conducted. The Internet allows dissemination of these positive psychology techniques throughout the world, anywhere participants have Web access. Internet programs have the potential to improve engagement, provide cost-effective and engaging programs, allowing participants to access content at their own pace. The effectiveness of online positive psychology interventions has been proved by many studies [30–33].

3   The Current Study

The proposed study has the aim to explore the effectiveness of an online positive psychology training, Positive Pregnancy, addressed to pregnant women. The primary objective of the program is to enhance and promote the well-being of the young mothers, and, in general, all pregnant women through the use of simple and daily Positive Psychology exercises. This training will be focused on activities related to some positive psychology dimensions as self-compassion, self-acceptance, savoring, satisfaction with life, social support, positive social relationships, and optimism.

Our first and principal hypothesis regards the construct of happiness. Since happiness is one of the principal well-being's construct [34–36], we hypothesize that participants will report a significant higher level of happiness at post-test, and follow-up. Secondly, we hypothesize that participants will report a significant increase in positive affect, optimism, life satisfaction, social support, self-compassion, and psychological well-being, and a reduction in depression, anxiety, and negative affect at post-test and follow-up. Tertiary study objective is to examine if particular subgroups (in term of ages, different week of pregnancy, relationship status, unwanted/wanted pregnancy, and different personality profile) will benefit differently than others from the training. In fact, specifically for pregnant adolescents, there is still not a general agreement about whether psychological well-being is compromised by young age alone, or whether emotional distress, depressive symptoms, and anxiety may be the result of other associated factors as single status or unwanted pregnancy [37].

4   Study Design

This study is characterized by a single experimental condition. After signing and sending to the researcher the consent form (in case of minor, the consent form has to be signed by one of the parents or a tutor of the girl), completing the screening and pre-assessment parts on the SurveyMonkey platform, participants will have free access to positivepregnancy.com. Every week, after a short assessment, they will receive free access to a new module. The training is composed by four modules, "Mindfulness and Self-Acceptance", "Savoring", "Connectedness", and "Best Possible Self", for a total length of five weeks (see Table 1). Each module is composed by two parts. The first one is dedicated to the psychoeducation about the particular positive psychology dimension of the module. In the second part, participants are invited to practice some activities, as for instance the "Best Possible Self" exercise [38], with the purpose to enhance the positive psychology dimension in question. All the modules are composed by different interactive elements as video, sounds, and images, which increase the engagement. At the end of the last module participants will receive by e-mail a link to complete the post-assessment on the SurveyMonkey platform. After one month from the post-assessment, participant will receive another link to complete the follow-up evaluation. The free access to the training will be guaranteed also after the follow-up, in order to permit to the woman to have access to the exercises and information available on http://pospre.wix.com/home at any time. Participant will always have access to an informative session which contains multimedia information about pregnancy, alimentation, and type of births.

Table 1. Modules of the Positive Pregnancy training

Week	Module	Dimensions	Exercises
1	Mindfulness and self-acceptance	Self-acceptance, and self-compassion	Psychoeducation about mindfulness Body scan exercise [39]
2	Savoring	Life satisfaction	Psychoeducation about savoring Three good things in life exercise [40, 41] Savoring the moment exercise [30, 42]
3	Connectedness	Positive relations with the others, and social support	Psychoeducation about connectedness Connectedness exercise
4	Best Possible Self (part 1)	Optimism	Best Possible Self exercise [38, 43]
5	Best Possible Self (part 2)	Optimism	Baby-steps exercise [43]

4.1   Inclusion and Exclusion Criteria

The training is open to all pregnant women, Spanish-speaking or Anglophone. The study, instead, will include pregnant women: (1) who are pregnant between the 12th and 28th week, (2) who have regular access to Internet, (3) who have decided to be the mother of the baby, and (4) who sign the consent form (for minors, the consent form has to be signed by a parent or a legal tutor).

5   Conclusion

The proposed study has the aim to explore the effectiveness of an online positive psychology training, Positive Pregnancy, addressed to pregnant women. Specifically, we hypothesize that participants will report a significant increase in positive affect, optimism, life satisfaction, positive social relations, self-acceptance, purpose in life, and psychological well-being, and a reduction in depression and negative affect at post-test and follow-up. Secondary study objective is to examine if particular subgroups (in term of ages, different month of pregnancy, and different personality profile) benefit differently than others from the training. If shown to be effective, the training could prove to be an affordable and valid tool to promote and improve well-being in young pregnant women and in general, in all pregnant women, and it could be translated in other languages in order to improve its accessibility.

References

1. Zuckerman, B., Bauchner, H., Parker, S., Cabral, H.: Maternal depressive symptoms during pregnancy, and newborn irritability. J. Dev. Biol. Behav. Pediatr. **11**(4), 190–194 (1990)
2. Buist, A., Gotman, N., Yonkers, K.A.: Generalized anxiety disorder: course and risk factors in pregnancy. J. Affect. Disord. **131**(1), 277–283 (2011)
3. Fisk, N.M., Glover, V.: Association between maternal anxiety in pregnancy and increased uterine artery resistance index: cohort based study. BMJ **318**(7177), 153–157 (1999)
4. Hertzberg, T., Wahlbeck, K.: The impact of pregnancy and puerperium on panic disorder: a review. J. Psychosom. Obstet. Gynaecol. **20**(2), 59–64 (1999)
5. Neziroglu, F., Anemone, R., Yaryura-Tobias, J.A.: Onset of obsessive-compulsive disorder in pregnancy. Am. J. Psychiatry **149**(7), 947–950 (1992)
6. Blais, M.A., et al.: Pregnancy: Outcome and impact on symptomatology in a cohort of eating-disordered women. Int. J. Eat. Disord. **27**(2), 140–149 (2000)
7. Kumar, R., Robson, K.M.: A prospective study of emotional disorders in childbearing women. Br. J. Psychiatry **144**(1), 35–47 (1984)
8. O'Hara, M.W.: Social support, life events, and depression during pregnancy and the puerperium. Arch. Gen. Psychiatry **43**(6), 569–573 (1986)
9. Stevenson, W., Maton, K.I., Teti, D.M.: Social support, relationship quality, and well-being among pregnant adolescents. J. Adolesc. **22**(1), 109–121 (1999)
10. Klein, J.D.: Adolescent pregnancy: current trends and issues. Pediatrics **116**(1), 281–286 (2005)
11. Ex, C.T., Janssens, J.M.: Young females' images of motherhood. Sex Roles **43**(11–12), 865–890 (2000)
12. Hudson, D.B., Elek, S.M., Campbell-Grossman, C.: Depression, self-esteem, loneliness, and social support among adolescent mothers participating in the new parents project. Adolescence **35**(139), 445–453 (2000)
13. Zachry, E.: Getting my education: teen mothers' experiences in school before and after motherhood. Teachers Coll. Rec. **107**(12), 2566–2598 (2005)
14. Kirby, D.: Emerging answers: research findings on programs to reduce teen pregnancy. National Campaign To Prevent Teen Pregnancy, 1776 Massachusetts Avenue, NW, # 200, Washington, DC 20036 (2001)

15. Martin, J.A., Park, M.M., Sutton, P.D.: Births: preliminary data for 2001. Nat. Vital Stat. Rep. **50**(10), 1–20 (2002)
16. Ventura, S.J., Mathews, T.J., Curtin, S.C.: Declines in teenage birth rates, 1991-97: national and state patterns. Nat. Vital Stat. Rep. **47**(12), n12 (1998)
17. UNICEF: A League of Teenage Births in Rich Nations. Innocenti Report Card No. 3. Florence, Italy: UNICEF Innocenti Research Centre (2011)
18. Key, J.D., Gebregziabher, M.G., Marsh, L.D., O'Rourke, K.M.: Effectiveness of an intensive, school-based intervention for teen mothers. J. Adolesc. Health **42**(4), 394–400 (2008)
19. McDonell, J.R., Limber, S.P., Connor-Godbey, J.: Pathways teen mother support project: longitudinal findings. Child Youth Serv. Rev. **29**(7), 840–855 (2007)
20. Rothenberg, A., Weissman, A.: The development of programs for pregnant and parenting teens. Soc. Work Health Care **35**(3), 65–83 (2002)
21. Lyubomirsky, S., Sheldon, K.M., Schkade, D.: Pursuing happiness: the architecture of sustainable change. Rev. Gen. Psychol. **9**(2), 111 (2005)
22. Seligman, M.E., Steen, T.A., Park, N., Peterson, C.: Positive psychology progress: empirical validation of interventions. Am. Psychol. **60**(5), 410 (2005)
23. Sheldon, K.M., Lyubomirsky, S.: How to increase and sustain positive emotion: the effects of expressing gratitude and visualizing best possible selves. J. Positive Psychol. **1**(2), 73–82 (2006)
24. Lyubomirsky, S.: The how of happiness: a scientific approach to getting the life you want. Penguin, London (2008)
25. Bolier, L., Haverman, M., Westerhof, G.J., Riper, H., Smit, F., et al.: Positive psychology interventions: a meta-analysis of randomized controlled studies. BMC Public Health **13**(1), 119 (2013)
26. Hone, L.C., Jarden, A., Schofield, G.M.: An evaluation of positive psychology intervention effectiveness trials using the re-aim framework: a practice-friendly review. J. Positive Psychol. **10**(4), 303–322 (2014)
27. Schueller, S.M.: Identifying and analyzing positive interventions: a meta-analysis. In: Paper presented at the 4th Annual European Conference on Positive Psychology, Rijeka, Croatia, July 2008
28. Sin, N.L., Lyubomirsky, S.: Enhancing well-being and alleviating depressive symptoms with positive psychology interventions: a practice-friendly meta-analysis. J. Clin. Psychol. **65**, 467–487 (2009)
29. Ryff, C.D.: Happiness is everything, or is it? explorations on the meaning of psychological well-being. J. Pers. Soc. Psychol. **57**(6), 1069 (1989)
30. Schueller, S.M.: Preferences for positive psychology exercises. J. Positive Psychol. **5**(3), 192–203 (2010)
31. Redzic, N.M., Taylor, K., Chang, V., Trockel, M., Shorter, A., Taylor, C.B.: An internet-based positive psychology program: strategies to improve effectiveness and engagement. J. Positive Psychol. **9**(6), 494–501 (2014)
32. Schueller, S.M., Parks, A.C.: Disseminating self-help: positive psychology exercises in an online trial. J. Med. Internet Res. **14**(3), e63 (2012)
33. Bolier, L., Abello, K.M.: Online positive psychological interventions: state of the art and future directions. In: The Wiley Blackwell Handbook of Positive Psychological Interventions, pp. 286–309 (2014)
34. Fordyce, M.W.: A review of research on the happiness measures: a sixty second index of happiness and mental health. Soc. Indic. Res. **20**(4), 355–381 (1998)

35. Hervás, G., Vázquez, C.: Construction and validation of a measure of integrative well-being in seven languages: the Pemberton Happiness Index. Health Qual. Life Outcomes **11**(1), 66 (2013)
36. Fordyce, M.W.: Development of a program to increase personal happiness. J. Couns. Psychol. **24**(6), 511 (1977)
37. Rowe, H.J., Wynter, K.H., Steele, A., Fisher, J.R., Quinlivan, J.A.: The growth of maternal-fetal emotional attachment in pregnant adolescents: a prospective cohort study. J. Pediatr. Adolesc. Gynecol. **26**(6), 327–333 (2013)
38. Meevissen, Y.M., Peters, M.L., Alberts, H.J.: Become more optimistic by imagining a best possible self: effects of a two week intervention. J. Behav. Ther. Exp. Psychiatry **42**(3), 371–378 (2011)
39. Williams, M., Penman, D.: Mindfulness: a practical guide to finding peace in a frantic world, vol. 360. Piatkus, London (2011)
40. Emmons, R.A., McCullough, M.E.: Counting blessings versus burdens: an experimental investigation of gratitude and subjective well-being in daily life. J. Pers. Soc. Psychol. **84**(2), 377 (2003)
41. Seligman, M.E., Ernst, R.M., Gillham, J., Reivich, K., Linkins, M.: Positive education: positive psychology and classroom interventions. Oxford Rev. Educ. **35**(3), 293–311 (2009)
42. Parks, A.C., Della Porta, M.D., Pierce, R.S., Zilca, R., Lyubomirsky, S.: Pursuing happiness in everyday life: the characteristics and behaviors of online happiness seekers. Emotion **12**(6), 1222 (2012)
43. Layous, K., Nelson, S.K., Lyubomirsky, S.: What is the optimal way to deliver a positive activity intervention? The case of writing about one's best possible selves. J. Happiness Stud. **14**(2), 635–654 (2013)

Help Me If You Can: Tech-Interventions for Mental Health

Rhythmic Reading Training (RRT)

A Computer-Assisted Intervention Program for Dyslexia

Alice Cancer[1]([✉]), Silvia Bonacina[1], Maria Luisa Lorusso[2],
Pier Luca Lanzi[3], and Alessandro Antonietti[1]

[1] Department of Psychology, Catholic University of the Sacred Heart, Milan, Italy
{alice.cancer,alessandro.antonietti}@unicatt.it
[2] IRCCS Eugenio Medea, Bosisio Parini, Italy
[3] Department of Electronics, Information and Bioengineering,
Polytechnic University, Milan, Italy

Abstract. Developmental dyslexia is a specific learning disorder of neurobiological origin that causes a reading impairment. Since music and language share common mechanisms and the core deficit underlying dyslexia has been identified in difficulties in dynamic and rapidly changing auditory information processing, it has been argued that enhancing basic musical rhythm perception skills in children with dyslexia may have a positive effect on reading abilities. Therefore, active engagement with music provides an enjoyable environment that may improve motivation of children and thus enhance the efficacy of the intervention. Taking these findings and hypotheses into account, a computer-assisted training, called Rhythmic Reading Training (RRT), was designed to implement a treatment which combines a traditional approach (sublexical treatment) with rhythm processing training. Some preliminary test-training-retest studies showed the efficacy of RRT intervention on reading abilities of children with dyslexia.

Keywords: Reading · Developmental dyslexia · Music · Rhythm · Auditory processing · Intervention · Personalized training

1 In Search of an Effective and Easy-to-Administer Training for Dyslexia

Developmental dyslexia (DD) is a specific learning disability of neurobiological origin, which causes an impairment in the ability of reading in spite of normal education, intellectual functioning and socio-cultural opportunity [1]. DD is one of the most common neuropsychological disorders affecting children. Studies conducted in English-speaking countries report a prevalence ranging from 5 to 17.5 % [2]. In Italy, due to the transparency of Italian orthography, the prevalence of DD is lower and ranges from 1.5 to 5 % [3]. The consequences of this impairment on learning and scholastic achievements are relevant and often causing a decrease of the motivation for learning, self-esteem and self-efficacy.

Although the core mechanism underlying DD is still under debate, a specific dysfunction in phonological processing is currently widely assumed to be the primary deficit, as confirmed by many evidences [4, 5]. It has also been showed that the impairment in

© Springer International Publishing Switzerland 2016
S. Serino et al. (Eds.): MindCare 2015, CCIS 604, pp. 249–258, 2016.
DOI: 10.1007/978-3-319-32270-4_25

phonological representation, which is the distinctive feature of DD, is associated to difficulties in rapidly changing auditory information processing [6, 7]. Children with DD are typically poor in basic auditory perceptual and timing skills, such as sensitivity to speech prosody, pitch perception and rhythm (sound attributes cued by amplitude, duration and frequency changes of the acoustic signal) [8, 9]. These auditory perception difficulties could contribute to the development of impaired phonological representation for words [10].

Regarding the Italian context, a meta-analysis [11] suggested that the most effective treatments for DD are the interventions aimed at improving the automatic decoding of sublexical and lexical stimuli, such as the Sublexical Treatment [12] and the visual hemispheric-specific stimulation inspired by the Balance-Model [13]. These treatments are characterized by some weaknesses in their application for the rehabilitation of DD. First, they require to be performed in a clinical setting by a therapist who is expert in the methodology, thus demanding a time-consuming and economic commitment of the patient's family. Moreover, the characteristics and the abilities of the therapist are crucial for the effectiveness of the treatment. Therefore it is difficult to ensure a standardized procedure and the outcomes are quite variable. Finally, since both of these treatments involve an intensive and repetitive reading training that has to stress decoding in order to be effective, they are often experienced as boring and tiring, causing a decrease of the participants' motivation.

These concerns point out the need for a rehabilitation methodology that could provide (a) a supervised usage at home, therefore not requiring the physical presence of an expert for every session; (b) a standardized procedure which could adapt to the specific needs of each participant planning the activities systematically and gradually increasing the exercises' difficulty; (c) the invariance of the effects in spite of therapist's personal characteristics and level of expertise; (d) engagement and motivation of participants throughout the whole intervention period.

Taking all these requirements into account, we designed a computerized training program whose characteristics help overcoming the limitations of traditional treatments while guaranteeing the effectiveness in improving reading abilities of children with DD. The use of information technology (IT) could provide some benefits in a rehabilitation setting. It has been proven that children with DD are more motivated and less stressed when they use IT tools for dealing with tasks involving reading [14]. Moreover, another feature of IT tools that facilitates reading training process is the multimodal presentation of stimuli, which can therefore be delivered simultaneously as auditory and visual.

Concerning the motivation issue, we thought about introducing music as a rehabilitation tool. Active engagement with music provides an enjoyable environment that may improve motivation and self-efficacy of children with DD. Moreover, many considerable studies support the hypothesis that music training could be effective in enhancing auditory perception abilities and consequentially improve language processing and reading skills.

1.1 Music as an Empowering Tool for the Development of Reading Skills

Many evidences about the existence of shared mechanisms supporting the processing of both music and language have been reported. Neuroimaging studies provided evidence of a significant overlap in the brain regions involved in processing the characteristic of both auditory speech and non-speech signals [15]. Furthermore, it has been proven that musical expertise has a positive effect on language and literacy abilities in normal-reading children, suggesting an association between music and reading skills [16]. In fact, music attributes discrimination abilities, assessed using tonal-melodic and rhythmic tasks, predict phonological and reading skills in both normal-reading children and children with DD [17]. These findings suggest that interventions aimed at enhancing basic auditory perception skills of children with DD may impact on reading abilities: improvements caused by music training might transfer to other domains, such as language, enhancing pitch, timing and timbre processing.

Some conjectures about how music could help children with DD have been put forward [18, 19]. So far, the attempts to improve reading skills through music training were carried out engaging poor readers, pre-schoolers or children with DD in activities involving mostly discriminating pitches, reproducing rhythmical patterns by tapping hands, foots or hitting the drums, evaluating the speed or the intensity of sounds and singing according to given instructions. In other words, music training occurred as a separate experience with no direct link to language and reading. It was expected that improvements produced by music activity in the basic auditory mechanisms in common between music and language should transfer from music to language.

A study conducted by Overy [18] examined the influence of a 15-week music training on reading skills of 9 children with DD. Music lessons were conducted 3 times per week in sessions of 20 min each. Reading skills were assessed across the music intervention period and the preceding 15-weeks control period. A significant improvement in phonological, spelling, rhythm copying and rapid auditory processing skills emerged, but reading skills were not significantly affected by the musical treatment. In a similar designed study, Register and colleagues [20] measured the efficacy of a short-term music curriculum, designed to target reading comprehension and vocabulary skills, on reading skills of second-grade students, some of which were diagnosed with DD. Significant improvements in word decoding, word knowledge and reading comprehension were found after the music intervention in the group of children with DD.

Even though the hypothesis of a positive effect of music training on the impaired auditory perception and timing processing of children with DD is supported by many studies, music education alone failed to produce improvements in reading skills comparable with those resulting from traditional intervention methods for DD, which hence should not be replaced [21]. We hence wondered if a more efficient way of taking advantage of music for the development of reading skills could be to incorporate the music dimension in the reading training. Better outcomes could be achieved if shared mechanisms between music and language are trained simultaneously through exercises involving both the musical and the linguistic dimensions. This combination should produce a synergy between the two dimensions, with both music sounds and verbal stimuli stressing the same elements (e.g., the rhythmical structure of language) and converging on the same results (such as hinting at temporal regularity in analysing and decoding the presented verbal stimuli).

For allowing the music and linguistic dimensions to interact and combine, IT appears to be the perfect choice. First, multimodal stimulation can be provided by a computerized application, presenting music and verbal materials simultaneously. Additional cues, such as visual elements aimed at highlighting the relevant part of the stimuli to be processes, can be easily included. Second, computerized exercises enable trainers to have control over timing and difficulty of the stimulus presentation. Finally, the perfect synchronisation of the concurrent presentation of sounds, verbal materials and visual cues is assured. All these outcomes cannot be reached without the use of IT, since the presentation of the stimuli performed by a human agent cannot be as accurate.

Taking all these considerations into account, a computerized training program which combines a traditional remediation approach (sublexical treatment) with rhythm processing training was designed and implemented. A rhythmic accompaniment provides readers a structure which helps them to organize temporal cues of speech sounds. Rhythm therefore should assume the role of an aid in rapid auditory processing which can support word decoding ability.

1.2   A Computerized Training Program: The Rhythmic Reading Training (RRT)

RRT is a child-friendly computerized reading program addressed to Italian students with DD aged 8–14 [22]. The software was developed using Unity as the game engine and therefore both a Windows and a Mac version of the software are available.

Concerning the content of the application, the training program is composed of three categories of exercises designed to improve reading skills, which can be selected from a user-friendly menu screen: "Syllables", "Merging" and "Words and Pseudo-words". Each category of exercises is aimed at training a specific reading ability. The section "Syllables" trains syllable recognition. The section "Merging" involves merging syllables for creating words. The goal of the section "Words and Pseudo-words" is to train word, pseudo-word and small phrases decoding.

All reading exercises include a rhythmical accompaniment with gradually increasing speed. Participants are taught to read the verbal stimuli (i.e., syllables, words, pseudo-words, phrases) presented on the screen in synchrony with the rhythmic accompaniment. The first time an exercise is presented, the stimulus (or the part of the stimulus) which has to be read is indicated by a visual cue (consisting in highlighting the target grapheme in red) synchronized with musical rhythm, so to allow trainees to understand clearly in which manner they had to read the verbal materials.

The software allows the trainer to modulate the speed of presentation of the verbal stimuli in the exercises depending on the reading level of each participant. In order to make the speed setting easier, the velocity is expressed in terms of syllables per second (in RRT, 1 syllable per second is equivalent to 60 beats per minute), which is the most common measure used in clinical setting for assessing reading speed. Also, the complexity of the verbal stimuli presented is gradually increasing along with speed modulation. The complexity is modulated by increasing the number of stimuli presented on the screen (and thus manipulating visual crowding), decreasing letter font size, removing the visual cue (so that children have to rely only on the auditory aid for maintaining reading speed) or introducing concurrent tasks, such as the detection of a specific verbal target while reading.

The software provides the possibility to adapt the exercises presentation to the specific characteristics of each participant. That is the reason why the software can target a quite wide range of participants' age and levels of reading impairment.

In order to provide a distractors-free environment, all the exercises were designed for having an extremely simple and clear setting, so that children could focus only on the task presented. The font chosen for the verbal stimuli is Helvetica, coloured in black (red when the letters are highlighted by the visual cue) on a white background. Finally, the easy-to-use interface and the intuitive settings of the software makes it extremely clear and easy to managed by any trainer, even a non expert one.

2   Evaluating RRT's Efficacy: Preliminary Studies

2.1   An Application of RRT in the School Setting

In order to evaluate the efficacy of RRT as a treatment for DD, a test-training-retest experimental design was applied. We measured possible changes in reading skills of a group of children with DD between the beginning (pre phase) and the end of the intervention period (post phase). Reading improvements were compared to the ones of a control group of children with DD. Reading skills of the control group were monitored before and after a period of the same length of the intervention during which no specific activity addressed to improve reading skills was carried out.

Twenty-eight students aged 11–14 (mean age = 12.07 yrs., SD = 1.14) with DD participated in the study. They attended a junior high school in Lecco (Lombardy, Northern Italy) and had been previously diagnosed with DD on the basis of standard inclusion and exclusion criteria (ICD-10: World Health Organization, 1992) and of the ordinary diagnosis procedure followed in the Italian context.

Two subgroups of the same size matched for gender, school grade and level of reading impairment were then created and randomly assigned either to the intervention or the control condition.

Reading and rhythmic perception skills were assessed before and after the intervention or control period. The assessment of reading skills was carried out using two different batteries of tests.

- "Prova di lettura di parole e non parole" (Word and pseudo-word reading test) [23], in which speed and accuracy scores were computed for single word (4 lists of 30 words each with different lengths and frequency of use) and pseudo-word reading (2 lists of 30 pseudo-words each with different lengths).
- "Nuove prove di lettura MT per la scuola media inferiore" (New MT reading tests for junior high school) [24], a set of tests providing accuracy and speed scores in reading aloud age-normed texts.

Both batteries are the most commonly used in Italy to assess reading abilities in students with DD. In both batteries z-scores for reading accuracy and reading speed were computed from raw scores (respectively, the number of errors and the reading time expressed in seconds). A decrease in speed and accuracy measures corresponds to an improvement of the reading performance.

Rhythm perception ability was assessed through the rhythm reproduction task [25], which consists in the request to reproduce a set of rhythmic patterns of increasing complexity performed by the examiner. Scores are computed by counting the number of errors in the reproduction of rhythmic patterns.

Participants assigned to the intervention condition took part in the training program for 9 biweekly sessions of 30 min in length each, resulting in a total of 4.5 h of intervention. Training sessions were individual and were managed by the same researcher in a quite room of the school. During the training session the child sat in front of the computer and performed the proposed reading exercises under the supervision of the researcher. The number of exercises performed in each session varied according to the difficulty and the speed of the exercises. All the tasks were repeated at least three times at gradually increasing speed. The researcher managed to set up the speed in which stimuli had been presented according to the student's performance in each exercise. The student had to fulfil at least a reading accuracy of 95 % of the verbal stimuli in each exercise in order to speed up and/or proceed to the next exercise.

A mixed factorial ANOVA was carried out in order to evaluate the effect of RRT on reading accuracy and reading speed. Condition (intervention vs. control) was considered as the independent between-subject variable and phase (pre vs. post) as the independent within-subject variable.

RTT improved participants' reading skills. Both reading speed and accuracy mean z-scores increased after the intervention and these gains were significantly higher in the intervention than in the control condition. Significant interaction effects were found in short pseudo-words reading speed ($F(1,26) = 4.411$, $p < .05$, $\eta^2 = .145$), long pseudo-words reading speed ($F(1,26) = 7.493$, $p < .05$, $\eta^2 = .224$), high-frequency long words reading accuracy ($F(1,26) = 5.387$, $p < .05$, $\eta^2 = .172$) and text reading accuracy ($F(1,26) = 10.020$, $p < .005$, $\eta^2 = .278$). In particular, the time required to read short pseudo-words and long pseudo-words decreased after the intervention respectively of 0.51 and 0.75 z-scores on average. Regarding accuracy, the numbers of reading errors was reduced of 0.39 z-scores for high-frequency long words and of 2.37 z-scores for text on average.

Concerning the rhythm reproduction task, no significant difference between the control and the intervention condition was found. After both the control and the intervention period participants performed the test slightly better: a decrease of 0.93 (SD = 2.81) mistakes on average after the control period and a decrease of 2.00 (SD = 2.04) mistakes on average after the intervention period were found.

2.2 An Application of RTT in the Rehabilitation Setting

The second study was carried out in a clinical setting. Participants were recruited among patients of the neuropsychiatry unit of the IRCCS "Don Gnocchi" in Milan, Italy. The main objective of the study was to test the efficacy of RRT in an actual rehabilitation setting and on a specific sample of participants, namely, children with a diagnosis of DD in comorbidity with other specific learning disabilities. The same experimental design of the first study was applied but – due to difficulties in recruiting in the same setting a control group of children with DD matched for age, IQ and level of reading impairment – it was decided to involve all the participants in the intervention condition and to measure possible improvements in reading skills between the pre and post phase. Seven students aged 9–11 (mean age = 9.77 yrs., SD = 0.71) with DD in comorbidity with at least one other specific learning disability (i.e., dyscalculia, dysgraphia or dysorthography) participated in the study. All of them were meant to start a speech-therapy intervention aimed at training their impaired learning abilities, as commonly offered to children with specific learning disabilities in Italian neuropsychiatry units. Regarding the pre and post assessments, besides reading and rhythm perception, a set of cognitive functions were also tested: visual sustained attention, auditory selective attention, verbal working memory and other auditory perception abilities.

Participants took part in the training program for 20 biweekly sessions of 20 min in length each, resulting in a total of 6.7 h of intervention. After each RRT session, children took also part in a traditional speech-therapy intervention session, during which other learning domains (e.g., mathematics, graphomotor skills, etc.) except reading were specifically trained for other 20 min. While RRT sessions were managed by a researcher using the same modality of the first study, traditional intervention was carried out by a speech-therapist belonging to the neuropsychiatric unit.

Because of the small sample size and the lack of a control group, it was not possible to carry out any statistical analysis. We compared the performances in the assessed skills before and after the participation in the intervention and found out the following improvements: pseudo-words and text reading speed increased after the intervention respectively of 0.22 and 0.19 z-scores on average; visual sustained attention increased of 0.66 z-scores on average; verbal working memory improved of 0.29 z-scores on average.

3   Discussion and Conclusions

The aim of the present article was to present an innovative computerized rehabilitation program for DD and to show preliminary results about its application in two different settings.

Previous research suggested that musical abilities play a role in reading and that musical training might improve reading skills. However, the musical intervention programs which have been tested so far included a variety of music activities (such as listening, singing, tapping, playing an instrument, etc.) which involved solely auditory and timing processing (e.g., pitch discrimination, reproduction of rhythmic patterns, etc.). The intervention approach that we are presenting, instead, combines a specific reading training, aimed at enhancing grapheme-phoneme connections, and music intervention, providing a simultaneous stimulation of the shared mechanisms between music and language. For implementing that, IT appeared to be the best choice: it provides multimodal (visual and auditory) stimulation as well as the perfect synchronisation of the concurrent presentation of sounds and visual stimuli and allows the trainer to have control over timing and difficulty of the stimulus presentation. Furthermore, the potentiality of music for boosting motivation and provide an enjoyable rehabilitation setting is well known and it is exploited in the training.

The results of the two preliminary studies reported suggest that RRT is effective in improving both reading speed and accuracy [26] and, thanks to the computerized version of the training, RRT can be easily applied in school and clinical rehabilitation settings.

In particular, significant improvements after the RRT were found on both short and long pseudo-words reading speed, as well as in high-frequency long words and in text reading accuracy. These results suggest that RRT is efficient in boosting accuracy in reading the kind of materials to which students are usually exposed to (namely, high frequently used words and text) and in enhancing speed when the grapheme-phoneme conversion mechanism is required, such as in pseudo-word reading. The effect of the training program seems to be specific on reading skills, since no significant improvement in rhythm reproduction was found.

Considering the duration of the intervention (4.5 h of intervention during a 5-week period), far shorter than traditional remediation treatments of DD, the fact that significant improvements of reading skills were found is promising. Regarding the clinical setting application, we found that besides improvements in short-words and text reading speed, also visual sustained attention and verbal memory were enhanced by RRT.

Results suggest that a combination of reading and rhythmic training could be an effective treatment for dyslexia and that the characteristic of the intervention can easily be adapted to different settings (i.e., scholastic and clinical settings).

However, the limited number of participants and the absence of a control group in the second study call for caution in evaluating the outcomes of the intervention. Another limitation of both of the studies is the use of the same battery of tests for both pre and post phase assessments, especially since the assessment sessions were only 5/10 weeks apart; this choice was the best for having a precise comparison of reading abilities.

Further research seems to be necessary to validate the effectiveness of RRT. In particular, it would be crucial to study the role of the rhythmic component in reading improvement. Although the hypothesis of a positive effect of music training on the impaired auditory perception and timing processing of children with DD is supported by experimental evidence, a comparison between RRT and traditional remediation treatments of DD would enable to understand the role of music in reading enhancement. Furthermore, a follow-up assessment should be carried out for evaluating the maintenance of reading improvements.

In conclusion, the combination of music and reading training allowed by the computerized version of RRT seems to be a promising rehabilitation strategy for improving reading skills in students with DD. Besides the effect on reading, this innovative treatment approach involves also an active engagement with music, which provides an enjoyable and pleasant experience for subjects with DD. Furthermore, the use of IT allows, for the reasons mentioned above, the training to be easily implemented also in home settings in a standardized and reliable way.

References

1. Lyon, G.R., Shaywitz, S.E., Shaywitz, B.A.: A definition of dyslexia. Ann. Dyslexia **53**, 1–14 (2003)
2. Démonet, J.F., Taylor, M.J., Chaix, Y.: Developmental dyslexia. Lancet **363**(9419), 1451–1460 (2004)
3. Cornoldi, C., Tressoldi, P.: Definizione, criteri e classificazione. In: Cornoldi, C., (ed.) Difficoltà e Disturbi Dell'apprendimento, (Bologna: Il Mulino), pp. 9–52 (2007)
4. Fraser, J., Goswami, U., Conti-Ramsden, G.: Dyslexia and specific language impairment: The role of phonology and auditory processing. Sci. Stud. Reading **14**, 8–29 (2010)
5. Farmer, M.E., Klein, R.M.: The evidence for a temporal processing deficit linked to dyslexia: A review. Psychon. Bull. Rev. **2**, 460–493 (1995)
6. Huss, M., Verney, P.J., Fosker, T., Mead, N., Goswami, U.: Music, rhythm, rise time perception and developmental dyslexia: Perception of musical meter predicts reading and phonology. Cortex **47**, 674–689 (2011)
7. Goswami, U., Fosker, T., Huss, M., Mead, N., Szűcs, D.: Rise time and formant transition duration in the discrimination of speech sounds: The Ba-Wa distinction in developmental dyslexia. Dev. Sci. **14**, 34–43 (2011)
8. Flaugnacco, E., Lopez, L., Terribili, C., Zoia, S., Buda, S., Tilli, S., Monasta, L., Montico, M., Sila, A., Ronfani, L., Schön, D.: Rhythm perception and production predict reading abilities in developmental dyslexia. Front. Hum. Neurosci. **8**, 392 (2014). doi:10.3389/fnhum.2014.00392
9. Goswami, U., Huss, M., Mead, N., Fosker, T., Verney, J.P.: Perception of patterns of musical beat distribution in phonological developmental dyslexia: Significant longitudinal relations with word reading and reading comprehension. Cortex **49**, 1363–1376 (2013)
10. Leong, V., Goswami, U.: Impaired extraction of speech rhythm from temporal modulation patterns in speech in developmental dyslexia. Front. Hum. Neurosci. **8**, 96 (2014). doi:10.3389/fnhum.2014.00096
11. Tressoldi, P.E., Vio, C., Lorusso, M.L., Facoetti, A., Iozzino, R.: Confronto di efficacia ed efficienza tra trattamenti per il miglioramento della lettura in soggetti dislessici [A comparison of the efficacy of the treatments to improve reading skills in dyslexic subjects]. Psicologia Clinica dello Sviluppo **7**, 481–494 (2003)
12. Cazzaniga, S., Re, A.M., Cornoldi, C., Poli, S., Tressoldi, P.E.: Dislessia e trattamento sublessicale [Dyslexia and sublexical treatment], Trento: Erickson (2005)
13. Bakker, D.J., Licht, R., Kappers, E.J.: Hemisphere-specific treatment of dyslexia. In: Tramontana, G., Hooper, S.R. (eds.) Advances in Child Neuropsychology, 3rd edn, pp. 144–177. Springer-Verlag, New York/Berlin (1995)
14. Elkind, J.: Computer Reading Machines for Poor Readers. Lexia, report 9801, 1-17 January 2015 (1998)
15. James, C.E.: Music and language processing share behavioral and cerebral features. Front. Psychol. **3**, 52 (2012). doi:10.3389/fpsyg.2012.00052
16. Anvari, S.H., Trainor, L.J., Woodside, J., Ann Levy, B.: Relations among musical skills, phonological processing, and early reading ability in preschool children. Exp. Child Psychol. **83**, 111–130 (2002)
17. Forgeard, M., Schlaug, G., Norton, A., Rosam, C., Lyengar, U., Winner, E.: The relation between music and phonological processing in normal-reading children and children with dyslexia. Music Percept. **4**, 383–390 (2008)
18. Overy, K.: Dyslexia and music: From timing deficits to musical intervention. Ann. NY Acad. Sci. **999**, 497–505 (2003)

19. Tallal, P., Gaab, N.: Dynamic auditory processing, musical experience and language development. Trends Neurosci. **7**, 290–382 (2006)
20. Register, D., Darrow, A.A., Swedberg, O., Standley, J.: The use of music to enhance reading skills of second grade students and students with reading disabilities. J. Music Ther. **44**, 23–37 (2007)
21. Kraus, N., Chandrasekaran, B.: Music training for developmental auditory skills. Nat. Rev. Neurosci. **11**, 599–605 (2010)
22. Germagnoli, S., Bonacina, S., Cancer, A., Antonietti, A.: Dislessia e musica: Dai meccanismi comuni ai trattamenti [Dyslexia and music: From common mechanisms to treatments], Dislessia. (in press)
23. Cornoldi, C., Colpo, G.: Nuove prove di lettura MT per la scuola media inferiore. Organizzazioni Speciali, Firenze (1995). [New MT reading tests for junior high school]
24. Zoccolotti, P., De Luca, M., Di Filippo, G., Judica, A., Spinelli, D.: Prova di lettura di parole e non parole [Test for reading of words and pseudo-words]. IRCCS Fondazione Santa Lucia, Rome (2005)
25. Stambak, M.: Problems of rhythm in the development of the child and in developmental dyslexia. Enfance **4**, 480–502 (1951)
26. Bonacina, S., Cancer, A., Lanzi, P.L., Lorusso, M.L., Antonietti, A.: Improving reading skills in students with dyslexia: the efficacy of a sublexical training with rhythmic background. Front. Psychol. **6**, 1–8 (2015). doi:10.3389/fpsyg.2015.01510

Designing Assistive Technologies for the ADHD Domain

Tobias Sonne[⊠] and Kaj Grønbæk

Department of Computer Science, Aarhus University, Aabogade 34, 8200 Aarhus N, Denmark
{tsonne,kgronbak}@cs.au.dk

Abstract. Assistive technologies have proven to support and empower people with a variety of mental diagnoses in performing self-care activities in their everyday lives. However, little research has explored the potentials for assistive technologies for people with Attention Deficit Hyperactivity Disorder (ADHD). In this paper, we identify a set of challenges that children with ADHD typically experience, which provides an empirical foundation for pervasive health researchers to address the ADHD domain. The work is grounded in extensive empirical studies and it is contextualized using literature on ADHD. Based on these studies, we also present lessons learned that are relevant to consider when designing assistive technology to support children with ADHD. Finally, we provide an example (CASTT) of our own work to illustrate how the presented findings can frame research activities and be used to develop novel assistive technology to empower children with ADHD and improve their wellbeing.

Keywords: Wearable computing · Assistive technology · Children · ADHD · Body sensor networks · Mental disorder management

1 Introduction

Recent developments in pervasive healthcare and related areas show great promise for technologies to assist people with e.g. chronic heart failure [1], freezing of gait [2] and children with autism [3]. However, only few researchers have investigated how technology can be designed to assist and empower people with ADHD. In contrast, research on assistive technologies, tools and methods for supporting people with Autism Spectrum Disorders (ASD) has received significant focus e.g. [3–5]. Even though patients can be diagnosed with both ASD and ADHD the two disorders are different. The diagnosis criteria for ASD include persistent impairments in social communication and social interactions, repetitive patterns of behavior and in some cases intellectual and language impairments [6]. In contrast the diagnosis criteria for ADHD relate to patterns of inattention and/or hyperactivity and impulsive behavior [6]. Therefore, assistive technologies for children with ASD cannot per se be used within the domain of ADHD.

ADHD is a highly heritable [7] childhood-onset neuro-developmental disorder with a worldwide prevalence of approximately 5 % among children and adolescents [8]. As a consequence of the difficulties (inattention, impulsivity, hyperactivity) caused by ADHD [6], there is a significant burden on those affected, their families and the society in general [9]. For instance, ADHD is associated with impaired academic performance

© Springer International Publishing Switzerland 2016
S. Serino et al. (Eds.): MindCare 2015, CCIS 604, pp. 259–268, 2016.
DOI: 10.1007/978-3-319-32270-4_26

[10, 11], difficulties in interacting with parents and teachers [12], increased risk of criminal convictions in adulthood [13, 14] as well as increased mortality [15]. Traditional ADHD treatment include prescribed medication [16], cognitive training [17] and parent training [18]. Furthermore, ADHD has shown to considerably affect the children's quality of life [7] and 70 % of children with ADHD in third grade report among other things that they have no close friends [7].

Due to the vast societal and personal losses caused by ADHD, it is important to investigate the potentials that pervasive assistive technologies can provide for this domain. In this regard, we have conducted multiple interdisciplinary studies within the domain of ADHD, including: Observations, in the wild evaluations together with children with ADHD and hands on training. Based on the insights from our empirical studies, we present challenges and experiences prevalent among children with ADHD. Furthermore, we present empirically grounded lessons we have learned are relevant to take into account when designing for this domain. Moreover, we present an example of one of our current research projects that build upon these findings as an example of how to explore the design space of assistive technologies for children with ADHD. Based on our experiences, we argue that assistive technologies can have great potentials for both novel research and for empowering children with ADHD.

2   Related Work

This section presents related research conducted on assistive technology for the domain of ADHD, according to their intended context i.e. the home, pervasive, and the school.

To start with, CogoLand is one of the existing projects that has investigated the effects of a neurofeedback game on ADHD symptoms, which has been evaluated in the home context [19]. The gameplay in CogoLand is based on an avatar in a 3D world, which has to complete a race as fast as possible. The speed of the avatar is controlled by the child's level of concentration, which is measured using an electroence-phalography (EEG) headband. 20 unmedicated children diagnosed with ADHD participated in the experiment that ran for 24 weeks. The parents filled out a baseline score based on an 18-question ADHD rating scale, before the experiment started. Eight weeks into the experiment the results showed a drop from a mean score of 33.4 to 24.1 in the combined score [19]. Similarly, Cogmed is a research based PC application that trains the child's working memory through various memory games in the home [20]. The recommended training period is minimum 25 sessions of 30–45 min over a six-week period. The level of difficulty is automatically adjusted as the child improves or worsens. Working memory training has shown to improve reasoning and response inhibition and to reduce the parent rated symptoms of ADHD [17]. In the medical domain, several studies [17, 21–23] indicate that both neurofeedback and working memory games can reduce ADHD symptoms.

Furthermore, a different example of an assistive technology is the ParentGuardian system that provides in situ Parental Behavioral Therapy (PBT) cues for parents of children with ADHD, in order to support parents to better manage stressful situations [24]. The ParentGuardian system uses changes in skin conductance, measured by an

Electro-Dermal Activity wristband, to estimate the stress level of the parent. When a high level of stress is detected, the parent is prompted with a combined textual and visual reflective strategy on their smartphone and on a peripheral display to remind them to use PBT strategies [24]. From their studies, Pina et al. found that in situ cues for parents could assist the parents to remember to use the PBT strategies during moments of need [24]. In addition, several commercial smartphone apps exist for providing structure and reminders for children with ADHD such as STRUKTUR[1]. The common concept for these apps is that a parent manually inputs a desired daily structure into a calendar like application, which is used to visualize the structure of the day for the child.

In particular, there are two examples of systems designed for the school context. For instance, McHugh et al. investigates if a wristwatch connected to a heart rate belt, could assist children to avoid emotional outburst in school contexts [25]. By analyzing sensor data from the heart rate belt, the system detects an approaching emotional outburst, and alerts the child to use self-calming techniques to prevent the upcoming emotional outburst. McHugh et al. found heart rate feedback a useful tool to assist children to calm themselves down, without the need of help from parents or teachers [25]. In addition, the Smart Pen prototype detects concentration lapses during reading, and remind the child about the current reading task in the school [26]. Via an embedded 3-axis accelerometer and a machine learning algorithm, the Smart Pen is able to recognize reading patterns. The Smart Pen discretely reminds children to (resume) reading, by either lighting a small LED or vibrating. Even though limited, the prior work shows great promises for assistive technologies within the ADHD domain. However, existing research focused on isolated systems, and do not provide explicit and practical directions for further research on how to design technology for the domain of ADHD. In this paper, we extend the related work by providing a set of challenges and design considerations as a foundation for designing assistive technologies for children with ADHD, and by identifying future directions within this domain.

3   Conducted Empirical Studies Within the ADHD Domain

To identify directions for IT-based research within the domain of ADHD, we set out to qualitatively understand the impairments caused by ADHD and how this affects the child, family and school. Thus, we conducted a broad range of empirical studies, including in the wild evaluations and intensive hands on training activities working with children with ADHD. The findings presented in this paper are based on more than one year of close collaboration with teachers, researchers within the field of ADHD and hands-on experience with children with ADHD, including:

- 10 h of observations in clinics with follow up interviews with child psychiatrists and psychologists.
- Following two psychologists under their observations of children being investigated for ADHD in school contexts for two full days.

---
[1] https://itunes.apple.com/kn/app/struktur/id692730085?mt=8.

- Extensive observations of children with ADHD (2nd–5th grade) and interviews with seven teachers from four different schools and two nurses, who had extensive experience working with children with ADHD.
- Two ideation workshops with a teacher and a pedagogue.
- More than 50 h (2.5–3.0 h each week for 20 weeks) of experience being together with, and taking care of children with ADHD, while their parents received parent training at Center for ADHD in Aarhus, Denmark. Furthermore, this training included weekly one-hour discussions with two psychologists working at Center for ADHD.
- Two one-hour phone interviews with parents of children with ADHD about sleep habits.
- A four-week and a three-week intervention experiment of our Healthy Sleep Habits (HSH) project with two families of children with ADHD including two one-hour follow up interviews in the home with parents and children.
- Five hours of in the wild studies with 11 children with ADHD in 4th–5th grade in three different schools in order to evaluate a wearable technology system for children with ADHD as presented in Sect. 6.

Through affinity diagrams, we have organized and analyzed the large amount of data (primarily field notes and transcribed interviews) together with literature from the ADHD domain. The most relevant themes from the analysis are presented in the following sections.

4 Challenges Caused by ADHD

This section presents challenges caused by ADHD in both school and home contexts, in order to provide HCI researchers and practitioners with a grounded set of design issues to take into account when developing assistive technologies for the ADHD domain:

1. *Remembering a Sequence of Instructions:* Holding a sequence of instructions depends on a person's working memory [17] and several studies have shown a link between ADHD and working memory deficits [17]. The consequences of these deficits affects both parents and teachers, as the child's forgets what to do next, and often instead does something else. This can cause stress for the parents and teachers as they often repeatedly have to remind the child of the current task.
2. *Handling Transitions Between Activities*: From our empirical studies we learned that one of the most challenging situations for children with ADHD is the transition from one activity to another. For example, in an interview with a mom she stated: "*[For the child] there can be a thousands inputs on your way [...], you always have your 'antennas' out so you cannot focus on the task originally planned*". From our classroom studies we often observed that transitions did cause conflicts between the child and other pupils or between the child and teacher.
3. *Sustained Attention:* Due to the nature of ADHD, children with ADHD suffer from various degrees of inability in sustaining attention, which "*most likely arises from poor interference control that allows other external and internal events to disrupt the executive functions that provide for self-control and task persistence*" [27].

Aligned with this study, our classroom observations are consistent and often show that even low sounds could distract the children from their current task.

4. *Impulsive Behavior:* Previous classroom observations reported that children with ADHD have a higher degree of off-task and disruptive behavior [28]. In our observational studies within classroom contexts we experienced several situations where a child with ADHD acted impulsively, in situations where such behavior is not normally expected.

5. *Perceiving Time:* Studies indicate that many children with ADHD exhibit impairments in perceiving time [29], which is consistent with our studies. This deficit often causes the children to loose focus, as they do not know how long they have to keep doing their current task. According to teachers this often results in disruptive behavior that causes disturbance in the classroom.

6. *Bedtime Resistance:* Sleep is important for a child's neurobehavioral functioning, and even a one-hour sleep restriction over six nights can manifests in increased hyperactivity, inattention, disruptive behaviors, poor concentration and poor school performance [30]. However, both existing research and our empirical studies indicate that children with ADHD show significant more bedtime resistance and longer sleep onset latency than children without ADHD [30].

The presented challenges are based on our analysis of our empirical data and supported with research from the ADHD domain. For a more complete diagnostic picture of the deficits related to ADHD, the reader is referred to the diagnostic criteria in [6]. The formulation of the above challenges will provide researchers and practitioners with a foundation for designing better assistive systems for the ADHD domain.

5 Lessons Learned from Evaluating Assistive Technologies with Children with ADHD

Based on our experiences with designing and evaluating assistive technologies for children with ADHD together with feedback from ADHD domain experts, we present the lessons learned that we find relevant to consider when designing for this domain.

5.1 Structure and Pictograms Maintains Focus

As identified in the previous section, children with ADHD struggle in remembering a sequence of instructions and perceiving time. From our observational studies we learned that pictograms placed on a wall are often used to visualize structure in schools and the homes as this helps the child to maintain focus. Our findings thus suggest that it is beneficial to design and incorporate a very simple and explicit structure, so the child is aware of what to do next and does not loose focus from the system. For instance, a dad from our HSH study expressed: *"It [the HSH prototype] is really good, especially for [the child's name], as it helps put things in system. That is really helpful when you tend to get many ideas from one task to another"*.

5.2 Rewards Influence Behavior

During our studies both parents, teachers and experts emphasized rewards as a way to influence the behavior and performance of a child with ADHD as seen below in Fig. 1, which is also documented in the ADHD literature e.g. [29]. Therefore, including explicit rewards in an assistive system for children with ADHD can both influence the behavior of the child and enhance the child's interest in the system itself. However, it should be clear what the child should do to earn the reward, like the reward also should be provided right after this action to get the best effect, due to their impairments in perceiving time as mentioned above.

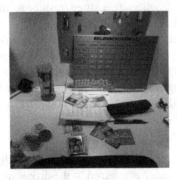 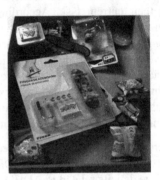

Fig. 1. Left, a reward board placed on the child's desk in the home. Right, a box of rewards from which the child can exchange "coins" for a reward.

5.3 Technology Fosters Interest and Responsibility

From our HSH pilot studies with two families we learned that using a smartphone instead of an analog counterpart (e.g. a paper based list of activities) increased the chances of successfully assisting the child to learn a new routine. After our four-week study we asked the parents what they perceived as the qualities and weaknesses of a smartphone based approach in contrast to a paper-based tool: *"[…] it creates an interest which you will not be able to create with a checklist on a piece of paper. Also, it [a paper-based tool] is not involving in the same way, I mean, a piece of paper appeals to something for adults right?"* (Interview with two parents). From the same interview we learned that technology made the child feel more responsible: *"He [the child] feels a responsibility in that it is he who is controlling the smartphone in another way than a child can take responsibility of a piece of paper."*

These three lessons learned constitute core design considerations for designing assistive technologies for children with ADHD based on our experiences working in this domain.

6   An Example of a Research Project

In this section, we present one of our current projects within the ADHD domain as a practical example on how to address the challenges children with ADHD experience (Sect. 4) and to incorporate our lessons learned (Sect. 5).

The objectives of our ongoing research on The Child Activity Sensing & Training Tool (CASTT) is to investigate the potential of using a wearable sensor system to provide in situ assistance to children with ADHD in regaining attention in school contexts. CASTT uses both physical and physiological data to detect when a child is having challenges in sustaining attention. When such a condition is detected, CASTT discreetly notifies the child through a smartphone-based quiz intervention that terminates with a clear guidance to the child to refocus on the school task in front of him (Fig. 2).

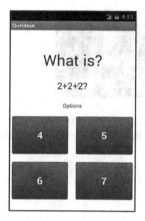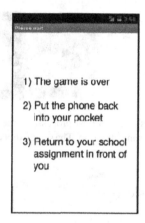

Fig. 2.   Screenshot from the quizz-based CASTT intervention. The termination screen to the right is the actual assistance for the child as it supports the child to regain attention of the school assignment.

In relation to above the presented empirically identified challenges children with ADHD experience, CASTT addresses the first three of these i.e. (1) Remembering a sequence of instructions by limiting the instructions to three clear action tasks, (2) Handling transitions between activities by displaying the three action tasks on termination of the quiz application, and (3) Sustained attention by detecting inattention and using the above presented technology and techniques to assisting the child to regain attention. Furthermore, we used rewards in the smartphone-based quiz intervention to motivate the child to play the game and to influence his behavior (Sect. 5.2).

So far we have evaluated the comfort of CASTT and its ability to collect relevant sensor data with 11 children with ADHD in school contexts. In addition we have evaluated the assistive component of CASTT with one child with promising results in lowering the child's hyperactivity and assisting the child to regain attention as seen on Fig. 3. In our study of the assistive component CASTT successfully assisted the child with ADHD to refocus his attention on the school assignment in front of him.

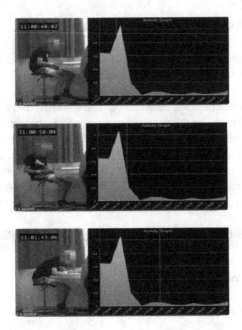

Fig. 3. Screenshots of a post processed video to show the effect of the CASTT on the child's physical activity and attention. The screenshots show the time before, during, and after the CASTT was triggered.

7   Conclusion

This paper discussed the challenges and opportunities uncovered from field studies in the domain of ADHD as well as the useful lessons learned for supporting user centered design of assistive technology for children with ADHD. Based on our studies and related research within pervasive technology and psychiatry, we presented an example of our own work on assistive technologies for children with ADHD, and showed how the empirical and theoretical findings presented in this paper were materialized into the CASTT prototype. Based on the empirical findings, we argue that there are many possibilities for IT-based research within the ADHD domain that may provide novel ways of empowering children with ADHD. Many challenges still remain and we hope that our outline of the design space of assistive technology for the ADHD domain will direct the relevant HCI communities into more and better pervasive technology for the ADHD domain.

References

1. Zhang, S., McCullagh, P., Nugent, C., Zheng, H.: A theoretic algorithm for fall and motionless detection. In: 3rd International Conference on Pervasive Computing Technologies for Healthcare, 2009, PervasiveHealth 2009, pp. 1–6 (2009)

2. Mazilu, S., Hardegger, M., Zhu, Z., Roggen, D., Troster, G., Plotnik, M., Hausdorff, J.M.: Online detection of freezing of gait with smartphones and machine learning techniques. In: 6th International Conference on Pervasive Computing Technologies for Healthcare (PervasiveHealth 2012), pp. 123–130 (2012)

3. Hayes, G.R., Hirano, S., Marcu, G., Monibi, M., Nguyen, D.H., Yeganyan, M.: Interactive visual supports for children with autism. Pers. Ubiquitous Comput. **14**, 663–680 (2010)

4. Hayes, G.R., Gardere, L.M., Abowd, G.D., Truong, K.N.: CareLog: a selective archiving tool for behavior management in schools. In: Proceedings of the SIGCHI Conference on Human Factors in Computing Systems, pp. 685–694. ACM, New York (2008)

5. Hirano, S.H., Yeganyan, M.T., Marcu, G., Nguyen, D.H., Boyd, L.A., Hayes, G.R.: vSked: evaluation of a system to support classroom activities for children with autism. In: Proceedings of the SIGCHI Conference on Human Factors in Computing Systems, pp. 1633–1642. ACM, New York (2010)

6. Diagnostic and Statistical Manual of Mental Disorders: Fifth Edition: DSM-5. American Psychiatric Pub (2013)

7. Wehmeier, P.M., Schacht, A., Barkley, R.A.: Social and emotional impairment in children and adolescents with ADHD and the impact on quality of life. J. Adolesc. Health **46**, 209–217 (2010)

8. Polanczyk, G., de Lima, M.S., Horta, B.L., Biederman, J., Rohde, L.A.: The worldwide prevalence of ADHD: a systematic review and metaregression analysis. Am. J. Psychiatry **164**, 942–948 (2007)

9. Harpin, V.A.: The effect of ADHD on the life of an individual, their family, and community from preschool to adult life. Arch. Dis. Child. **90**(Suppl 1), i2–i7 (2005)

10. Goldman, L.S., Genel, M., Bezman, R.J., Slanetz, P.J.: Diagnosis and treatment of attention-deficit/hyperactivity disorder in children and adolescents. Council on Scientific Affairs, American Medical Association. JAMA **279**, 1100–1107 (1998)

11. Massetti, G.M., Lahey, B.B., Pelham, W.E., Loney, J., Ehrhardt, A., Lee, S.S., Kipp, H.: Academic achievement over 8 years among children who met modified criteria for attention-deficit/hyperactivity disorder at 4-6 years of age. J. Abnorm. Child Psychol. **36**, 399–410 (2008)

12. Storebø, O.J., Skoog, M., Rasmussen, P.D., Winkel, P., Gluud, C., Pedersen, J., Thomsen, P.H., Simonsen, E.: Attachment competences in children with ADHD during the social-skills training and attachment (SOSTRA) randomized clinical trial. J. Atten. Disord. (2014). doi: 10.1177/1087054713520220

13. Dalsgaard, S., Mortensen, P.B., Frydenberg, M., Thomsen, P.H.: Long-term criminal outcome of children with attention deficit hyperactivity disorder. Crim. Behav. Ment. Health CBMH **23**, 86–98 (2013)

14. Mannuzza, S., Klein, R.G., Moulton, J.L.: Lifetime criminality among boys with ADHD: a prospective follow-up study into adulthood using official arrest records. Psychiatry Res. **160**, 237–246 (2008)

15. Barbaresi, W.J., Colligan, R.C., Weaver, A.L., Voigt, R.G., Killian, J.M., Katusic, S.K.: Mortality, ADHD, and psychosocial adversity in adults with childhood ADHD: a prospective study. Pediatrics **131**, 637–644 (2013)

16. Hechtman, L., Greenfield, B.: Long-term use of stimulants in children with attention deficit hyperactivity disorder: safety, efficacy, and long-term outcome. Paediatr. Drugs **5**, 787–794 (2003)

17. Klingberg, T., Fernell, E., Olesen, P.J., Johnson, M., Gustafsson, P., Dahlström, K., Gillberg, C.G., Forssberg, H., Westerberg, H.: Computerized training of working memory in children with ADHD: a randomized, controlled trial. J. Am. Acad. Child Adolesc. Psychiatry **44**, 177–186 (2005)
18. Anastopoulos, A.D., DuPaul, G.J., Barkley, R.A.: Stimulant medication and parent training therapies for attention deficit-hyperactivity disorder. J. Learn. Disabil. **24**, 210–218 (1991)
19. Lim, C.G., Lee, T.S., Guan, C., Fung, D.S.S., Zhao, Y., Teng, S.S.W., Zhang, H., Krishnan, K.R.R.: A brain-computer interface based attention training program for treating attention deficit hyperactivity disorder. PLoS One **7**, e46692 (2012)
20. Cogmed Working Memory Training. http://www.cogmed.com/
21. Heinrich, H., Gevensleben, H., Strehl, U.: Annotation: neurofeedback – train your brain to train behaviour. J. Child Psychol. Psychiatry **48**, 3–16 (2007)
22. Lubar, J.F., Swartwood, M.O., Swartwood, J.N., O'Donnell, P.H.: Evaluation of the effectiveness of EEG neurofeedback training for ADHD in a clinical setting as measured by changes in T.O.V.A. scores, behavioral ratings, and WISC-R performance. Biofeedback Self-Regul. **20**, 83–99 (1995)
23. Monastra, V.J., Monastra, D.M., George, S.: The effects of stimulant therapy, EEG biofeedback, and parenting style on the primary symptoms of attention-deficit/hyperactivity disorder. Appl. Psychophysiol. Biofeedback **27**, 231–249 (2002)
24. Pina, L., Roseway, A., Czerwinski, M., Rowan, K.: In situ cues for ADHD parenting strategies using mobile technology. Presented at the May 2014
25. McHugh, B., Dawson, N., Scrafton, A., Asen, E.: "Hearts on their sleeves": the use of systemic biofeedback in school settings. J. Fam. Ther. **32**, 58–72 (2010)
26. DePrenger, M., Shao, Y., Lu, F., Fleming, N., Sikdar, S.: Feasibility study of a smart pen for autonomous detection of concentration lapses during reading. Eng. Med. Biol. Soc. EMBC **2010**, 1864–1867 (2010)
27. Barkley, R.A.: Behavioral inhibition, sustained attention, and executive functions: constructing a unifying theory of ADHD. Psychol. Bull. **121**, 65–94 (1997)
28. Lauth, G.W., Heubeck, B.G., Mackowiak, K.: Observation of children with attention-deficit hyperactivity (ADHD) problems in three natural classroom contexts. Br. J. Educ. Psychol. **76**, 385–404 (2006)
29. McInerney, R.J., Kerns, K.A.: Time reproduction in children with ADHD: motivation matters. Child Neuropsychol. **9**, 91–108 (2003)
30. Sadeh, A., Gruber, R., Raviv, A.: The effects of sleep restriction and extension on school-age children: what a difference an hour makes. Child Dev. **74**, 444–455 (2003)

The Effect of tDCS on EEG Profile During a Semantic Motor Task Divided in a Correct and Incorrect Ways

Cristina Liviana Caldiroli[1]([✉]) and Michela Balconi[2]

[1] Centre for Studies in Communication Science – CESCOM,
University of Milan-Bicocca, Milan, Italy
c.caldiroli@unimib.it
[2] Laboratory of Cognitive Psychology, Department of Psychology,
Catholic University of the Sacred Heart, Milan, Italy

Abstract. In this experimental we investigated the cortical neuromodulation during a tDCS (transcranial direct current stimulation) section to induce a temporary inhibition of the frontal area. The induced effect of brain modulation was tested on the EEG (electroencephalography) and ERPs (event-related potentials) profile when subjects performed a task in which they had to respond if the object represented in the sequence was correctly or incorrectly used. It was shown that an increased negative peak deflection (N400) is observable in case of semantic anomalies. We attended a significant reduction of this ERPs deflections when tDCS was applied to frontal area. During the detection task, participants were asked to evaluate the semantic correctness of some motor sequences that manipulated simple objects. EEG were registered during the tDCS or no tDCS stimulation. Significant differences between the two conditions and a reduction of the peak amplitude were observed in case of tDCS stimulation.

Keywords: tDCS · Action · N400 effect · Non-invasive brain stimulation

1 Introduction

In the present study, we explored the representation of an incongruent action (instrumentally incorrect use of an object) in comparison with sentences ending with an incongruent action word (Balconi et al. 2014; Balconi and Caldiroli 2011). This activity was appositely modulated by tDCS (transcranial direct current stimulation). Moreover, we considered the cortical response (N400) to the semantic incongruence induced by a final anomalous object-related action within an actions' sequence. It can be argued that the N400-like effect is similar in nature to the N400 which is generally evoked by linguistic stimuli (Maffongelli et al. 2015; Amoruso et al. 2013). When perception of plausible or implausible actions within a context is performed a specific semantic process is activated, that was showed to be similar in nature to the processing of anomalous linguistic information (Ganis and Kutas 2003). Indeed, this link was well demonstrated by the cognition of language: seeing a verb with an action content may modulate the motor area (Rizzolatti and Craighero 2004). Nevertheless, an analogous process has been reported for action processing because it has

© Springer International Publishing Switzerland 2016
S. Serino et al. (Eds.): MindCare 2015, CCIS 604, pp. 269–273, 2016.
DOI: 10.1007/978-3-319-32270-4_27

been hypothesized that the mechanisms involved in the perception of action sequences may be similar to those associated with the processing of semantic information in language (Reid et al. 2008; Bach et al. 2009). Taken together, these findings are consistent with the hypothesis that people store information within semantic memory in a structured and amodal fashion and that the N400 reflected a process whereby the meaning of an incoming stimulus was mapped into the corresponding field in semantic memory. During the experiment, we sought to analyzed the direct effect of tDCS on the ERPs profile in response to the semantic task. The effect of tDCS when subjects processed congruent/incongruent object-related actions or sentences was verified by measuring changes in the ERPs in N400. The stimulation effect (a cathode applied to the DLPFC and an anode to the right supraorbital region) was analyzed by comparing the ERPs profiles before and after stimulation (or sham treatment).

2   Methods and Materials

2.1   Subjects

Thirty undergraduate students took part in the experiment (18 women and 12 men, age range = 20–28 years, M = 24.22 years, SD = 2.77 years). They were all right handed, with normal or corrected-to normal visual acuity. Handedness was assessed using the Italian version of the Edinburgh Handedness Inventory (Salmaso and Longoni 1985). The exclusion criteria were history of psychopathology for the subjects or immediate family.

2.2   Stimuli

Three sets of 60 action sequences (four action-frames), were presented to the participants, respectively with a congruous (30 sequences) or incongruous (30 sequences) final frame. The stimulus sequences were constructed, taking into account some general data sets previously validated (Balconi and Caldiroli 2011; Balconi and Vitaloni 2012). Frames were shown without sound for 1.5 s, with an inter-frame interval of 250 ms. Each frame was composed of a real-world scene that represented a subject and an object within a neutral background. The semantic incongruence consisted of an object that was not correctly used with respect to the instrumental properties required for the central action-goal (grasping a bat upside-down).

The inter-sequence interval was 5 s. For each set of stimuli, the scene material was then organized into two sets, each consisting of half congruous and half incongruous

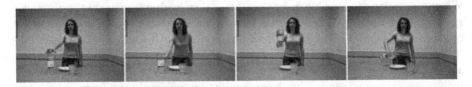

Fig. 1. Example of stimulus with incongruous final frame

sequences. Each set contained only one of the two versions of the final target action frame. Half of the participants viewed the first set, and half viewed the second set (the order of the sequence was counterbalanced across participants) Fig 1.

2.3 Procedure

The procedure was subdivided in two phases. Prior to tDCS stimulation, the pre-stimulation task was conducted, and EEG was registered (phase 1, baseline task). The participants were required to press a left or right pulse of the mouse depending on whether the final target action represented a congruous or an incongruous ending scene. The stimulus material was presented on a PC monitor (by using the software STIM 2.2), and the participants sat on a comfortable chair in front of the PC. They were instructed to gaze at the center of the screen, where a small cross served as fixation point. They were also required to minimize blinking. A familiarization phase preceded the phase 1 (10 min with eleven trials). The EEG was recorded with a 64-channel DC amplifier (SYNAMPS system) and acquisition software (NEUROSCAN 4.2) during task executions. The data were recorded using sampling rate of 500 Hz, with a frequency band of 0.1 to 50 Hz. Successively (two days later) the subjects took part in the phase 2. Firstly, tDCS/sham stimulation was induced on the subjects by a battery-driven, constant current stimulation through a pair of saline-soaked sponge electrodes (7 cm $\times$ 5 cm). A constant current of 2 mA was applied for 15 min. The cathode was placed above the left DLPFC with the center above F3 and the anode above the right supraorbital region, the site was chosen based on the results obtained in phase 1. For sham tDCS a custom-built placebo stimulator was used (indistinguishable from the active tDCS device). The impedance was controlled by the device, normally ranging below 5 kΩ. All subjects underwent single sessions of active tDCS and sham tDCS in randomized order with both conditions counterbalanced across subjects. Finally, immediately after tDCS/sham stimulation (10 min later) subjects were submitted to the same experimental task of phase 1 (EEG was registered using the same procedure adopted in phase 1).

3 Results

A significant reduction of the N400 was observed for incongruent stimuli in the case of cathodal (inhibitory) stimulation of the DLPFC compared with pre-stimulation conditions. It was suggested that perturbation of the DLPFC may limit the ability to analyzed a semantically anomalous action sequence, with a reduced N400 ERPs effect and increased random responses being observed.

For the phase 1 (baseline task), to estimate the localization of the source of the cortical differences between congruent/incongruent conditions, morphological analysis on ERPs was performed. A significant difference was revealed between congruent versus incongruent conditions for the selected mean N400 peak.

ERPs data were entered into three-ways repeated measure ANOVA, with factors congruence (2 = congruence; incongruence) x localization (4) x lateralization (3) applied to the peak deflection variable. For localization, the data were averaged over frontal (Fz, F3, F4), central (Cz, C3, C4), temporo-parietal (T5, T6, Pz, P3, P4) and occipital (Oz, O1, O2) electrode location; for lateralization were averaged over left (F3, C3, P3, T5,

O1), central (Fz, Cz, Pz, Oz) and right (F4, C4, P4, T6, O2) regions. Significant main effects were found for congruence (F(1,29) = 9.08, P = 0.001, η2 = .37) and congruence x localization (F(3,29) = 7.79, P = 0.001, η2 = .26). An ampler ERP negativity was found in response to incongruous than congruous condition. Moreover, as shown by the post-hoc analysis (contrast analysis, with Bonferroni corrections for multiple comparisons) a more frontal distribution in comparison with temporo-parietal ($F(1,29) = 10.09$, $P = 0.001, \eta^2 = .39$) and occipital ($F(1,29) = 9.45, P = 0.001, \eta^2 = .36$) distribution was found for incongruous stimuli.

For the phase 2 (post-stimulation task), a negative deflection was observed within the 300–400 ms temporal window, similar to the previously analyzed N400 component (phase 1). The ERPs data were subjected to a four-way repeated measures ANOVA, in which the factors Congruence (2) × Stimulation (2) × Lateralization (3) × Localization (4) were applied to the peak deflection. Significant main effects were found for congruence, stimulation, and localization factors.

Specifically an ampler N400 effect was observed in response to incongruous condition ($F(1,29) = 6.60, P = 0.001, \eta^2 = .25$), when sham effect was performed in comparison with tDCS ($F(1,29) = 7.08, P = 0.001, \eta^2 = .27$), and it was more frontally localized in respect to temporo-parietal and occipital area.

Interaction effects showed also a significant stimulation x congruence ($F(1,29) = 10.09, P = 0.001, \eta^2 = .31$) and stimulation x congruence x localization ($F(3,29) = 9.13, P = 0.001, \eta^2 = .30$) significant effects. Specifically, a higher peak deflection was revealed in case of sham more than tDCS stimulation in response to incongruous stimuli ($F(1,29) = 6.24, P = 0.001, \eta^2 = .27$), whereas no significant differences were found in response to congruous stimuli ($F(1,29) = 9.13, P = 0.001$, $\eta^2 = .33$). Moreover, whereas congruous and incongruous condition did not differ in case of tDCS stimulation ($F(1,29) = 1.24, P = 0.35, \eta^2 = .14$). About the three-ways interaction, it was shown an ampler N400 effect in response to incongruous condition within the frontal area in case of sham in comparison with tDCS stimulation ($F(1,29) = 8.10, P = 0.001, \eta^2 = .29$).

4   Discussion

A significant reduction of the N400 was observed for incongruent stimuli in the case of cathodal (inhibitory) stimulation of the DLPFC compared with sham conditions. It was suggested that perturbation of the DLPFC may limit the ability to analyzed a semantically anomalous action sequence, with a reduced N400 ERPs effect and increased random responses being observed.

On the basis of the localization data, the prefrontal site (medial frontal gyrus) was responsible for incongruence processing, as revealed by the presence of a more anteriorly distributed N400 effect. This area could support semantic anomaly representation for an object-related action inserted into sequential frames. This increased N400 effect for incongruent conditions was found in previous studies (Amoruso et al. 2013; Balconi and Caldiroli 2011; Proverbio et al. 2010; Sitnikova et al. 2008). In another study, the DLPFC was found to be responsive to action semantic anomalies tested by brain oscillations (Balconi et al. 2014). However, the present research introduced an innovative approach by directly exploring the effect of tDCS on the DLPFC within a specific time interval: the 300–400 ms successive to the anomaly presentation. Partial inhibition of the frontal cortical region by tDCS reduced the standard "semantic incongruence effect," as indicated by the decreasing of N400. The reduction of the N400 component in frontal area in the case of tDCS inhibition may suggest a relevant role of the prefrontal area in this semantic process. In fact, the decrease in the N400 amplitude may be related to a subjective partial inability to process the semantic anomaly induced by an incongruent action as a consequence of the temporary inhibition of the left DLPFC. It was suggested that perturbation of the DLPFC may limit the ability to analyzed a semantically anomalous action sequence, with a reduced N400 ERPs effect and increased random responses being observed. To summarize, the incidence that neurostimulation may have on electrophysiological measures was verified, with a direct impact on the functional level. Observing ERPs changes enables the understanding of the direct effect of tDCS over the brain functions. Moreover, this measures may be the basis for the deeply comprehension of the characteristic and the potential of tDCS.

References

Amoruso, L., Gelormini, C., Aboitiz, F., González, M.A., Manes, F., Cardona, J.F., Agustín, I.: N400 ERPs for actions: building meaning in context. Front. Hum. Neurosci. **4**, 7–57 (2013)

Balconi, M., Caldiroli, C.L.: Semantic violation effect on object-related action comprehension. N400-like ERP in a non linguistic task. Neurosci. **197**, 191–199 (2011)

Balconi, M., Vitaloni, S.: The tDCS effect on alpha brain oscillation for correct vs. incorrect object use. The contribution of the left DLPFC. Neurosci. Lett. **517**, 25–29 (2012)

Balconi, M., Canavesio, Y., Vitaloni, S.: Activation of the prefrontal cortex and posterior parietal cortex increases the recognition of semantic violations in action representation. Brain Stimul. **7**, 435–442 (2014)

Bach, P., Gunter, T.C., Knoblich, G., Prinz, W., Friederici, A.D.: N400-like negativities in action perception reflect the activation of two components of an action representation. Soc. Neurosci. **4**, 212–232 (2009)

Ganis, G., Kutas, M.: An electrophysiological study of scene effects on object identification. Cogn. Brain. Res. **16**, 123–144 (2003)

Maffongelli, L., Bartoli, E., Sammler, D., Kölsch, S., Campus, C., Olivier, E., Fadiga, L., D'Ausilio, A.: Distinct brain signatures of content and structure violation during action observation. Neuropsychologia **75**, 30–39 (2015)

Proverbio, M.A., Riva, F., Zani, A.: When neurons do not mirror the agent's intentions: Sex differences in neural coding of goal-directed actions. Neuropsychologia **48**, 1454–1463 (2010)

Reid, V.M., Hoehl, S., Grigutsch, M., Groendahl, A., Parise, E., Striano, T.: The neural correlates of infant and adult goal prediction: evidence for semantic processing systems. Dev. Psychol. **45**, 620–629 (2008)

Rizzolatti, G., Craighero, L.: The Mirror-neuron system. Annu. Rev. Neurosci. **27**, 169–192 (2004)

Salmaso, D., Longoni, A.M.: Problems in the assessment of hand preference. Cortex **21**, 533–549 (1985)

Sitnikova, T., Holcomb, P.J., Kiyonaga, K.A., Kuperberg, G.R.: Two neurocognitive mechanisms of semantic integration during the comprehension of visual real-world events. J. Cogn. Neurosci. **20**, 2037–2057 (2008)

An Ambient Medication Display to Heighten the Peace of Mind of Family Caregivers of Older Adults: A Study of Feasibility

Ernesto Zárate-Bravo[✉], Juan-Pablo García-Vázquez, and Marcela D. Rodríguez

Engineering School, Autonomous University of Baja California, UABC, Mexicali, Mexico
{ernesto.zarate,juan.pablo,marcerod}@uabc.edu.mx

Abstract. Older adults relatives, playing the role of primary caregivers, face an emotional burden as elderly dependence increments. Interventions to help older adults to maintain activities of daily living, such as managing their medications, may alleviate family caregivers' burden. Medication adherence supported by ambient computing technologies has been previously explored for improving older adults' medication compliance. However, their impact has not been evaluated on family caregivers. In this study we assessed the utilization feasibility and acceptance of a Medication Ambient Display for supporting elderly to autonomously medicate. The system was placed in the homes of two seniors-caregivers dyads during 4 weeks. The attitudes and preferences of these volunteers were assessed through survey instruments. Overall experiences were consistently positive even though some usability issues were also reported. Responses from our participants indicated that they appreciated the potential of this technology to make older adults more responsible for taking their medications, which provided caregivers with peace of mind.

Keywords: Ambient display · Family caregivers · Older adults · Medication

1 Introduction

Approximately 50 % of chronically ill older adults do not adhere to their prescribed medication regimens [1]. One of the most common reasons for non-adherence among older adults is forgetfulness, which has been associated with the fact that multiple cognitive processes (associated with prospective memory) are involved in remembering to follow a medication regimen [1, 2]. Thus, prospective memory, the ability to remember future intentions, is crucial to maintain older adults functional independence. Problems with prospective memory cause more deficits in basic and instrumental activities of daily living, such as taking medications, which increments caregiving demands [3]. Older adults relatives, playing the role of primary caregivers, face an emotional burden as elderly dependence increments due normal ageing and cognitive decline increases (4). It has been found that caregiver burden had a stronger association with functional impairment than that of cognitive functioning [4, 5]. Therefore, interventions to help maintain activities of daily living in older adults may

© Springer International Publishing Switzerland 2016
S. Serino et al. (Eds.): MindCare 2015, CCIS 604, pp. 274–283, 2016.
DOI: 10.1007/978-3-319-32270-4_28

alleviate family caregivers burden and improve their well-being [4]. For instance, evaluations of tele-health technologies for the remote monitoring of older adults' activities have showed that help to cope with the caregiving burden [6]. Similarly, qualitative evidence showed that peripheral displays which present the status of older adults' activities, help adult children to maintain a sufficient awareness of their parents' well being [7, 8].

Ambient computing has focused on motivating older adults to follow their medication regimens, for which persuasive strategies have been used. For instance, MoviPill, a mobile phone app that gamifies the medication activity by awarding adherent users and promoting social competition [9]. Similarly, dwellSense is an ambient display that shows representations of users' medication adherence to encourage reflection about their medication errors [10]. Medication adherence supported by these ambient computing technologies has been assessed for improving older adults' medication compliance; however, their impact on family caregivers has not been evaluated [9, 10].

In this paper, we present a qualitative study conducted with older adults and family caregivers to assess the feasibility and acceptance of our Medication Ambient Display to support older adults medication taking. In the next section we present the Medication Ambient Display. Section 3 presents the design of our study. In Sect. 4, we discuss about the study insights. Finally, Sect. 5 presents our conclusions and future work.

2 Medication Ambient Display

An ambient display is characterized by presenting information useful and relevant to the users in the intended setting; it should be unobtrusive, unless it requires the user's attention; additionally, users should be able to easily monitor the display to obtain the desirable information [11]. To reach this end, ambient displays uses information representational modalities that encode data into abstract representations based on pictures, words, sounds, movement, and patterns. We decided to use three ambient modalities to represent information:

- auditory notifications to call the older adults attention when they have to take medications;
- pictograms-based notifications that encourage elders to implement their intention to take the correct medication doses;
- abstract representations of the daily medication taking.

The Medication Ambient Display was implemented for Android tablet to be placed as a portrait in the older adult's home. It shows a virtual cage of birds, which has the aim of raising elders' consciousness about how they have to take the responsibility for caring for their own health, in a similar way that they gladly take care of their pets. A detailed description of the ambient display design is presented elsewhere [12]. As depicted in Fig. 1b, the abstract representation is a parakeet that symbolizes the daily medication compliance. Each day, a newborn pet grows to represent the medication compliance. The parakeet provides auditory reminders (a parakeet whistle) and presents the visual reminders. These are pictograms that present critical information of the medication regimen which includes: (a) medication to take, (b) the health problem addressed, and (c) doses to take (e.g. Fig. 1a shows the morning visual reminder denoting to take 1 pill of Losartan, for controlling blood pressure). After the older adult takes his pill, he should move the tablet closer to the pills container to register that the medication was taken. As depicted in Fig. 1c, the container has a Near Field Communication (NFC) tag that is detected by the tablet's NFC reader. By touching the parakeet, a history of the daily medication compliance is presented. For instance, Fig. 1d shows that 4 medicines need to be taken during the day, 3 of them has to be taken 3 times: morning, afternoon and night; and 1 of them, 2 times. All morning doses of each medicine have already been taken.

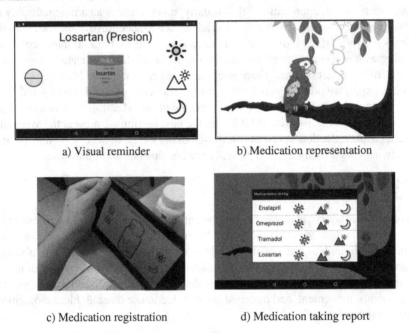

a) Visual reminder   b) Medication representation

c) Medication registration   d) Medication taking report

Fig. 1. Functionalities of the Medication Ambient Display

3   Study Design

We conducted a study to assess the feasibility of our approach by determining: (1) if the system is perceived as useful for supporting elderly to medicate and reducing the burden of their family caregivers; and (2) if the system is ease to use. To reach this ends, we designed our study as an observational study which enabled us to obtain qualitative evidence about factors that represent the subjective nature of patient care (e.g. patient satisfaction, feelings of wellbeing) [13]. It consisted of three phases: recruitment (4 weeks approximately), pre-intervention (2 weeks) and intervention (4 weeks).

3.1 Participants Recruitment

The target population was dyads of an elder and a family caregiver (i.e. a spouse or children who helps elder to manage their medications) and preferably living together. Older adults had to be over the age of 65, taking at least three medications, and presenting mild cognitive impairment (MCI). We decided to include seniors in a mild stage since the concern that prospective memory is often disrupted, is greater than the concern generated in the context of normal adult aging [14]. MCI is "characterized by subjective and objective cognitive decline greater than expected for an individual's age and education level; however, it does not cause significant functional impairment" [14].

We generated a pamphlet announcing the need for recruiting participants for the study, which was disseminated through social web sites. Elected dyads were provided with a gift certificate ($35 dlls) every week during the pre-intervention and intervention

Table 1. Data collected from the 8 contacted dyads during the recruitment phase

Dyad	Presence of MCI?	Auto-effi-cacy?	Medication defi-ciencies	Additional informa-tion	Included?
1	No	Yes	Elder needs to be reminded when to buy more medi-cines.		No
2	Yes	Yes	Caregiver reminds elder to medicate and refill medi-cines	Caregiver not reach-able	No
3	**Yes**	**No**	**Overmedication and forgetful-ness**		**Yes**
4	Yes	Yes	The caregiver reminds the adult to take the medi-cines.	Elder not accepted to participate	No
5	**Yes**	**No**	**Caregiver reminds elder, and helps refilling medi-cine**		**Yes**
6	No	No	The adult doesn't know medication names.		No
7	Yes	Yes	Elder doesn't know medicines names. Someone else reminds him.	Caregiver not reach-able	No
8	Yes	Yes	The adult doesn't know the medi-cines names.	Not a complex med. Regimen	No

phases, and a tablet (w/value of $80 dlls) when they completed the study. Eight relatives of seniors-caregivers dyads contacted us. We visited them to assess potential subjects' eligibility and confirm their interest in participating. We used medical instruments for measuring the elders' cognitive decline (MMSE); for identifying the deficiencies of elders for medicating (MedMaIDE [15] and for determining the self-efficacy for medicating (SEAMS [16]). To understand how caregivers involved on the older adults' medication administration and how it stresses them, we designed a semi-structured interview. We initially considered to use the results of the Zarit Burden Interview [17]) which was designed for assessing the burden of caregivers of patients with dementia; however it was not appropriate since the contacted older adults did not present severe cognitive disabilities and behavioral problems. Table 1 summarizes the results of the recruitment phase and emphasizes the two dyads (3 and 4) included in the study: a daughter-mother and a wife-husband.

3.2 Pre-intervention

During two weeks, we daily collected data from the two selected caregivers. They answered a survey which made questions about: the seniors' medications problems; the reasons for which seniors might not have taken medications; the assistance provided to seniors; and if caregivers feel worry about seniors' medication taking. The caregivers (daughter-mother dyad) accepted to answer an on-line version of the survey, while the second one (wife-husband dyad) answered a printed version. We weekly visited them to collect the data, reviewed them and asked additional questions regarding the survey responses.

3.3 Intervention

Seniors used the system during four weeks. The first day, we introduced the system to the older adults (in the presence of caregivers) by using the "spaced retrieval" approach, (i.e. teach, ask, wait, ask again, wait ask again) [2]. This approach has been used to support the encoding, retention, and retrieval processes involved in interventions designed to support medication taking [2]. Thus, we explained older participants how to conduct their medication taking by using the system. Afterwards, we asked them to recall the system's functionalities we have just presented. To do this, we activated each of the system's functionalities and asked seniors to explain them (e.g. registering medications, consulting their medication compliance). Then we waited 1 min and asked them to recall the system's functionalities again. Then we asked again in 15 min. When the session ends, we asked participants once again. After the completion of the teaching session (which lasted 40 min approximately), we used the information gathered during the recruitment and pre-intervention phases to agree with the participants about the appropriate schedule for presenting the reminders. Finally, we placed the system on a bedside table as they kept and took their medications in the bedroom.

During this phase, caregivers continue answering the survey used during the pre-intervention phase. Additionally, we conducted weekly in-home semi-structured interviews to the caregivers and seniors. We asked them about the problems faced for using the system; which system's functionalities they perceived as more useful and easy to use, and which ones were perceived as less useful and more difficult to use.

4   Results

Based on the recruitment and pre-intervention phases, we developed the following scenarios. They describe the complexity of medication regimens and how seniors adapt the medication regimens to daily routines. On the other side, caregivers act as facilitators of the seniors' medication regimens either by reminding or providing medications.

4.1   Participants Medication Scenarios

Daughter-mother dyad. "Mrs Rosy, an 82 years old woman, lives with her husband and her adolescent grandson. The rest of her grandchildren and her three children frequently visit her. Her 42 years daughter is attentive to Rosy's health and her medication taking. She visits Mrs Rosy every day to help preparing meals, and asks her if she has taken her medications. Mrs Rosy daily takes 7 medicines for coping with diabetes, hypertension and glaucoma. She associates most of her medications intake with her daily routines, such as: when waking up (around 7:00 am), after taking breakfast (around 8:00 am), and at night before going to bed (around 11:00 pm), The eye drops for her glaucoma disease is the only medication that she did not associate with routines since she needs help for instilling them; so she waits for her daughter or grandson to be able to help her (e.g. when her daughter visits her everyday, which happens between 10:00 am to 12:00 pm). When Mrs. Rosy spends time socializing with her neighbors at night, she may go to bed later than usual. This situation may cause she forgets to take the insulin doses at night".

Wife-husband dyad. "Ruben is 69 years old; he takes 10 medications for controlling his blood pressure, for the pain he feels due his permanent physical trauma condition, and for coping with medications side effects (digestive disorders). As he spends most of the day lying down on his bed, he maintains the medications on a bedside table (location). He follows a complicated medication schedule, which he associates with daily routines. For instance, he takes Enalapril and Lozartan pills for blood pressure early morning (6:00 or 7:00 am) and two hours before taking breakfast; afterwards, along with the breakfast (8:00 or 9:00 am) he takes omeprazole for chronic digestive disease; and two hours later (10:00 or 11:00 am), he should take the sulindaco to ameliorate pain. Sometimes, his 56 years-old wife reminds him to medicate; but other times he asks her if he took medications since he is afraid of forgetting them".

4.2   System's Usefulness and Ease of Use

Table 2 summarizes the system functionalities perceived as useful for supporting the medication of the older adults and for supporting the caregiving role. It also presents the functionalities for which older adults faced usability problems.

Table 2. Usability aspects weekly reported regarding each system's functionality

	System functionality	Rosy	Daughter	Ruben	Wife		Rosy	Ruben
Usefulness	Auditory reminder	week 1-4	week 1	week 1-4	week 4	Usability Problems	week 1	
	Visual reminder	week 1-4	-	week 1	-		-	-
	Medication taking report	week 1	week 1-4	week 1	week 1,2,4		-	-
	Medication registration	-	-	week 3	week 3		week 2,3	week 1-4

Thus, the most useful functionality was the auditory reminder, since it was consistently reported as useful for the seniors throughout the study; while the medication taking report was most useful for caregivers. Most usability problems were associated with the medication registration functionality, which was due: some NFCs stop working (which were immediately replaced) and due the size font of the messages feedback were not appropriate for Ruben.

4.3 Perceived Benefits

The comments given by participants for explaining their answers about the system usefulness, enabled us to identify the system's benefits for the participants:

Older adults are more responsible and independent for taking medications. Mrs Rosy's daughter emphasized the importance that her mother was able to hear the reminders from any place at home, since she is not always near of the portrait (e.g. the patio). This system limitation, and Rosy's worry for registering the medication to make the parakeet grow, increased her responsibility for taking medications. She reported to be more alert to the auditory reminders: *"it has helped me a lot; before [using the system] I missed the times for taking medications, and now, the parakeet's reminder is very precise.... [she did not hear some reminders during week 1] but now, I hear it even though I am in the kitchen"* (Week 3).

For Mrs Ruben, who used to take several medications for pain relief, the system helped him to realize about the importance of taking them on time, and not under-medicating (which increases his physical pain) or overmedicating which worried his wife since he is not following the timetables established by his medical doctor. Regarding this, Mr Ruben reported: *"I am more responsible, before [using the system] I used to skip the doctor instructions; now I obey the system and I feel more supported.....Additionally, the parakeet helps me to know if I miss the time for taking medications"* (Week 2). His wife complemented Ruben's comment by mentioning: *"[the system] reminds him that he should not take his pills for pain relief before the parakeet whistle... however, unless the pain is very intense, then he does not wait for the reminder"* (Week 2).

Involvement of relatives (not primary caregivers) was increased. Mrs. Rosy's relatives became conscious about the importance of taking medications timely. She reported that her grandkids, who frequently visit them, showed curiosity about the system functionality and started to be aware of the auditory reminders: *"Now nobody has to worry about if I medicate on time... When my grandkids hear the parakeet whistle, then they tell me: 'grandma it is time to take your pills!' And then, they want to use the tablet to register the medication in order to see how the parakeet grows" (Week 4)*. A more relevant result was that the system made Mrs Rosy's adolescent grandchild to get more involved in her medication routine. During the first week, he helped her to solve system's technical problems; in addition to he got familiarized with the system functionality. During the four weeks, the afternoon auditory notification made him aware about instilling her eye-drops on time.

Peace of mind for primary caregivers. The system made caregivers to feel less worry and to be aware about the elders' medication compliance. Both caregivers reported that the system's functionality that they most used was the Medication taking report. Ruben's wife perceived that the system helped Ruben to reduce over-medication of the pills for his pain. She felt calmer, since the system encouraged Ruben to follow the medication schedule whenever his pain allowed it. Similarly, Rosy's daughter felt more confident that her mother was forgetting less, as she stated: *"Now the system establishes the times she should medicate; and before, [using the system] my mother used to say: 'did I take it [a medication]?' Now she can notice [in the system] if she took it"*. Rosy's daughter considered that the elder improved the compliance of the glaucoma eye-drops, which was the main situation that worried her. Finally, she reported consulting the system once a day, every day: *"If I don't check it in the morning, I check it in the afternoon; now I don't have to ask my mom about their medications"*. These results suggested that the system helped caregivers to be aware of older adult medication intake.

4.4 Caregivers Suggestions

We received several recommendations from the caregivers to improve the system. Their recommendations indicates how they envisioned new ways to assist elderly and to heighten their own peace of mind:

Provide historical reports of medication compliance. Rosy's daughter wanted to be able to consult older adult's medication compliance of any day in the past (e.g. weekly reports) as she sometimes is not able to visit her mother.

Remind to execute daily routines relevant for elders' medication taking. When Rosy's daughter is not able to visit her mother at noon, she calls her to remind her preparing meals, as she needs to take it before the insulin. So, she suggested providing elderly with reminders for preparing meals.

Augment the system's auditory modalities. Both older adults and their caregivers suggested to enhance the system with auditory modalities: in order for reminders being perceived from anyplace in the home (reported by Rosy's daughter) and to complement the system's text messages (as suggested by Ruben's wife).

5   Conclusions and Future Work

Our feasibility study provides preliminary evidence of the potential of our approach and that it could be useful and accepted by older adults. Specifically, our results showed that the Ambient Medication Display supports older adults to self-medicate, and impacts on family primary caregivers by reducing some of the caregiving hassles. Overall experiences were consistently positive even though several usability issues were also reported. Responses from our participants indicated that they appreciated the potential of the ambient display to make older adults more independent and responsible for taking their medications, which provided caregivers with peace of mind.

Even though using a time-based scheme for presenting the reminders were considered useful, the system showed limitations for supporting medications regimens based on the seniors routines. As illustrated in the scenarios of Sect. 4.1, older adults tend to use daily routines for remembering their medication. We need to analyze how the system may naturally support elders' medication regimens. That is, the system should facilitate elders to associate critical routines with medication taking, such as Mrs Rosy, who needs to remember to take her meals before taking the insulin.

Further research is needed to quantitatively measure the system's impact on the older adults' medication adherence and caregivers' burden. As a future work we plan to evaluate the effectiveness of the AC displays to support older adults' medication adherence and to reduce caregiver burden. We plan to recruit 20 seniors-caregivers dyads (10 for using the ambient display and 10 for the control group), who will be monitored during four months (including pre-intervention and intervention phases). To overcome the difficulties of recruiting participants, we will conduct this evaluation by collaborating with the Nursing School of our University. Additionally, nursing students will make weekly visits to assess the elders' medication adherence (pills counting), their self-efficacy for medicating and the family caregivers' burden.

Acknowledgments. We thank to CONACyT and UABC for the funding provided and the scholarship provided to the first co-author. We thank to the study's participants.

References

1. Murray, M.D., Morrow, D.G., Weiner, M., Tu, W., Deer, M.M., Brater, D.C., Weinberger, M.: A conceptual framework to study medication adherence in older adults. Am. J. Geriatr. Pharmacother. **2**, 36–43 (2004)
2. Insel, K.C., Einstein, G.O., Morrow, D.G., Hepworth, J.T.: A multifaceted prospective memory intervention to improve medication adherence: design of a randomized control trial. Contemp. Clin. Trials **34**, 45–52 (2013)
3. Chasteen, A.L., Park, D.C., Schwarz, N.: Implementation intentions and facilitation of prospective memory. Psychol. Sci. **12**, 457–461 (2001)
4. Kang, H.S., Myung, W., Na, D.L., Kim, S.Y., Lee, J.H., Han, S.H., Choi, S.H., Kim, S., Kim, S., Kim, D.K.: Factors associated with Caregiver Burden in patients with Alzheimer's disease. Psychiatry Investig. **11**, 152–158 (2014)

5. Smith, G., Della Sala, S., Logie, R.H., Maylor, E.A.: Prospective and retrospective memory in normal ageing and dementia: a questionnaire study. Mem. Cogn. **8**, 311–321 (2000)

6. Reder, S., Ambler, G., Philipose, M., Hedrick, S.: Technology and Long-term Care (TLC): a pilot evaluation of remote monitoring of elders. Gerontechnology **9**(1), 18–31 (2010)

7. Mynatt, E.D., Melenhorst, A.S., Fisk, A.D., Rogers, W.A.: Aware technologies for aging in place: understanding user needs and attitudes. IEEE Pervasive Comput. **3**(2), 36–41 (2004)

8. Consolvo, S., Roessler, P., Shelton, B.E., LaMarca, A., Schilit, B., Bly, S.: Technology for care networks of elders. IEEE Pervasive Comput. Mag. Successful Aging **3**(2), 22–29 (2004)

9. Lee, M., Dey, A.: Real-time feedback for improving medication taking. In: CHI 2014 Proceedings of the SIGCHI Conference on Human Factors in Computing Systems, pp. 2259–2268. ACM Press, New York (2014)

10. Oliveira, R., Cherubini, M., Oliver, N.: MoviPill: improving medication compliance for elders using a mobile persuasive social game. In: Proceedings of the 12th ACM International Conference on Ubiquitous Computing – Ubicomp 2010, pp. 251–260. ACM Press, New York (2010)

11. Mankoff, J., Dey, A.K., Hsieh, G., Kientz, J., Lederer, S., Ames, M.: Heuristic evaluation of ambient displays. In: Proceedings of the SIGCHI Conference on Human Factors in Computing Systems (CHI 2003), pp. 169–176. ACM Press, New York (2003)

12. García-Vázquez, J.P., Rodríguez, M.D., Andrade, A.G., Bravo, J.: Supporting the strategies to improve elders' medication compliance by providing ambient aids. Pers. Ubiquit. Comput. **15**(4), 389–397 (2011)

13. Kooistra, B., Dijkman, B., Einhorn, T.A., Bhandari, M.: How to design a good case series. J. Bone Joint Surg. Am. **91**, 21–26 (2009)

14. Thompson, C., Henry, J.D., Rendell, P.G., Withall, A., Brodaty, H.: Prospective memory function in mild cognitive impairment and early dementia. J. Int. Neuropsychol. Soc. **16**, 318–325 (2010)

15. Orwig, D., Brandt, N., Gruber-Baldini, A.L.: Medication management assessment for older adults in the community. Gerontologist **46**, 661–668 (2006)

16. Risser, J., Jacobson, T.A., Kripalani, S.: Development and psychometric evaluation of the Self-efficacy for Appropriate Medication Use Scale (SEAMS) in low- literacy patients with chronic disease. J. Nurs. Meas. **15**(3), 203–219 (2007)

17. Zarit, S.H., Reever, K.E., Bach-Peterson, J.: Relatives of the impaired elderly: correlated of feelings of burden. Gerontologist **20**, 649–655 (1980)

The Design of an Immersive Mobile Virtual Reality Serious Game in Cardboard Head-Mounted Display for Pain Management

Xin Tong[✉], Diane Gromala, Ashfaq Amin, and Amber Choo

School of Interactive Arts and Technology, Simon Fraser University,
250 - 13450 102 Avenue Surrey, Burnaby, BC V3T 0A3, Canada
{tongxint,gromala,aamin,achoo}@sfu.ca

Abstract. Researchers have proved immersive Virtual Reality (VR) to be an effective method and non-pharmacological analgesic for distracting acute pain and chronic pain, and for reducing anxiety levels. VR has been developed and deployed in pain management contexts in medical settings for dental and medical procedures, as well to manage cancer and burn pain. Often, what patients are distracted by can typically be described as immersive VR games. Although this is promising, and although the cost of VR has dramatically fallen in the past few years, most VR systems are still comparatively expensive in terms of accessibility for patients in their everyday contexts, such as at home or at work. For most patients — especially chronic pain patients — it is important that pain-related VR is accessible when it is needed, or "just" needed. However, the so-called Cardboard VR is affordable enough for everyday use. It provides a low-cost stereoscopic display that patients attached to smartphones. Therefore, a mobile VR game has been designed, developed and tested for this purpose. This paper describes the game design and game mechanics of *Cryoblast*, a mobile VR game for self-managing pain. We introduce the design of the gameplay and pain metaphors, and believe it will inspire more mobile VR games for healthcare.

Keywords: Immersive virtual reality · Pain management and distraction · Cardboard head-mounted display · Mobile health game · Serious game

1 Introduction

Virtual Reality (VR) — defined as three-dimensional, stereoscopic, interactive computer graphics — is a technology that has recently regained popularity since its introduction to the public sphere in the mid- to late 1990s. The VR technology, often referred to as immersive multimedia, is a computer-generated environment that can simulate physical presence in virtual worlds by recreating human sensory experiences. In health research, it has been demonstrated to be a successful method for mitigating pain in numerous research studies, initially for acute pain from burn injuries. The VR simulation, typically designed as a game, helps to distract patients away from their physical pain and reduces their perceived pain as well as related anxiety.

© Springer International Publishing Switzerland 2016
S. Serino et al. (Eds.): MindCare 2015, CCIS 604, pp. 284–293, 2016.
DOI: 10.1007/978-3-319-32270-4_29

Studies of VR use for acute pain distraction initially involved burn injuries among veterans. *SnowWorld* [1], for example, was an desktop VR simulation developed by Hunter Hoffman et al. It drews patients' attention away from their pain experience and redirected it to the immersive 3D environment. This virtual environment (VE) featured a snowy landscape where patients could "throw" or fire snowballs at snowmen, and in later iterations, at animals. The initial *SnowWorld* study demonstrated that patients undergoing burn debridement reported less pain when provided VR distraction via the immersive environment. The VR system comprised a stereoscopic head-mounted display (HMD) equipped with position and orientation trackers that changed the visual field in response to head movement. Other researchers such as Steele et al. [2], used an HMD with a tracking device that controlled the movement of the gun inside 3D game. They also obtained reductions in self-reported pain in a 16-year-old boy with cerebral palsy undergoing painful physical therapy. Subsequently, numerous studies, though small in the number of patients tested, reported that VR reduced acute pain.

VR pain distraction methods have been shown to be superior to other forms of pain distraction. In a study of two adults undergoing painful dental procedures, Hoffman, Garcia-Palacios, et al. [3] demonstrated that an immersive VE resulted in lower subjective pain ratings during painful dental procedures than watching a movie without VR technology. Hoffman [4] also found that immersive VR distraction using *SpiderWorld* resulted in lower subjective pain ratings in two adolescents undergoing wound care for severe burns, compared to trials in which they played *Mario Kart* or *Wave Race* on a Nintendo without the addition of any VR technology. Another study concluded "VR is a uniquely attention-grabbing medium capable of maximizing the amount of attention drawn away from the real world, allowing patients to tolerate painful dental procedures" [3]. All of these studies involved acute or short term pain. However, more recently, VR has also been implemented in patients who suffer from long term or chronic pain. Here too, VR combined with mindfulness-based stress reduction (MBSR) proved to be effective in short period pain reductions by Gromala et al. [13].

However, all of the VE and VR games were based on a desktop platform and required professional operations and VR hardware in medical settings. Taking into account the relative expense of an HMD, these factors together make VR inaccessible to patients' everyday interactions and varying needs. The currently most popular technical configuration of VR relies on a stereoscopic HMD, such as the Oculus Rift or Samsung Gear. Although the Oculus Rift quickly became a commercially viable HMD, other approaches to VR displays have also been growing. One example is Google's *Cardboard VR* HMD, which is cardboard that the consumer folds up into an HMD-like viewer and includes plastic lenses. Compared to higher-end VR devices like Oculus Rift, the cardboard is significantly less expensive by a factor of ten, and therefore has the potential for mass consumer use. It relies on a user's smartphone, which the user inserts into the cardboard viewer. This is only one example of a number of similar, inexpensive devices that are being referred to as "DIY VR" or "Cardboard VR".

Therefore, to design VR game as interventions for pain management, to make them accessible to more patients and to allow patients to interact with VR as often as they need, we designed the mobile VR game, *Cyroblast*. Based on a Cardboard VR HMD, *Cryoblast* is a serious game designed specifically as a form of pain distraction for acute and chronic pain patients. Our prior research demonstrated significant decreases of patients' pain levels after the patients tried a desktop VR game that has a similar gameplay and game components as *Cryoslide's*. Therefore, we developed this mobile game, *Cryoblast*, to make it possible for patients to bring and use their VR at home. We believe that VR pain distraction games are an effective non-drug approach for managing spikes in chronic pain, and that mobile VR may provide more accessible tools for the dissemination of VR interventions.

2   Head-Mounted Display vs. Cardboard Mobile VR

Immersive VR, developed primarily in research labs and popularized by the media in the 1990s, built upon a number of technologies and approaches to computer graphics that were initially described and tested in Ivan Sutherland's *Sword of Damocles*. At that time, VR was described as a version of Star Trek's *Holodeck* [5] and as a "consensual hallucination" [6]. However, because the hardware for VR was extremely expensive and limited, and because 3D software and programming VR was so complex, it didn't become commercially viable in the 1990s. Therefore, VR's popularity was eclipsed by the advent of the worldwide web and a number of other more accessible computational devices, networks and software.

After decades of commercially failed products and unfulfilled promises, Oculus Rift brought back life to the VR industry and made people again became excited about immersing themselves in a computer-generated world. Advanced HMDs like Samsung Headgear are also now in the VR market. Although these devices are significantly cheaper than HMDs were a few years ago, these are possibly still not inexpensive enough for large-scale mass consumption, since their prices range from $350 to $1,500. The concept of DIY VR aims at closing this gap. Since the number of smartphone consumers are increasing at a geometric rate, the potential for DIY VR devices are tremendous.

Although the Oculus Rift (Fig. 1, left) and Samsung Gear (Fig. 1, right) quickly became commercially viable VR displays, other approaches to VR displays have also been emerging. One example is Google's Cardboard VR (Fig. 2, right), which is cardboard that the consumer folds up into a viewer and includes plastic lenses. Another example are plastic VR HMDs designed for mobile phones like Archos Mobile VR (Fig. 2, left). These are less expensive than Samsung Gear, but still provide a sense of immersion for VR applications.

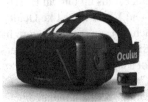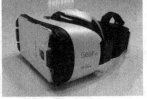

Fig. 1. The Oculus Rift HMD (left) and the Samsung Gear mobile HMD (right).

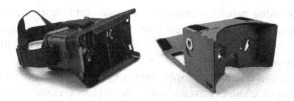

Fig. 2. Economical mobile VR HMDs: ARCHOS mobile HMD (left), and Do-It-Yourself Cardboard mobile HMD (right).

Cardboard VR is a do-it-yourself (DIY) kit that utilizes a piece of cardboard with a magnet, a rubber band and a couple pieces of plastic. It has been manufactured by various companies and are priced from $3. to $30., according to cardboard quality. Although these cardboard or DIY VR displays are described as inexpensive alternatives to more traditional immersive VR HMDs, they differ from traditional HMDs in their design, construction materials, optics and reliance on smartphones. Moreover, their methods of interaction are quite different from more traditional VR HMDs that rely on handheld input devices (joysticks, mice, data-gloves) and desktop or laptop computers.

Despite limitations, the Cardboard-like DYI VR system has an immense potential of having a larger consumer base than do the traditional HMDs since these are affordable and easy to carry. With a large user base, it has the possibility of becoming a regular device, which promises to give a taste of VR to users in everyday life. In our case, our users have acute or chronic pain, and a percentage are disabled; therefore, expense is a considerable factor that determines whether or not an HMD is viable for home use.

3   Design Concepts and Principles

Distraction Principle: Cognitive Load. The theoretical basis upon which we designed the game is Cognitive Load, including Continuous Action and Attention Switching. All work together in the form of tasks that we present players with throughout the length of the game. This provides continuous action and constantly captures and maintains the players' attention. Cognitive Load serves as stimulants of the users' working memory. Continuous Action keeps the users' attention constantly focused forward, and Attention Switching stimulates the users' cognitive and sensory capacities to effectively distract them from their pain.

Consistent with capacity theories of attention, Dahlquist et al. [7] suggests that although interactive and passive distraction are effective, interactive distraction is significantly better than passive distraction. This is because the interactive games stimulate visual and auditory sensations, but can also provoke tactile and kinesthetic sensations as the game is played, thus increasing attentional demand. They used a VR HMD for a distraction procedure, which may also have blocked sensory awareness from much of the surrounding input.

Given that an individuals' attentional capacity is finite, a distracting task that requires a great deal of the person's attentional resources should leave little attentional capacity available for processing painful stimuli. Moreover, multiple resource theories suggest that attentional resources within different sensory systems can function relatively independently. For instance, an activity that involves one sensory modality may not deplete the attentional resources in another sensory modality. Thus, an engaging and interactive distraction activity that involves multiple sensory systems is likely to be more effective than a more passive distractor, or even a distractor that involves only one or two sensory systems.

In addition, although Dalquist et al. argue that interactive distraction is more effective in terms of the kinds of sensations that may be involved, the role of agency that interactive games may also play a role, as other game theorists suggest [14].

The Distraction Principle: Sense of Immersion.   Jennett et al. defines immersion as a "lack of awareness of time, a loss of awareness of the real world, involvement and a sense of being in the task environment" [8]. Immersion in this sense relates to how present the user feels in the simulated world and how real (or engaging) the virtual environment seems. When a sense of immersion is strong, much of the user's attention is focused in the VE, leaving little of it to notice other things such as pain. Therefore, users need a sense of immersion in order to be captivated enough to feel as they're part of or "in" the VE. Immersion is one of the concepts that are believed to enable VR environments to distract patients undergoing various medical procedures in ways that go above and beyond other techniques and media forms explored in prior research.

Affective Changes: Relaxation and Anxiety Control in VR.   Immersive Virtual Reality (VR) has become more popular and widely accepted as a non-pharmacological analgesic in clinical settings. In a number of research studies, VR has been considered successful as a method for distracting patients and reducing their perceived bodily pain, as well as managing emotional disorders, such as overcoming anxiety [9].

Research showed that the use of VR for relaxation [15] and stress-reduction also represents a promising approach in the treatment of generalized anxiety disorders since it enhances the quality of the relaxing experience through the elicitation of the sense of presence [10]. The visual presentation of a calm virtual scenario can facilitate patients' practice and mastery of relaxation [13], making the experience more vivid and real, especially for subjects who have difficulty "visualizing" – that is, using their own imagination and memory [15].

4   The VR Game Design and Game Mechanics: *Cryoblast*

In broad terms, VR games such as *Cryoblast* build on early VR pain distraction work that was initiated by Hunter Hoffman et al. [1]. *Cryoblast* itself is a direct outgrowth from a more recent VR pain distraction game, *Mobius Floe*. The aim of *Cryoblast* is to improve on VR pain distraction games by enabling patients to use them on mobile platforms. This is because VR games that run on mobile platforms may provide an effective source of pain distraction without the use of analgesics, and because cardboard VR is inexpensive enough to be used not just in hospitals, but also in the comfort of the patients' own homes.

First Person Shooter (FPS) Game in a Cave Adventure.   The genre of the First-Person Shooter (FPS) was chosen to be the main game mechanic and game type in this cardboard mobile VR scenario. In FPS games, the player can identify with the game character represented only by weapons and/or hands which are seen as virtual prostheses that reach into the game environment [11]. This means that in an FPS, the player virtually turns into the game character as they feel as if they are acting directly in the virtual game world.

Patients are immersed in the virtual wintry cave setting where they wander through cave landscape paths and trails where they experience action-packed encounters. The tasks in *Croblast* stimulate the patients' working memory and keep their attention constantly focused forward, in turn stimulating cognitive and sensory capacities to effectively distract them from their short-term pain. The beginning screen is depicted in Fig. 3.

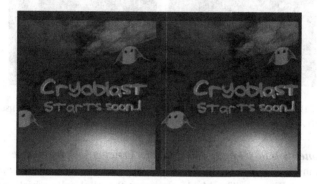

Fig. 3.   The beginning scene of *Cryoblast* HMD scene with two lens view (in cardboard VR).

Game Components and Design: The Caves.   To constantly engage patients' attention inside the cave and to avoid repetition, we designed 6 different caves, each of which differs in terms of size, textures and landscapes (Fig. 4). Thus, the players have diverse caves to explore, offering them an opportunity to stay engaged in the adventure gaming mode. Two main game objects were implemented in each cave: the Mushi and the coins. The goal is to collect as many coins as possible.

Fig. 4.   A view from far outside of *Cryoblast's* cave landscape, where six caves are connected.

However, in each cave, the layout of both the Mushi creatures and the amounts of coins vary considerably in order to provide some level of uncertainty in the gameplay deployment as well as to inspire the players to create their own strategies in response to differing types of targets. For instance, in the left of Fig. 5, the cave has only coins, and the amount of coins were exact enough to keep players focused on the virtual world and shooting actions. It is the fifth cave, which was created to generate more flow for the players with a feast of coins. In contrast to the fifth cave the last cave is populated with a lot of Mushi creatures, but has fewer coins, as depicted in the right side in Fig. 5. The goal here is also to capture players' attention to shoot as many Mushis as possible. Figure 7 shows a cave has more of a blance between the number of coins and Mushis.

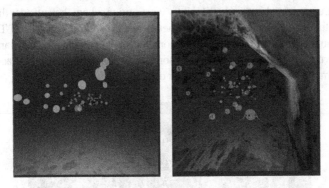

Fig. 5. Two of the six caves in *Cryoblast*: the CoinCave (left), and the Intense Mushi Cave *Cryoblast* (right).

Game Components and Design: The Mushi. Patients find themselves under threat from little "monsters" — the Mushis — which appear to be half neuron, and half flying ball-like character (Fig. 6). The Mushi represent the glial cells which are thought to regulate the human neurological systems that are responsible for the pain experience.

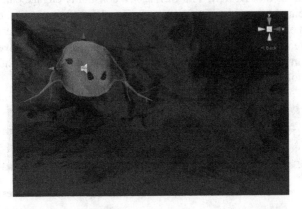

Fig. 6. Design of the Mushi. Half glial cell and half ball, the flying Mushis represent regulator compnents of an abstracted neurological process thought to result in peristent pain.

There are analgesic 'drugs' that the player can use as weapons to shoot the Mushis: morphine and gabapentin. Patients are able to calm the Mushis down by aiming them, and throwing these abstract 'drugs' or analgesics with the cardboard's magnetic button. Each drug has functions differently in how it calms the Mushis. Figure 7 demonstrates Mushis who turn from red/magenta to green when they are shot.

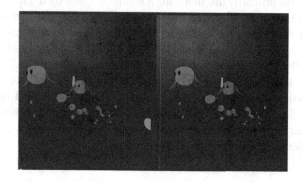

Fig. 7. When the aggressive Mushi is hit, it changes to another state — green and calm (Color figure online)

Game Components and Design: Game Victory Points–Coins. Coins are the final victory points. The player is able to assess how many coins s/he has and the percentage of Mushis s/he has shot. Although the players cannot control their initial moving speed in the cave, shooting the Mushis decreases the speed so that players can slow down and have more time collecting coins. Coins are designed to be smaller than Mushi so that they are more difficult to target and to shoot. But the more coins a player has collected, the quicker the player's speed will be so that s/he needs to shoot more Mushis with the "drugs" to calm them down. The reason for creating two things — the Mushis and the coins — and a feedback loop is to keep patients more engaged in the gameplay and thinking about their strategy of what to shoot and how to deploy the drugs.

The whole journey through the six caves is an embodied way that the players — patients who have persistent or chronic pain — self-manage their bodily pain by distracting themselves from it, and attend instead to interacting in the immersive virtual worlds. The game components were designed to stimulating patients' working memory. Moreover, the metaphor of the neurological processes that are involved in persistent pain may function as a kind of abstract VR visualization — by shooting 'drugs' or analgesics at the Mushis, these neuron-like monsters that have caused pain are calmed, offering the players greater agency in their speed and movements in the game.

5   Conclusions and Future Work

Combined with an Android smartphone, the Cardboard VR works as a more accessible albeit new kind of virtual reality gaming platform. The concept of DIY VR is very new and has the potential to grow a large consumer base because of its low cost. *Cryoblast* is an immersive VR game created for this platform, designed to help both chronic and acute pain patients lower their pain and anxiety, especially when professional medical VR devices are not available to them. Moreover, the Cardboard VR is accessible enough to be used at home, thereby increasing its utility to be used when and where patients may need it.

In this paper, we primarily discussed the potential of Cardboard VR as a more accessible VR HMD for patients, as well as the design metaphor and gameplay of *Cryoblast*. The pain distraction metaphors and how they may be translated by patients immersed in *Cryoblast* differentiates this VR game from others. Currently, the cardboard VR game is available on the Andriod mobile phone platform with Cardboard HMD. In our future work, this VR game will be tested with chronic pain patients to evaluate the sense of immersion and engagement it provides for the specialized needs of these patients. In addition, we will compare how this VR platform differs from others, such as Samsung Gear and Oculus Rift, in terms of the effectiveness of VR pain distraction and pain management as a everyday design application.

References

1. Hoffman, H.G., Chambers, G.T., Meyer, W.J., Arceneaux, L.L., Russell, W.J., Seibel, E.J., Richards, T.L., Sharar, S.R., Patterson, D.R.: Virtual reality as an adjunctive non-pharmacologic analgesic for acute burn pain during medical procedures. Ann. Behav. Med. **41**(2), 183–191 (2011). Publ. Soc. Behav. Med.
2. Steele, E., Grimmer, K., Thomas, B., Mulley, B., Fulton, I., Hoffman, H.: Virtual reality as a pediatric pain modulation technique: a case study. Cyberpsychol. Behav. **6**(6), 633–638 (2003)
3. Hoffman, H.G., Garcia-Palacios, A., Patterson, D.R., Jensen, M., Furness, T., Ammons, W.F.: The effectiveness of virtual reality for dental pain control: a case study. Cyberpsychol. Behav. **4**(4), 527–535 (2001). Impact Internet Multimed. Virtual Real Behav. Soc.
4. Carlin, A.S., Hoffman, H.G., Weghorst, S.: Virtual reality and tactile augmentation in the treatment of spider phobia: a case report. Behav. Res. Ther. **35**(2), 153–158 (1997)
5. Rheingold, H.: Virtual Reality: The Revolutionary Technology of Computer-Generated Artificial Worlds-And How It Promises to Transform Society. Simon & Schuster, New York (1992). Reprinted edn
6. Gibson, J.J.: The Senses Considered as Perceptual Systems, New edition edn. Praeger, Westport (1983)
7. Das, D.A., Grimmer, K.A., Sparnon, A.L., McRae, S.E., Thomas, B.H.: The efficacy of playing a virtual reality game in modulating pain for children with acute burn injuries: a randomized controlled trial. BMC Pediatr. **5**(1), 1 (2005)
8. Jennett, C., Cox, A.L., Cairns, P., Dhoparee, S., Epps, A., Tijs, T., Walton, A.: Measuring and defining the experience of immersion in games. Int. J. Hum. Comput. Stud. **66**(9), 641–661 (2008)
9. Gold, J.I., Kant, A.J., Kim, S.H., Rizzo, A.S.: Virtual anesthesia: the use of virtual reality for pain distraction during acute medical interventions. Semin. Anesth. Perioper. Med. Pain **24**(4), 203–210 (2005)
10. Gorini, A., Riva, G.: The potential of virtual reality as anxiety management tool: a randomized controlled study in a sample of patients affected by generalized anxiety disorder. Trials **9**(1), 25 (2008)

11. Grimshaw, M., Charlton, J., Jagger, R.: First-person shooters: immersion and attention. Eludamos J. Comput. Game Cult. **5**(1), 29–44 (2011)
12. Mcmahan, A.: Immersion, engagement, and presence: a method for analyzing 3D videogames. In: Wolf, M., Perron, B. (eds.) The Video Game Theory Reader, pp. 67–86. Routledge, New York (2003)
13. Gromala, D., Tong, X., Choo, A., Karamnejad, M., Shaw, C. D.: The virtual meditative walk: virtual reality therapy for chronic pain management. In: CHI 2015, pp. 521–524, April 2015
14. Salen, K., Zimmerman, E.: Rules of Play: Game Design Fundamentals. MIT Press, Cambridge (2003)
15. Shaw, C. D., Gromala, D., Seay, A. F.: The meditation chamber: enacting automatic senses. In: Proceedings of ENACTIVE/07 (2007)

Author Index

Printed in the United States
By Bookmasters